Atlas of EEG Patterns

Atlas of EEG Patterns

John M. Stern, M.D.

Assistant Professor of Neurology
Geffen School of Medicine at the University of California, Los Angeles
Los Angeles, California

Consulting Editor

Jerome Engel, Jr., M.D., PH.D.

Jonathan Sinay Professor of Neurology and Neurobiology
Geffen School of Medicine at the University of California, Los Angeles
Los Angeles, California

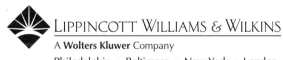
LIPPINCOTT WILLIAMS & WILKINS
A **Wolters Kluwer** Company
Philadelphia · Baltimore · New York · London
Buenos Aires · Hong Kong · Sydney · Tokyo

Acquisitions Editor: Anne M. Sydor
Developmental Editor: Joanne Bersin
Production Editor: Emily Lerman
Manufacturing Manager: Benjamin Rivera
Marketing Manager: Adam Glazer
Cover Designer: Christine Jenny
Compositor: Graphic World Publishing Services
Printer: Edwards Brothers

© 2005 by LIPPINCOTT WILLIAMS & WILKINS
530 Walnut Street
Philadelphia, PA 19106 USA
LWW.com

Library of Congress Cataloging-in-Publication Data
Stern, John M.
    Atlas of EEG patterns / John M. Stern ; consulting editor, Jerome Engel Jr.
       p. ; cm.
    Includes bibliographical references and index.
    ISBN 0-7817-4124-6
    1. Electroencephalography—Atlases.   I. Engel, Jerome.   II. Title.
    [DNLM: 1. Electroencephalography—methods—Atlases.   WL 17 S839a 2005]
RC386.6.E43S74 2005
616.8′047547—dc22
                                                                                          2004048379

Care has been taken to confirm the accuracy of the information presented and to describe generally accepted practices. However, the authors and publisher are not responsible for errors or omissions or for any consequences from application of the information in this book and make no warranty, expressed or implied, with respect to the currency, completeness, or accuracy of the contents of the publication. Application of this information in a particular situation remains the professional responsibility of the practitioner.

The authors and publisher have exerted every effort to ensure that drug selection and dosage set forth in this text are in accordance with current recommendations and practice at the time of publication. However, in view of ongoing research, changes in government regulations, and the constant flow of information relating to drug therapy and drug reactions, the reader is urged to check the package insert for each drug for any change in indications and dosage and for added warnings and precautions. This is particularly important when the recommended agent is a new or infrequently employed drug.

Some drugs and medical devices presented in this publication have Food and Drug Administration (FDA) clearance for limited use in restricted research settings. It is the responsibility of the health care provider to ascertain the FDA status of each drug or device planned for use in their clinical practice.

10   9   8   7   6   5   4   3   2   1

For my sons, Peter and Joel, and my wife, Rebecca.

Contents

Acknowledgments

I am thankful to many individuals for their contributions to this book. Jeff Nicholl, Jason Soss, and Marc Nuwer were instrumental in refining the pattern categorization approach and crucial in the transition of the approach from concept to book. Alan Shewmon, Lara Schrader, Jeffrey Chung, James Chen, Jack Lin, and Jennifer Hopp attentively and enthusiastically identified figures from the many clinical EEGs they interpreted. Tony Fields, Kirk Shattuck, and Chris Barnhart provided skillful technical assistance in the figure preparation. David Millett's and Frisca Yan-Go's comments on portions of the manuscript were very helpful. Sabrina Hubbard, Doug Hawkins, Rowena Concepcion, Joanne Chiu, Dale Booth, and Sandra Dewar from the UCLA Seizure Disorder Center provide outstanding professional support and assistance on a daily basis. My editors Anne Sydor, Joanne Bersin, and Cassie Carey deserve special recognition for their efforts and commitment to the book and its underlying approach. The figures were prepared with Insight II EEG review software (Persyst Development Corporation, Prescott, AZ), and I appreciate the use of Persyst's excellent software and equally excellent technical support.

I am especially thankful to Pete Engel who has been an extraordinary mentor as well as a friend. His critical review of the manuscript substantially improved this book.

More than anyone else, I have enormous gratitude to my wife, Rebecca. Her encouragement and enthusiasm from the start of this project to its completion sustained me. In exchange, I express my love and devotion. Her creative energy remains an inspiration to me. My sons, Peter and Joel, bring childhood wonder, exuberance, and joy to my life. I am most grateful for them.

SECTION I
Introduction

CHAPTER 1

How to Use This Book

Pattern recognition, as it is applied to the interpretation of electroencephalograms (EEGs), usually refers to the familiarity of the interpreter with the appearance of EEG waves. This skill is typically taught with the teacher and student reviewing EEGs together, and the teacher identifying the patterns then providing their names and significance. Pattern recognition in this sense is based on visual recognition of the wave as a whole and eventually becomes automatic, but it always remains constrained to the interpreter's personal experience. Identifying an unfamiliar wave is only possible with the assistance of someone who already has familiarity with it. Indeed, a search for an unfamiliar wave in a conventional EEG text is not straightforward because texts are organized by the names of the patterns, which is the very thing the interpreter is seeking. Such searches become dependent on the interpreter's self-generated list of named patterns and, therefore, are inadequate if the list is not comprehensive.

The problem that follows from this viewing of EEG patterns only as wholes may be circumvented by approaching EEGs with the type of pattern recognition that is commonly used when approaching a clinical diagnosis. Although expert clinicians may reach a diagnosis after an automatic assembly of clinical information, this process is easily deconstructed into a systematic narrowing of diagnostic possibilities with the stepwise inclusion of basic findings. The ultimate diagnosis results from the combined findings (the pattern) and a familiarity with diseases according to their patterns of presenting findings. This assembling of findings is flexible and allows diagnostic reference books to be organized in such a way that clinicians may identify diagnostic possibilities solely from the clinical findings. Such books include the differential diagnoses for common and uncommon clinical presentations, and provide distinguishing features for the diseases among the diagnostic possibilities. Approaching EEGs in an analogous fashion depends on describing the EEG patterns as a pattern of basic wave features and using these features as the findings that are used in the clinical diagnosis.

This reference uses the standard language used to describe EEG waves to deconstruct the established EEG patterns. To keep this system as straightforward as possible, it does not include the additional physiologic measures of a neonatal EEG. Therefore, this reference may be applied only to EEGs recorded from patients who are 2 months post term or older. Once deconstructed, the patterns are grouped according to their features. Each group is defined by a collection of EEG features and includes all of the patterns that may manifest with those features. To include the variations in how patterns may appear, most patterns appear in more than one group. Therefore, each group is an EEG differential diagnosis based on pattern appearance. These groups constitute the Categorization by Pattern Features section. The differential diagnoses are then narrowed with the addition of secondary features, and the remaining possibilities are evaluated using the Patterns section. The Patterns section includes descriptions of each pattern with an emphasis on distinguishing the pattern from patterns that have a similar appearance.

ORIENTATION TO ELECTROENCEPHALOGRAMS

A detailed discussion of theories for the generation of EEGs is beyond the scope of this reference; however, an understanding of the physical principles behind an EEG is necessary for accurate interpretation and full understanding of the descriptions contained in the Patterns section. The following is a basic review of fundamentals.

Routine, clinical electroencephalography is the recording of electrical potentials on the scalp; however, it provides a highly limited view of cerebral activity because of inherently poor spatial resolution and insensitivity to electrical fields that are either not perpendicular to the scalp's surface or distant from it. The spatial resolution limitation partly results from the electrical field insensitivity. To have an amplitude that is detectable at the level of the scalp, neuronal potentials must be sufficiently synchronized with neighboring neuronal potentials over distances of several square centimeters. Nevertheless, electroencephalography has excellent temporal resolution, which is in the millisecond order of magnitude.

Recording the low-amplitude cerebral potentials, especially in the context of the larger amplitude potentials of muscle and ambient electrical noise, requires differential recording, which is also called common mode rejection. This technique produces an EEG wave by subtracting the electrical field detected by one electrode from the field detected by another electrode. Because the subtraction cancels any electrical field that is present at both electrodes, extracerebral electrical noise is minimized and cerebrally generated fields that are local to one electrode remain visible despite their much lower voltage. However, this cancellation is nonspecific and, therefore, also minimizes the amplitude of any broad cerebrally generated activity that is identical at the two electrode locations. The other major limitation of this technique is the absence of any external reference against which the field of one electrode may be compared. Without an external reference, every wave represents a combination of focal activities. Thus, viewing activity with multiple pairs of electrodes is necessary to best understand its location.

For reasons of standardization, the locations of the electrodes used in recording EEGs are defined by international agreement as the "10-20 system" of electrode placement (Fig. 1-1). This system uses measurements of the head referenced to visible anatomic landmarks to minimize the variation in electrode placement among recording technologists and to provide the maximal uniformity in electrode to brain structure correspondence among patients. The nasion and inion define the midline sagittal line, and the superior attachment of the ears to the scalp defines the midline coronal line. Using increments of 10% and 20% along these principal lines, additional lines are drawn. Electrodes are placed at the 10% and 20% increments of both the principal and additional lines.

A standard nomenclature is used for the electrode locations based on a letter prefix, which indicates the region of the head, and a number suffix, which indicates the exact location within that region. The common letter prefixes are as follows: **F** for the frontal region, **C** for the central region, **P** for the parietal region, **T** for the temporal region, **O** for the occipital region, and **A** for the ears. The most commonly used numbering system is illustrated in Fig. 1-1. As is evident, an odd number suffix indicates the left side of the head, an even number suffix indicates the right side, the suffix **z** indicates the sagittal midline, and a suffix that includes **p** indicates the frontal pole. For example, F3 is over the left frontal lobe and Cz is at the vertex, that is, the intersection of the midline sagittal and coronal lines. In the commonly used 10-20 system, higher numbers generally indicate greater distance from the sagittal midline. The T electrodes are the exception to this because C electrodes that are close to the vertex have the same suffix. A revised system, sometimes called the "10-10 system," corrects this inconsistency and also includes names for electrode locations between the standard locations of the 10-20 system (Fig. 1-2). This corrected naming system is not used universally.

The EEG record, also called a **tracing,** truly is a polygraph composed of multiple horizontal lines, each of which is generated by two electrode inputs and is called a **channel.** The channels are named for their respective electrodes. Currently, a routine EEG usually includes at least 16 channels, and with the advent of digital EEG the number of channels has become flexible and often greater than 20. The specific electrode locations used for the creation of each channel depend on the procedures of the laboratory performing the EEG, but certain EEG page organizations are common. These organizations are termed **montages** and are divided into two general approaches—**bipolar** and **referential** (Figs. 1-3 and 1-4). The channels in a bipolar montage are created from electrodes that are typically adjacent to one another. This contrasts with a referential montage, which uses a minimal number of electrodes in the second position of the electrode pair. One often-used referential montage compares all of the electrodes to the ipsilateral ear's electrode, thus using two references to maximize the symmetry of the comparisons. A **common reference** montage uses the same electrode input as the second in the pair. Cz, an input comprising A1 and A2 combined, and an input that is an average of all the electrodes are three often-used common references. On closer inspection, the terms bipolar and referential are misleading because referential montages are technically bipolar through the use of two electrodes, and bipolar montages include two electrodes that each act as a reference for the other.

The depiction of polarity is based on a convention that specifies a downward deflection of the wave when either the first electrode becomes more positive or the second electrode becomes more negative. Inversely, greater negativity at the first electrode or greater positivity at the second produces an upward deflection. When waves are referred to as either positive or negative, a tacit simplification has the second electrode as neutral; thus, a "positive wave" is down and a "negative wave" is up. However, each electrode in the pair truly is active; thus, a positive wave does not necessarily indicate that the corresponding cortical surface is electropositive at the first electrode. In reality, it may be negative at the first electrode and even more negative at the second. Thus, the polarity of the surface's electrical field at one location can be assessed only by comparison to fields present at other regions.

Following this polarity convention and the usual format for referential montages, channels within a referential montage deflect downward when the first electrode is more positive than the reference and deflect upward when it is more negative, and the amplitude of the deflection indicates the relative amplitudes of the fields. Because the electrodes constituting each channel in a referential montage usually are distant from each other, the amplitude measurement is not affected by local field shape. Polarity and amplitude are manifested differently in bipolar montages. Channels in bipolar montages are organized on the page in **chains,** which is a series of channels that each share one electrode with the preceding channel and one electrode with the following channel. For example, one chain in a bipolar montage has the following series of channels: Fp2-F8, F8-T4, T4-T6, T6-O2. This organization deliberately changes the location of each duplicated electrode between its two channels. This is demonstrated by F8 being in the second position of Fp2-F8 and in the first position of F8-T4. This position change takes advantage of the system for depicting polarity to assist in the localization of waves. If the cortical surface beneath the F8 electrode briefly becomes negative compared to both the Fp2 and T4 electrodes, then the EEG signal will deflect downward in the Fp2-F8 channel and deflect upward in the adjacent F8-T4 channel. This opposing alignment of the same potential is called a **phase reversal** and provides an easily observed means to identify the point of maximum negativity or positivity across a chain (Fig. 1-5). Phase reversals that occur across two channels that are separated by a channel that is **isoelectric** (flat) indicate a broader area of maximum polarity. An isoelectric channel is produced when the two electrodes record from fields with equal potentials. The possibility of isoelectric channels provides an example for the limitation of bipolar montages in their depiction of local amplitudes. When two electrodes produce an isoelectric channel, comparison of each to a more distant region, such as with a referential montage, is necessary to better assess their local amplitudes.

USING THIS REFERENCE

Definitions

Identifying the name of an unfamiliar wave begins with the categorization of the pattern according to basic descriptors. Combinations of these descriptors are the headings in the Categorization section, which contains the differential diagnoses. Before outlining this reference's process of pattern identification, a review of standard definitions may be helpful. The portion of each definition that is within quotes originates from the International Federation of Clinical Neurophysiology's glossary (1). The text that follows a quotation is intended to clarify or slightly modify the definition for the purposes of this reference. The definitions are presented in an order that builds a conceptual framework instead of the alphabetical order of the glossary.

Wave—"Any change of the potential difference between pairs of electrodes in EEG recording. May arise in the brain or outside it." Waves have a morphologic difference from the ongoing background activity that gives them a distinct duration.

Pattern—"Any characteristic EEG activity." The term pattern differs from the term wave by emphasizing the existence of particular wave features and referring to a wave type and not a singular wave.

Background activity—"Any EEG activity representing the setting in which a given normal or abnormal pattern appears and from which such pattern is distinguished." Background activity is defined by its morphologic difference from a wave receiving attention. Thus, generalized slowing could be a background activity for another type of wave or could be a collection of individual slow waves.

Morphology "1) The study of the form of EEG waves. 2) The form of EEG waves." This specifically refers to the features of a wave, such as amplitude, contour, and duration. These features are what characterize an overriding wave pattern.

Waveform—"The shape of an EEG wave." This is synonymous with the second definition of morphology.

Baseline—"1) Strictly: line obtained when an identical voltage is applied to the two input terminals of an EEG amplifier or when the instrument is in the calibrate position but no calibration signal is applied. 2) Loosely: imaginary line corresponding to the approximate mean values of the EEG activity assessed visually in an EEG derivation over a period of time." One should note that baseline and background are not synonymous.

Attenuation—"1) Reduction in amplitude of EEG activity. 2) Reduction of sensitivity of an EEG channel." The second definition allows for attenuation to be caused by deliberate changes in the amplifier's gain; however, the first definition is the only one used for the purpose of this reference's descriptor system. One should note that the amount of attenuation is not defined.

Attenuation is characterized by a relatively low amplitude, regardless of the absolute amplitude of the attenuated segment.

Transient—"Any isolated wave or complex, distinguished from background activity."

Complex—"A sequence of two or more waves having a characteristic form or recurring with a fairly consistent form, distinguished from background activity."

Monophasic wave—"Wave developed on one side of the baseline." A monophasic transient is a wave that does not cross the imaginary baseline.

Diphasic wave—"Wave consisting of two components developed on alternate sides of the baseline." A diphasic transient is a complex of two waves that may be either similar or different from each other.

Triphasic wave—"Wave consisting of three components alternating about the baseline." Like the diphasic wave, triphasic waves are complexes. One should note that triphasic wave also is used in reference to a specific EEG pattern with particular clinical significance, as is described under the Triphasic Wave heading of the Patterns section.

Polyphasic wave—"Wave consisting of two or more components developed on alternating sides of the baseline." Polyphasic waves are diphasic waves, triphasic waves, and any complex that includes an even greater number of waves.

Spike—"A transient, clearly distinguished from the background activity, with a pointed peak at conventional paper speeds and a duration from 20 to less than 70 msec. . . Amplitude is variable. . . " See sharp wave.

Sharp wave—"A transient, clearly distinguished from the background activity, with a pointed peak at conventional paper speeds and a duration of 70–200 msec. . . Amplitude is variable. . . " As a deviation from the standard definition, sharp waves are defined for the purpose of this reference by their duration alone. Therefore, any wave lasting between 70 to 200 msec is considered a sharp wave, regardless of morphology or the further restrictions in the glossary definition that exclude specific waves, such as the vertex sharp transient, from the sharp wave category.

Slow wave—"Wave with duration longer than alpha waves." Based on this definition, waves that are not pointed and have a duration longer than 125 msec are considered slow waves. Because this may allow overlap between sharp waves and slow waves, slow waves often are defined as waves lasting longer than 200 msec. This alternate definition is used in this reference.

Regular—"Applies to waves or complexes of approximately constant period and relative uniform appearance." By definition, a regular pattern must include a repeating wave or complex in order for the period and appearance to be unchanging.

Rhythm—"EEG activity consisting of waves of approximately constant period." Because they are not composed of complexes, rhythms have simple, sometimes sinusoidal, morphologies.

Periodic—"Applies to: 1) EEG waves or complexes occurring in a sequence at an approximately regular rate. 2) EEG waves or complexes occurring intermittently at approximately regular intervals, generally of 1 to several seconds."

In addition to the standard terms, the descriptors used for categorization include the following terms that were created for this reference.

Repetition—Any transient that recurs one or more times without interruption by background activity. A repetition may be an isolated wave that recurs and thereby forms a rhythm, or it may be a complex that recurs such as a series of spike and slow wave complexes in immediate succession. Because the definition for periodic allows for intervals between occurrences, a more specific term is used.

Evolution—Applies to repetitions in which the transients change over time in their period, appearance, or distribution across the scalp. Evolving is the opposite of regular.

Focal—An electrical field of an attenuation, transient, or repetition that is limited in its distribution to one electrode location and its immediate neighbors.

Hemispheric—An electrical field of an attenuation, transient, or repetition that is unilateral, extends to include electrode locations that are both anterior and posterior to the coronal midline, and has a distribution across more than two interelectrode distances.

Bilateral—An electrical field of an attenuation, transient, or repetition that extends to include electrode locations across more than two interelectrode distances and on both sides of the sagittal midline, but does not extend to include electrode locations that are both anterior and posterior to the coronal midline.

Generalized—An electrical field of an attenuation, transient, or repetition that is bilateral and extends to include electrode locations that are both anterior and posterior to the vertex, except if the field meets the definition of focal for the vertex. A focal field at the vertex includes Cz and only the electrode locations immediately adjacent to Cz, which are Fz, C3, C4, and Pz.

Polarity—The polarity of a complex is defined by the polarity of the fastest component wave. Therefore, the polarity of a triphasic complex that includes a spike and slow wave is defined for the purpose of categorization as the polarity of the spike.

Categorization with Descriptors

The categorization of a pattern begins with its classification into one of three types: **Attenuation, Transient,** or **Repetition.** These three types constitute the three major headings in the Categorization by Pattern Features section. Following the classification by type, the distribution of the pattern's field is defined as **Focal, Hemispheric, Bilateral,** or **Generalized,** and this descriptor leads to a subheading. Below each of the subheadings is a comprehensive differential diagnosis that includes all of the EEG patterns having features matching the subheading's descriptors. However, the three pattern types vary in how many descriptors are present in its subheadings. Attenuations have no categorization other than field distribution. Transients are further classified by whether the wave is **monophasic, diphasic,** or **triphasic** and whether it is a **spike, sharp wave,** or **slow wave.** With the addition of these two findings, each subheading under transient has three descriptors. Repetitions are further classified by whether the transient that repeats within the wave is **monophasic** or **polyphasic;** thus, two descriptors form each repetition subheading. To demonstrate this process, a phase reversing, temporal discharge lasting 100 msec is categorized as "Transient/Focal/Monophasic/Sharp Wave," and 3-Hz rhythmic activity across the frontal lobes is categorized as "Repetition/Bilateral/Monophasic."

Narrowing the Possibilities

Because some subheadings have extensive differential diagnoses, qualifiers follow each pattern to narrow the lists. Specific location is a qualifier that applies to transients and repetitions with the locations divided into **Frontal, Temporal, Parietal, Central, Occipital,** and **Anywhere.** Anywhere means that the pattern may occur at any location, and this applies to all attenuations. The locations refer to the regions where the pattern are centered and are relevant to even generalized patterns because generalized is defined in this system as bilateral and including both sides of the coronal midline. Thus, a frontal pattern that extends past the vertex is considered generalized for the purpose of categorization and is qualified as frontal to distinguish it from an occipital pattern that also extends past the vertex.

With the location qualifier, patterns in the differential diagnosis are eliminated when their specific location does not match the location of the unfamiliar wave.

For example, among the 12 patterns on the differential for "Transient/Focal/Monophasic/Sharp Wave," there are cardiac artifact, vertex sharp transient, lambda wave, and interictal epileptiform discharge. However, the occurrence of the unfamiliar wave over the temporal lobe eliminates vertex sharp transient and lambda wave from the list because they do not have temporal locations.

The transients include polarity as a second qualifier. The polarity options are **positive, negative,** and **either positive or negative.** Similar to the location qualifier, polarity eliminates patterns from the differential when the polarity does not match the polarity of the unfamiliar wave. If the unfamiliar wave mentioned previously is negative, this qualifier does not further reduce the list of possibilities because both cardiac artifact and interictal epileptiform discharges may be negative. The second feature for the repetitions is whether the pattern is regular or evolving. The repetition patterns are qualified as **evolving, regular,** or having the potential to **either evolve or remain regular.** The repetition pattern categorized previously as Repetition/Bilateral/Monophasic was frontal and not evolving. These two qualifiers eliminate 9 patterns from the total differential of 26.

Identifying the Pattern

Once the differential diagnosis is as short as the categorization and narrowing allows, each of the remaining candidate patterns is compared to the unfamiliar wave. These comparisons use the Pattern section. The Pattern section alphabetically lists all of the patterns contained in the Categorization section. Some of the patterns in the Categorization section have subheadings, and these follow their specific heading in the Pattern section in their own alphabetical order.

The comparison of the unfamiliar wave to each pattern that remains in the differential diagnosis may be accomplished several different ways, and each approach is discussed separately within a pattern's section. Each pattern is described in detail first, and this includes attention to unique features. The morphologic description is followed by a direct contrast between the pattern and other patterns that have similar features. This contrast includes specific features that distinguish the patterns from each other. Next, patterns that may occur around the same portion of the EEG record are listed to use the context of a pattern to help in its identification. Finally, examples of the patterns are provided for a visual comparison. The clinical significance of each pattern also is discussed in this section. These comparisons lead to determination if the unfamiliar wave is the pattern being described and is analogous to using a more detailed clinical reference to verify the diagnosis that is reached from an assembly of the presenting clinical findings.

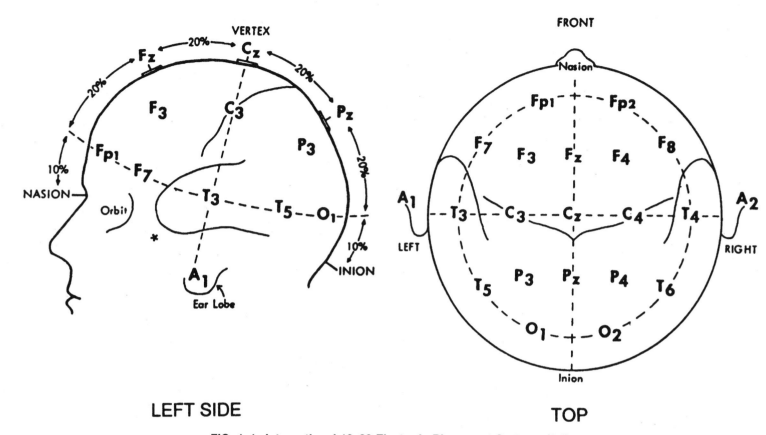

LEFT SIDE   **TOP**

FIG. 1–1. International 10–20 Electrode Placement System. (2,4)

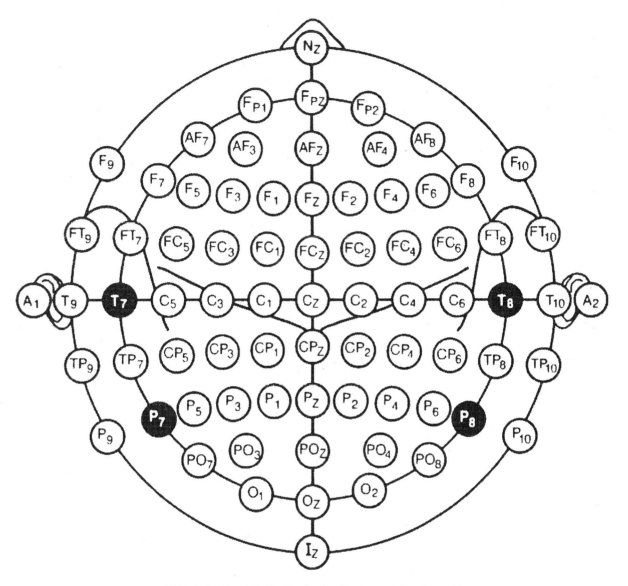

FIG. 1–2. The 10–10 Electrode Placement System. (5)

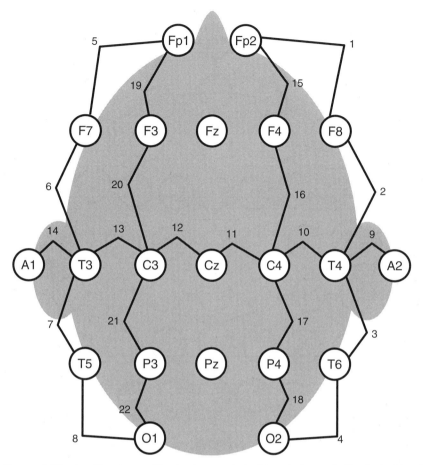

FIG. 1–3. One Type of Bipolar Montage. Electrodes are in bold and channels illustrated by lines linking the electrodes. The channels are labeled with number indicating order of the channels as presented on an EEG page.

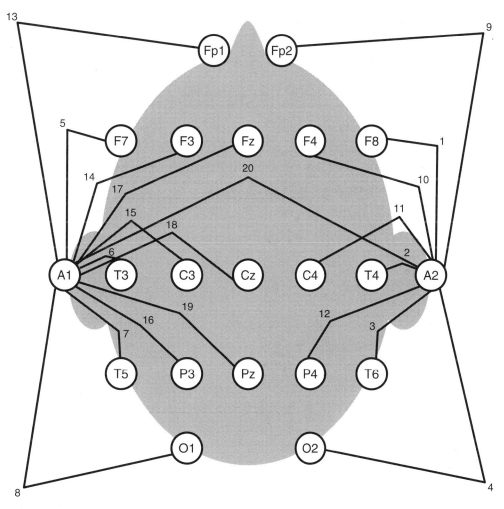

FIG. 1–4. One Type of Referential Montage. An "ipsilateral ear" montage with the channels listed as they may appear on an EEG page.

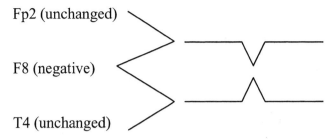

Fp2 (unchanged)

F8 (negative)

T4 (unchanged)

FIG. 1–5. Phase Reversal. With an increased negative field at F8 compared to Fp2, Fp2-F8's resulting wave has a downward deflection. Because F8 is in the opposite position in the F8-T4 channel, convention produces an upward deflection with the increased negative field at F8. Thus, the location of the focal negative field is easily visualized as where the two waves have opposite phase.

SECTION II
Categorization by Pattern Features

CHAPTER 2

Pattern Feature Tables

DEFINITIONS AND ABBREVIATIONS

Focal, field limited to one electrode and its immediate neighbors

Hemispheric, unilateral field that is larger than focal

Bilateral, bilateral field that is limited to either anterior or posterior to the vertex

Generalized, a bilateral field that is both anterior and posterior to the vertex, except if centered at the vertex.

F, frontal
T, temporal
P, parietal
C, central

O, occipital
A, anywhere

For transients:
  p, positive polarity
  n, negative polarity
  p/n, either polarity
For repetitions:
  e, evolves
  r, regular (does not evolve)
  e/r, either

	Location	Page Number
ATTENUATIONS		
Focal		
1. Artifact, electrode	A	61
2. Ictal pattern, focal	A	143
3. Low-voltage EEG	A	195
Hemispheric		
1. Artifact, electrode	A	61
2. Burst-suppression pattern	A	107
3. Ictal pattern, focal	A	143
4. Low-voltage EEG	A	195
Bilateral		
1. Artifact, electrode	A	61
2. Burst-suppression pattern	A	107
3. Ictal pattern, focal	A	143
4. Ictal pattern, generalized	A	154
5. Low-voltage EEG	A	195

	Location	Page Number
ATTENUATIONS *(continued)*		
Generalized		
1. Artifact, electrode		61
2. Burst-suppression pattern		107
3. Low-voltage EEG/Electrocerebral inactivity		195
4. Ictal pattern, generalized		154

	Location	Polarity	Page Number
TRANSIENTS			
Focal/Monophasic/Spike			
1. Alpha activity, mu rhythm fragment	C	n	44
2. Alpha activity, wicket rhythm fragment	T	n	49
3. Artifact, cardiac	A	p/n	55
4. Artifact, electrode	A	p/n	61
5. Artifact, external device	A	p/n	67
6. Artifact, muscle	F/T/C	p/n	73
7. Artifact, ocular (lateral rectus spike)	F	p/n	79
8. Benign epileptiform transients of sleep	F/T	p/n	87
9. Breach effect fragment	A	p/n	101
10. Fourteen & six positive burst fragment	T/P/O/C	p	129
11. Interictal epileptiform discharge, focal	A	p/n	161
12. Occipital spike of blindness	O/P	n	203
Focal/Monophasic/Sharp			
1. Alpha activity, mu rhythm fragment	C	n	44
2. Alpha activity, wicket rhythm fragment	T	n	49
3. Artifact, cardiac	A	p/n	55
4. Artifact, electrode	A	p/n	61
5. Benign epileptiform transient of sleep	F/T	p/n	87
6. Interictal epileptiform discharge, focal	A	p/n	161
7. Lambda wave	O	p	191
8. Positive occipital sharp transients of sleep	O	p	243
9. Theta activity, Cigánek rhythm fragment	C/F	p/n	269
10. Theta activity, polymorphic	A	p/n	273
11. Theta activity, rhythmic midtemporal theta fragment	T	p/n	276
12. Vertex sharp transient	C	n	287

	Location	Polarity	Page Number
TRANSIENTS *(continued)*			
Focal/Monophasic/Slow			
1. Artifact, cardiac	A	p/n	55
2. Artifact, electrode	A	p/n	61
3. Artifact, external device	A	p/n	67
4. Cone wave	O	p/n	113
5. Delta activity, polymorphic	A	p/n	115
6. Lambda wave	O	p	191
7. Theta activity, Cigánek rhythm	C/F	p/n	269
8. Theta activity, polymorphic	A	p/n	273
9. Theta activity, rhythmic midtemporal theta	T	p/n	276
Focal/Diphasic/Spike			
1. Alpha activity, mu rhythm fragment	C	n	44
2. Alpha activity, wicket rhythm fragment	T	n	49
3. Artifact, cardiac	A	p/n	55
4. Artifact, external device	A	p/n	67
5. Artifact, muscle	F/T/C	p/n	73
6. Artifact, ocular (lateral rectus spike)	F	p/n	79
7. Benign epileptiform transient of sleep	F/T	p/n	87
8. Fourteen & six positive burst fragment	T/P/O/C	p	129
9. Interictal epileptiform discharge, focal	A	p/n	161
10. Occipital spike of blindness	O/P	n	203
11. Periodic epileptiform discharges, lateralized (PLEDs)	A	n	213
Focal/Diphasic/Sharp			
1. Alpha activity, mu rhythm fragment	C	n	44
2. Alpha activity, wicket rhythm fragment	T	n	49
3. Artifact, cardiac	A	p/n	55
4. Artifact, muscle	F/T/C	p/n	73
5. Benign epileptiform transient of sleep	F/T	p/n	87
6. Interictal epileptiform discharges, focal	A	p/n	161
7. K complex	C	p/n	185
8. Lambda wave	O	p	191
9. Periodic epileptiform discharges, lateralized (PLEDs)	A	n	213
10. Positive occipital sharp transient of sleep (POSTS)	O	p	243
11. Vertex sharp transient	C	n	287
Focal/Triphasic/Spike			
1. Artifact, cardiac	A	p/n	55
2. Artifact, external device	A	p/n	67
3. Artifact, muscle	F/T/C	p/n	73
4. Artifact, ocular (lateral rectus spike)	F	p/n	79

	Location	Polarity	Page Number

TRANSIENTS (continued)

	Location	Polarity	Page Number
5. Benign epileptiform transient of sleep	F/T	p/n	87
6. Interictal epileptiform discharge, focal	A	p/n	161
7. Periodic epileptiform discharges, lateralized (PLEDs)	A	n	213

Focal/Triphasic/Sharp

	Location	Polarity	Page Number
1. Artifact, cardiac	A	p/n	55
2. Artifact, external device	A	p/n	67
3. Artifact, muscle	F/T/C	p/n	73
4. Benign epileptiform transient of sleep	F/T	p/n	87
5. Interictal epileptiform discharge, focal	A	p/n	161
6. K complex	C	p/n	185
7. Lambda wave	O	p	191
8. Periodic epileptiform discharges, lateral (PLEDs)	A	n	213
9. Vertex sharp transient	C	n	287

Hemispheric/Monophasic/Spike

	Location	Polarity	Page Number
1. Artifact, cardiac	A	p/n	55
2. Artifact, external device	A	p/n	67
3. Benign epileptiform transient of sleep	F/T	p/n	87
4. Breach effect fragment	A	p/n	101
5. Fourteen & six positive burst fragment	T/P/O/C	p	129

Hemispheric/Monophasic/Sharp

	Location	Polarity	Page Number
1. Artifact, cardiac	A	p/n	55
2. Benign epileptiform transient of sleep	F/T	p/n	87
3. Theta activity, polymorphic	A	p/n	273
4. Theta activity, rhythmic midtemporal theta	T	p/n	276

Hemispheric/Monophasic/Slow

	Location	Polarity	Page Number
1. Delta activity, polymorphic	A	p/n	115
2. Delta activity, rhythmic fragment	F/O/T	p/n	122
3. Theta activity, polymorphic	A	p/n	273
4. Theta activity, rhythmic midtemporal theta	T	p/n	276

Hemispheric/Diphasic/Spike

	Location	Polarity	Page Number
1. Artifact, cardiac	A	p/n	55
2. Artifact, external device	A	p/n	67
3. Benign epileptiform transient of sleep	F/T	p/n	87
4. Fourteen & six positive burst fragment	T/P/O/C	p	129
5. Interictal epileptiform discharge, focal	A	n	161
6. Periodic epileptiform discharges, lateralized (PLEDs)	A	n	213

	Location	Polarity	Page Number
TRANSIENTS *(continued)*			
Hemispheric/Triphasic/Spike			
1. Artifact, cardiac	A	p/n	55
2. Benign epileptiform transient of sleep	F/T	p/n	87
3. Interictal epileptiform discharge, focal	A	n	161
4. Periodic epileptiform discharges, lateralized (PLEDs)	A	n	213
Bilateral/Monophasic/Spike			
1. Artifact, cardiac	A	p/n	55
2. Artifact, external device	A	p/n	67
3. Benign epileptiform transient of sleep	F/T	p/n	87
4. Fourteen & six positive burst fragment	T/P/O/C	p	129
5. Interictal epileptiform discharge, focal	F/C/P/O	p/n	161
6. Interictal epileptiform discharge, generalized	F/C	n	174
7. Photic stimulation response, photic driving	O	p/n	233
Bilateral/Monophasic/Sharp			
1. Artifact, cardiac	A	p/n	55
2. Artifact, ocular	F	p/n	79
3. Benign epileptiform transient of sleep	F/T	p/n	87
4. Fourteen & six positive burst fragment	T/P/O/C	p	129
5. Interictal epileptiform discharge, focal	F/C/P/O	p/n	161
6. Interictal epileptiform discharge, generalized	F/C	n	174
7. Positive occipital sharp transient of sleep	O	p	243
8. Theta activity, Cigánek rhythm	C/F	p/n	269
9. Theta activity, polymorphic	A	p/n	273
10. Vertex sharp transient	C	n	287
Bilateral/Monophasic/Slow			
1. Artifact, electrode	A	p/n	61
2. Artifact, ocular	F	p/n	79
3. Cone wave	O	p/n	113
4. Delta activity, polymorphic	A	p/n	115
5. Hypersynchrony and hypersynchronous slow fragment	A	p/n	133
6. Lambda wave	O	p	191
7. Mitten	F	p/n	201
8. Posterior slow wave of youth	O	p/n	247
9. Theta activity, Cigánek Rhythm	C/F	p/n	269
10. Theta activity, polymorphic	A	p/n	273
Bilateral/Diphasic/Sharp			
1. Artifact, cardiac	A	p/n	55
2. Artifact, external device	A	p/n	67

	Location	Polarity	Page Number
TRANSIENTS *(continued)*			
3. Benign epileptiform transient of sleep	F/T	p/n	87
4. K complex	C	p/n	185
5. Interictal epileptiform discharge, focal	F/C/P/O	p/n	161
6. Interictal epileptiform discharge, generalized	F/C	n	174
7. Lambda wave	O	p	191
8. Mitten	F	p/n	201
9. Periodic epileptiform discharges, bilateral (BiPEDs)	F/C/P/O	n	223
10. Positive occipital sharp transient of sleep	O	p	243
11. Posterior slow wave of youth	O	p/n	247
12. Theta activity, Cigánek rhythm	C/F	p/n	269
13. Vertex sharp transient	C	n	287
Bilateral/Triphasic/Spike			
1. Artifact, muscle (photomyogenic)	F	p/n	73
2. Artifact, external device	A	p/n	67
3. Benign epileptiform transient of sleep	F/T	p/n	87
4. Interictal epileptiform discharge, focal	F/C/P/O	p/n	161
5. Interictal epileptiform discharge, generalized	F/C	n	174
6. Periodic epileptiform discharge, bilateral (BiPED)	FC/P/O	n	223
7. Phantom spike and wave	F/O	n	229
8. Photic stimulation response, photoparoxysmal	O	n	238
Bilateral/Triphasic/Sharp			
1. Artifact, cardiac	A	p/n	55
2. Benign epileptiform transient of sleep	F/T	p/n	87
3. Interictal epileptiform discharge, focal	F/C/P/O	p/n	161
4. Interictal epileptiform discharge, generalized	F/C	n	174
5. K complex	C	p/n	185
6. Lambda wave	O	p	191
7. Periodic epileptiform discharge, bilateral (BiPED)	FC/P/O	n	223
8. Phantom spike and wave	F/O	n	229
9. Posterior slow waves of youth	O	p/n	247
10. Triphasic waves	F/O	p	281
11. Vertex sharp transient	C	n	287
Generalized/Monophasic/Spike			
1. Artifact, external device	A	p/n	67
Generalized/Monophasic/Sharp			
1. Artifact, electrode	A	p/n	61
2. Artifact, external device	A	p/n	67
3. Theta activity, polymorphic	A	p/n	273

	Location	Polarity	Page Number
TRANSIENTS *(continued)*			
Generalized/Monophasic/Slow			
1. Artifact, electrode	A	p/n	61
2. Delta activity, polymorphic	A	p/n	115
3. Hypersynchrony and hypersynchronous slowing	A	p/n	133
4. Theta activity, polymorphic	A	p/n	273
Generalized/Diphasic			
1. Interictal epileptiform discharge, generalized	F/C	n	174
2. Periodic epileptiform discharge, bilateral (BiPED)	F/C/P/O	n	223
Generalized/Triphasic			
1. Interictal epileptiform discharge, generalized	F/C	n	174
2. Periodic epileptiform discharge, bilateral (BiPED)	F/C/P/O	n	223
3. Triphasic waves	F/O	p	281

	Location	Regular/Evolving	Page Numbers
REPETITIONS			
Focal/Monophasic			
1. Alpha activity, alpha rhythm (Bancaud's phenomenon)	O/T/P	r	27
2. Alpha activity, mu rhythm	C	r	44
3. Alpha activity, wicket rhythm	T	r	49
4. Artifact, electrode	A	r	61
5. Artifact, external device	A	r/e	67
6. Beta activity, frontocentral	F/C/P	r	93
7. Breach effect	A	r	101
8. Delta activity, polymorphic	A	r	115
9. Delta activity, rhythmic	F/T/O	r	122
10. Interictal epileptiform discharges, focal	A	r	161
11. Ictal pattern, focal	A	e	143
12. Paroxysmal fast activity	A	r	207
13. Photic stimulation response, photic driving	O	r	233
14. Posterior occipital sharp transients of sleep	O	r	243
15. Saw-tooth waves of REM sleep	C/F	r	251
16. Spindles	C/F	r	255
17. Subclinical rhythmic electrographic discharge of adults (SREDA)	T/P/O/C	e	263
18. Theta activity, Cigánek rhythm	C/F	r	269
19. Theta activity, polymorphic	A	r	273
20. Theta activity, rhythmic midtemporal theta	T	r	276
21. Vertex sharp transients	C	r	287

	Location	Regular/Evolving	Page Number
REPETITIONS (continued)			
Focal/Polyphasic			
1. Artifact, electrode	A	r	61
2. Artifact, external device	A	r	67
3. Artifact, muscle	F/T/C	r/e	73
4. Interictal epileptiform discharge, focal	A	r	161
5. Ictal pattern, focal	A	e	143
6. Theta activity, Cigánek rhythm	C/F	r	269
7. Theta activity, rhythmic midtemporal theta	T	r	276
Hemispheric/Monophasic			
1. Alpha activity, alpha rhythm	O/T/P	r	27
2. Alpha activity, mu rhythm	C	r	44
3. Alpha activity, wicket rhythm	T	r	49
4. Artifact, electrode	A	r/e	61
5. Breach effect	A	r	101
6. Burst-suppression pattern	A	r/e	107
7. Delta activity, polymorphic	A	r	115
8. Delta activity, rhythmic	T/F/O	r	122
9. Fourteen & six positive bursts	T/P/C/O	r/e	129
10. Hypersynchrony and hypersynchronous slowing	A	r/e	133
11. Ictal pattern, focal	A	e	143
12. Paroxysmal fast activity	A	r	207
13. Spindles	C/F	r	255
14. Subclinical rhythmic electrographic discharge of adults (SREDA)	T/P/O/C	e	263
15. Theta activity, polymorphic	A	r	273
16. Theta activity, rhythmic midtemporal theta	T	r	276
Hemispheric/Polyphasic			
1. Artifact, electrode	A	r/e	61
2. Artifact, muscle	F/T/C	r	73
3. Burst-suppression pattern	A	r/e	107
4. Ictal pattern, focal	A	e	143
5. Theta activity, rhythmic midtemporal theta	T	r	276
Bilateral/Monophasic			
1. Alpha activity, alpha rhythm	O/T/P	r	27
2. Alpha activity, mu rhythm	C	r	44
3. Alpha activity, wicket rhythm	T	r	49
4. Artifact, electrode	A	r/e	61
5. Artifact, external device	A	r	67
6. Artifact, muscle	F/T/C	r	73
7. Artifact, ocular	F	r	79

	Location	Regular/Evolving	Page Number
REPETITIONS *(continued)*			
8. Beta activity, frontocentral	F/C/P	r	93
9. Burst-suppression pattern	A	r/e	107
10. Delta activity, rhythmic	F/O	r	122
11. Delta activity, polymorphic	A	r	115
12. Fourteen & six positive bursts	T/P/C/O	r/e	129
13. Hypersynchrony and hypersynchronous slowing	A	r/e	133
14. Ictal pattern, focal	A	e	143
15. Ictal pattern, generalized	A	r/e	154
16. Paroxysmal fast activity	F/C	r	207
17. Phantom spike and wave	F/O	r	229
18. Photic stimulation response, driving response	O	r	233
19. Positive occipital sharp transients of sleep	O	r	243
20. Posterior slow waves of youth	O	r	247
21. Saw-tooth waves of REM sleep	C/F	r	251
22. Spindles	C/F	r	255
23. Subclinical rhythmic electrographic discharge of adults (SREDA)	T/P/O/C	e	263
24. Theta activity, Cigánek rhythm	C/F	r	269
25. Theta activity, polymorphic	A	r	273
26. Vertex sharp transients	C	r	287
Bilateral/Polyphasic			
1. Artifact, cardiac	A	r	55
2. Artifact, muscle	F/T/C	r	73
3. Burst-suppression pattern	A	r/e	107
4. Ictal pattern, generalized	A	r/e	154
5. Interictal epileptiform discharge, focal	F/C/P/O	r	161
6. Interictal epileptiform discharge, generalized	F/C	r/e	174
7. Periodic epileptiform discharges, bilateral (BiPEDs)	F/C/P/O	r	223
8. Phantom spike and wave	F/O	r	229
9. Photic stimulation response; photoparoxysmal response	O	r/e	238
10. Posterior slow waves of youth	O	r	247
11. Theta activity, Cigánek rhythm	C/F	r	269
12. Triphasic waves	F/O	r	281
Generalized/Monophasic			
1. Alpha activity, generalized	A	r	42
2. Artifact, external device	A	r/e	67
3. Beta activity, frontocentral	F/C/P	r	93
4. Beta activity, generalized	A	r	98
5. Burst-suppression pattern	A	r/e	107
6. Delta activity, polymorphic	A	r	115
7. Fourteen & six per second positive bursts	T/P/C/O	r/e	129

	Location	Regular/Evolving	Page Number
REPETITIONS *(continued)*			
8. Hypersynchrony and hypersynchronous slowing	A	r/e	133
9. Ictal pattern, generalized	A	r/e	154
10. Interictal epileptiform discharges, generalized	F/C	r/e	174
11. Paroxysmal fast activity	F/C	r	207
12. Phantom spike and wave	F/O	r	229
13. Saw-tooth waves of REM sleep	F/C	r	251
14. Subclinical rhythmic electrographic discharge of adults (SREDA)	T/P/C/O	e	263
15. Theta activity, polymorphic	A	r	273
Generalized/Polyphasic			
1. Artifact, cardiac	A	r	55
2. Artifact, electrode	A	r/e	61
3. Artifact, external device	A	r/e	67
4. Artifact, muscle	F/T/C	r/e	73
5. Burst-suppression pattern	A	r/e	107
6. Ictal pattern, generalized	A	r/e	154
7. Interictal epileptiform discharge, generalized	F/C	r/e	174
8. Periodic epileptiform discharges, bilateral (BiPEDs)	F/C/P/O	r	223
9. Phantom spike and wave	F/O	r	229
10. Photic stimulation response; photoparoxysmal response	O	r/e	238
11. Triphasic waves	F/O	r	281

SECTION III

Patterns

CHAPTER 3

Alpha Activity

ALPHA RHYTHM

Other Names and Types
Occipital alpha rhythm
Posterior dominant rhythm
Posterior basic rhythm
Alpha squeak
Squeak effect

Description
With Hans Berger's 1929 publication on the human electroencephalogram (EEG), the Alpha rhythm (AR) was the first EEG pattern to be described, and it continues to be the most commonly noted rhythm in clinical EEG interpretation because it is reproducible and easily recognized. According to the International Federation of Societies for Electroencephalography and Clinical Neurophysiology (IFSECN) definition, the AR has a frequency of 8 to 13 Hz and is present over the posterior head regions in a state of relaxed wakefulness with the eyes closed (1) (Figs. 3–1 and 3–2). It blocks, that is, attenuates or disappears with drowsiness, concentration, stimulation, or visual fixation. Thus, the AR may be present with the eyes opened if the environment is devoid of light. Drowsy individuals who awaken and open their eyes without immediate visual fixation may have a paradoxical AR in which the AR is absent with eyes closed and briefly present with eyes opened (6,7). This is most common in the context of sedation (8).

The extent of the AR's blocking varies among individuals and, along with amplitude and persistence, tends to decrease with aging (7). However, the complete absence of blocking with either visual fixation or concentration is abnormal (9–11). Unilateral blocking also is abnormal and is termed Bancaud's phenomenon (12) (Fig. 3–3). In such instances, the side lacking the blocking response is abnormal.

The AR's amplitude varies among individuals and usually is between 40 and 50 μV in adults. An amplitude greater than 60 μV occurs in only 6% of adults, and an amplitude greater than 100 μV is exceedingly rare (6). Overall, children have higher amplitude ARs (13). Adults commonly have a low-amplitude AR with 30% having an amplitude less than 20 μV. An amplitude between 5 and 10 μV is not rare, and the AR is not present in up to 10% of healthy individuals (10,14). The AR commonly extends over a smaller distribution or is absent when blindness has been present since early in life (15,16). Its absence also may be genetic with autosomal dominant inheritance (17). Because of the AR's large and uniform field, its amplitude is most accurately measured with a referential montage.

The AR's morphology usually is sinusoidal but may be arceau with a sharply contoured negative component. Regardless of the morphology for the individual waves, the rhythm as a collection of waves occurs as spindles with amplitudes that build and fall over periods of about 1 second. This spindle pattern is due to superimposition of two frequencies, which also produces the arceau morphology if one of the frequencies is in the beta frequency range (9). The frequency within the spindle's packet typically is 9 or 10 Hz in healthy adolescents and adults.

During childhood, a rhythm is present that is similar to the AR in its location and reactivity but has a frequency below the alpha frequency range. Because it is not alpha activity, it is better termed the posterior dominant rhythm (PDR); however, it commonly is referred to as the AR because of its similar significance. Similarly, the AR in adults may be referred to as the PDR, especially when it is abnormally slow. The PDR first develops at 3 or 4 months in 75% of infants and at this age has a frequency of 4 Hz (6,18). By 1 year, its frequency is 5 or 6 Hz in 70% of children. By 3 years, 80% have a true AR because the PDR has reached a frequency of 8 Hz. By 9 years, 65% have a frequency of 9 Hz; by 15 years, 65% have a frequency of 10 Hz (7,14). The AR's frequency in early childhood is highly variable with frequencies between 5 and 10 Hz commonly occurring during the second year (13). Frequencies less than 8.5 Hz are abnormal in adults regardless of age (19). The AR's frequency commonly declines by 1 Hz between early and late adulthood, but a decrease below 8.5 Hz is a sign of cerebral dysfunction even in centenarians (20–22). Frequency assessment should not include the first 0.5 to 1 second after eye closure because this period may have a brief, higher frequency, which is termed alpha squeak or the squeak effect (23) (Fig. 3–4).

The AR's frequency may occur as two normal variants, the slow alpha variant and the fast alpha variant. Both of the variants have the same location and reactivity as the AR (7,9). The slow alpha variant is a subharmonic of the AR that may be due to a fusion of adjacent waves (9) (Fig. 3–5). Its frequency usually is 4 to 5 Hz , that is, half of the AR frequency present at other times in the same EEG. The waves within the slow alpha variant may or may not have a minor bifurcation indicating the two component waves that constitute the normal AR frequency (13,14). The slow alpha variant typically first occurs around age 8 years (7). The fast alpha variant is a harmonic of the AR and usually has a frequency between 16 and 20 Hz (7) (Fig. 3–6). It also may have a bifurcated morphology, but the bifurcation for the fast alpha variant is of the waves in the normal AR. Both variants occur as brief repetitions among the typical AR or, occasionally, in place of it, and both block in the same way as the AR.

The AR's distribution always includes the occiput and commonly extends to include the posterior temporal and occipital parietal regions. This extension should be symmetric, and asymmetry in this indicates abnormality on the side with a larger field. The normal frequency asymmetry between the sides is less than 1 Hz (10). Frequency asymmetries greater than this are due to the superimposition or admixture of slower activity; thus, the side with the lower frequency is abnormal (9).

Some amplitude asymmetry is present for 60% of individuals, and this asymmetry rarely is greater than 20 μV. About 80% of those who have an AR asymmetry have greater amplitude on the right side (24). This asymmetry is not related to handedness and may be due to asymmetry in the skull's thickness (7). When the right side has a higher amplitude, the asymmetry is abnormal when the left is less than 50% of the right (7,9,10,13). Only 1.5% of those with amplitude asymmetry have more than a 50% difference between the sides. Because greater amplitude on the left side is much less common, the maximum allowable asymmetry is for the right to be less than 67% of the left (14), that is, the left should not be greater than 150% of the right. As with all amplitude measurements for the AR, assessment of symmetry should be done with a referential montage (9) (Figs. 3–7, 3–8, and 3–9). When the amplitude has a greater asymmetry that is not caused by a breach effect, the side of lower amplitude usually is abnormal side. Occasionally, a space-occupying lesion within the occiput may produce an abnormal increase in the ipsilateral AR.

During drowsiness, the AR disappears with a transition that includes a decrease in amplitude, extension of the field anteriorly, a loss of clearly sinusoidal or arceau morphology, and inclusion of more theta frequency range activity (9,25) (Fig. 3–10). Eventually, the rhythm's overall frequency reaches the theta frequency range (26). The anterior extension may reach the central and midtemporal regions and becomes frontal in rare instances (7). With arousal from drowsiness, alpha activity sometimes is briefly present with a frontal predominance. This most commonly occurs in children and has a duration of up to 20 seconds (27).

Distinguishing Features
Versus Generalized Alpha Activity

In drowsiness, the AR may resemble generalized alpha activity because of its extension into the temporal and frontocentral regions; however, it remains distinguishable by its occipital predominance and reactivity to either visual fixation or levels of alertness. Generalized alpha in the context of coma, regardless of its cause, does not respond to either condition.

Versus Phi Rhythm

The phi rhythm is a brief, paroxysmal, bisynchronous, occipital delta rhythm that occurs within 2 seconds of eye closure and lasts 1 to 3 seconds (28). Because of these features, it has similarity to the slow alpha variant. It differs from this AR through its consistent occurrence only with eye closure and absence during periods of sustained lack of visual fixation. The slow alpha variant typically occurs throughout the time that the AR is present.

Co-occurring Waves
The AR is present only in wakefulness; thus, it always is accompanied by other EEG signs of wakefulness. This includes both eye blink artifact and muscle

artifact. However, the AR is absent in wakefulness when blinks are frequent, which indicates that the eyes are open, and when muscle artifact is considerable, which indicates a relaxed state is not present. Further evidence that a pattern in the AR arises from the pattern's change or disappearance with EEG signs of drowsiness, such as increased theta frequency activity, vertex sharp transients, and positive occipital sharp transients of sleep (POSTS). Lambda waves also occur during wakefulness and have an occipital distribution. However, they occur when the eyes are open and are therefore independent to the AR (6).

Clinical Significance

The AR is a normal pattern that likely is due to rhythmic cellular interactions between occipital and some parietal cortex and the pulvinar region of the thalamus (29–34). Its function likely relates to gated levels of attention, perhaps as an active stand-by state (35). Within individuals who are adolescent or older, its frequency is highly reproducible among EEG recordings of the same state. Because drowsiness increases the slowing within the AR, ascertainment of whether the EEG includes the best waking state is important in determining whether abnormal slowing is present. Thus, a consistently slow AR within an EEG that does not include the best possible waking state should not be interpreted as abnormal. Notation from the technologist describing the observed behavioral state and responses to stimulation are the preferred source of waking state information, but observing movement and ocular artifact also is helpful.

Apparent slowing of the AR with inclusion of greater theta activity commonly occurs with encephalopathy, regardless of whether the condition is reversible (Fig. 3–11). Therefore, a slow AR (better termed PDR) in the best waking state is a nonspecific finding that may indicate either posterior or generalized cerebral dysfunction. Abnormal changes to the AR also may occur in the absence of encephalopathy. Hypoperfusion may produce asymptomatic slowing of the AR by up to 2 Hz, which may be reversed by improvement in cardiac output (14). Fever and hypermetabolic states, including hyperthyroidism and amphetamine intoxication, may increase the AR's frequency (6,36) (Fig. 3–12). In contrast to adults, high fever in children may increase or decrease the frequency (7). Hypothyroidism and antiepileptic medications may produce an asymptomatic and minor decrease in the AR frequency (37). Marijuana may produce an increase or a decrease in the AR frequency, depending on the psychologic effect of the drug (36).

Failure of the AR to be blocked either unilaterally (Bancaud's phenomenon) or bilaterally usually is due to a structural abnormality but also may occur transiently with migraines or transient ischemic attacks (27). When unilateral, the pathology is ipsilateral to the side that fails to block and usually within occipital lobe or its subcortical gray matter connections (7). However, it sometimes occurs with lesions of the parietal or temporal lobes (27). The absence of blocking bilaterally may be due to an occipital or a pontine lesion (6,38,39).

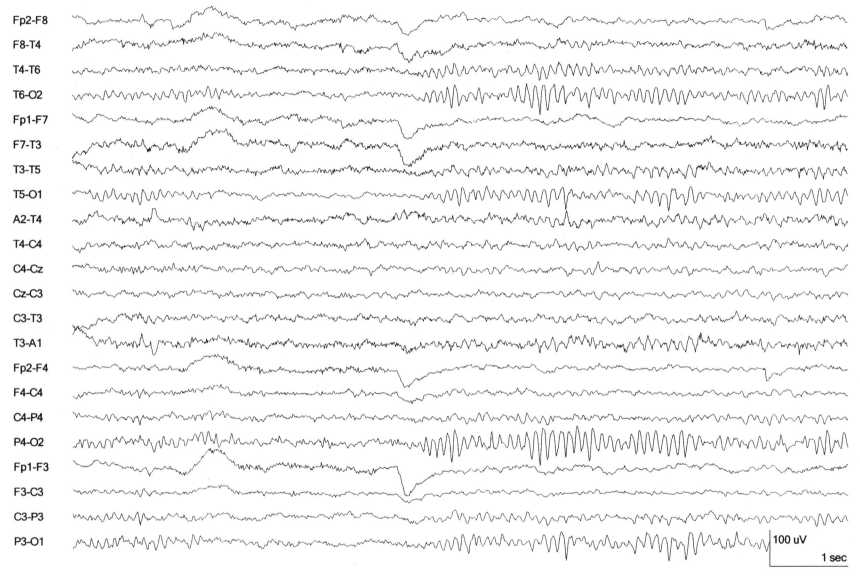

FIG. 3–1. Normal Alpha Rhythm. The alpha rhythm appears immediately following the eye-blink artifact and has the typical spindle pattern. (LFF 1 Hz, HFF 70 Hz)

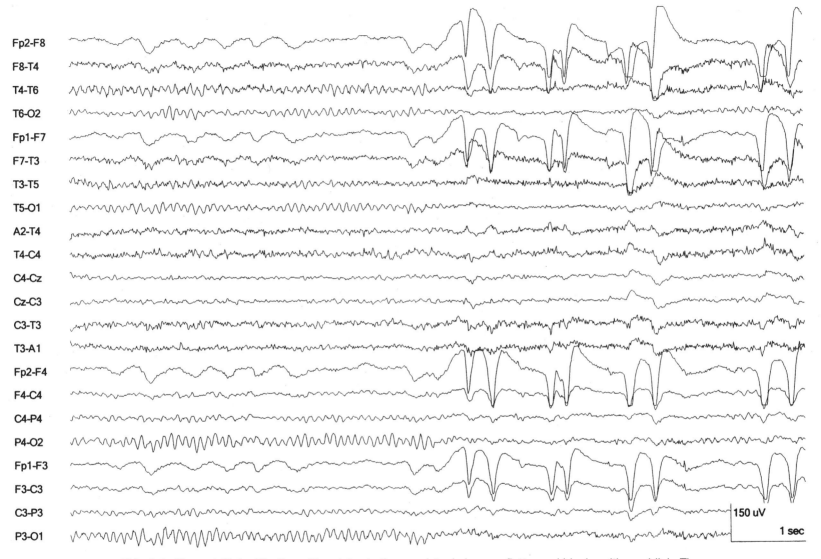

FIG. 3–2. Normal Alpha Rhythm. The alpha rhythm persists during eye flutter and blocks with eye blink. The spindle pattern is less apparent than in Fig. 3–1. (LFF 1 Hz, HFF 70 Hz)

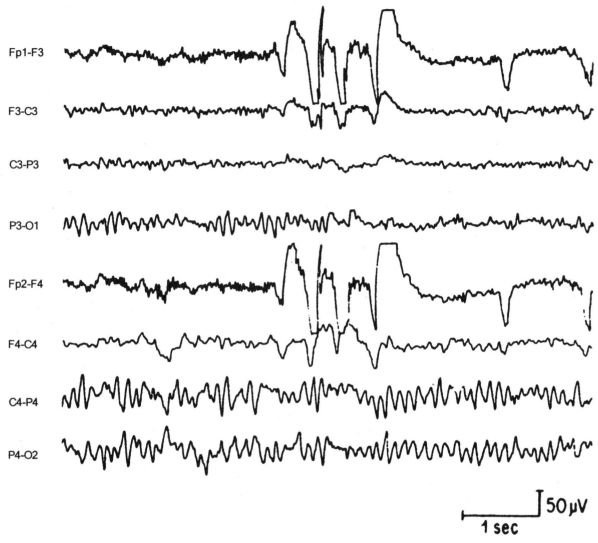

FIG. 3–3. Bancaud's Phenomenon. With eye opening, the alpha rhythm blocks on the left side but continues unchanged on the right. The EEG corresponds to a right posterior cerebral infarction. (From Westmoreland BF, Klass DW. Unusual EEG patterns. *J Clin Neurophysiol* 1990;7:209–228, with permission.)

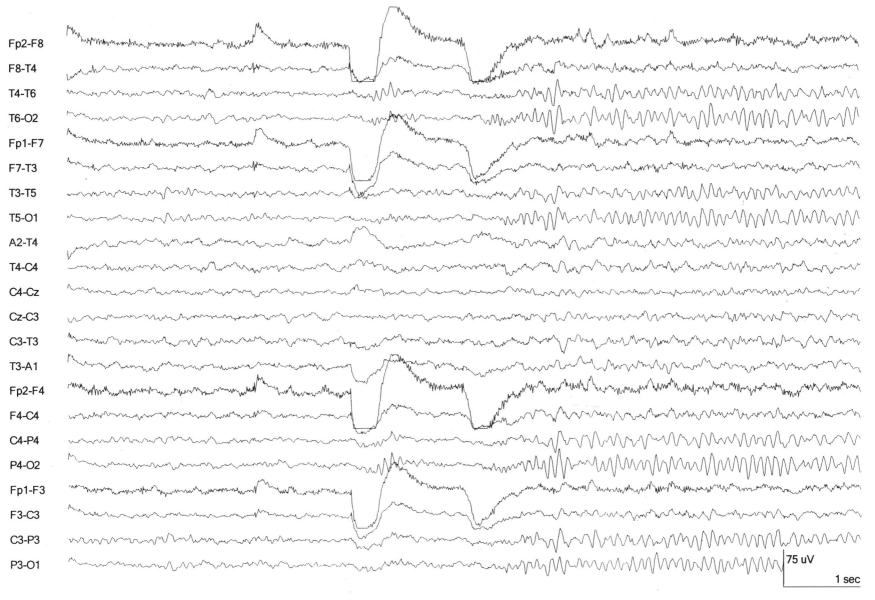

FIG. 3–4. Alpha Squeak. The alpha rhythm's frequency is slightly higher as it first appears following the eye-blink artifact. (LFF 1 Hz, HFF 70 Hz)

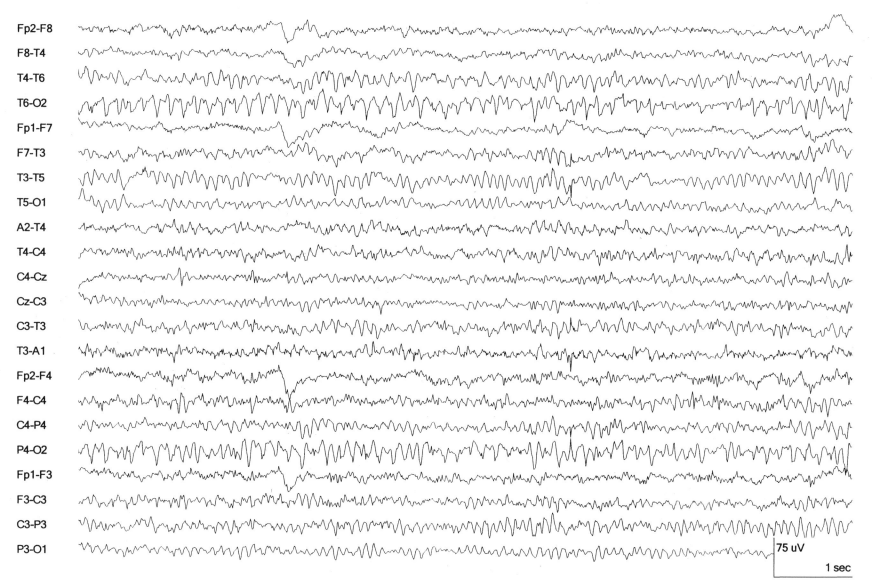

FIG. 3–5. Slow Alpha Variant. The alpha rhythm's component waves are bifurcated, indicating that the apparent frequency is a subharmonic of the true frequency. (LFF 1 Hz, HFF 70 Hz)

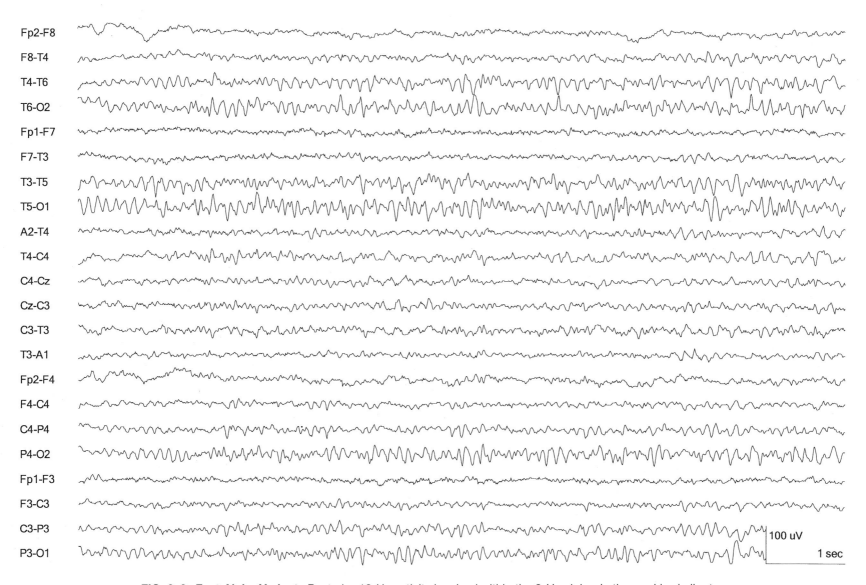

FIG. 3–6. Fast Alpha Variant. Posterior 18-Hz activity is mixed within the 9-Hz alpha rhythm and is similar to the two component waves of the bifurcated alpha rhythm waves. (LFF 1 Hz, HFF 70 Hz)

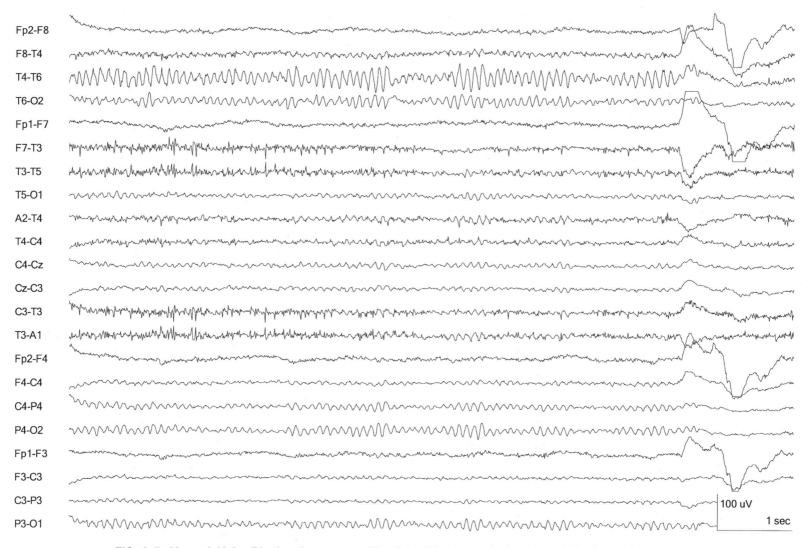

FIG. 3–7. Normal Alpha Rhythm Asymmetry. The right-sided alpha rhythm is 47 μV in the T6-O2 channel, and the left-sided is 22 μV in the T5-O1 channel. As illustrated in Fig. 3–8, this asymmetry is due to a broad and isoelectric field across the left side with loss of amplitude due to the common mode rejection recording technique. The alpha rhythm attenuates with eye opening at the end of the segment. (LFF 1 Hz, HFF 70 Hz)

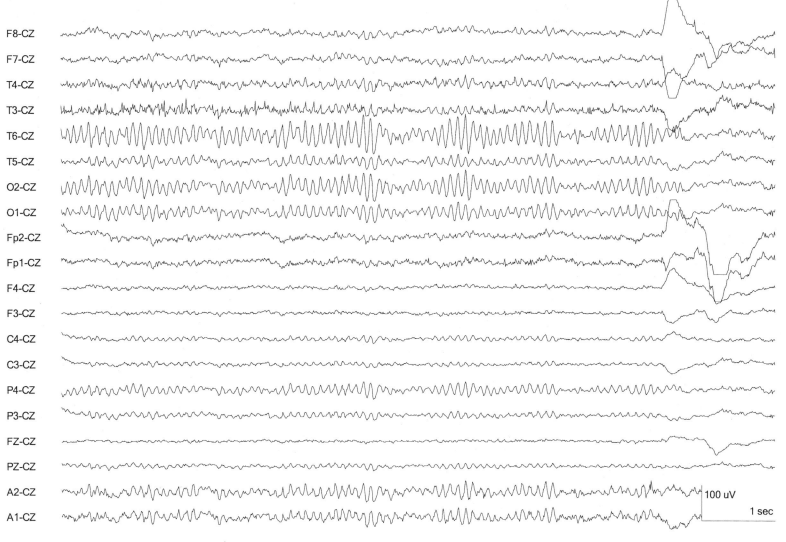

FIG. 3–8. Normal Alpha Rhythm Asymmetry. Referenced to the vertex, the alpha rhythm is 89 μV in the O2 channel and 62 μV in the O1 channel, which is within the limits of normal asymmetry. The similarity between the O1 and T5 channels leads to the low-amplitude T5-O1 channel in Fig. 3–7. (LFF 1 Hz, HFF 70 Hz)

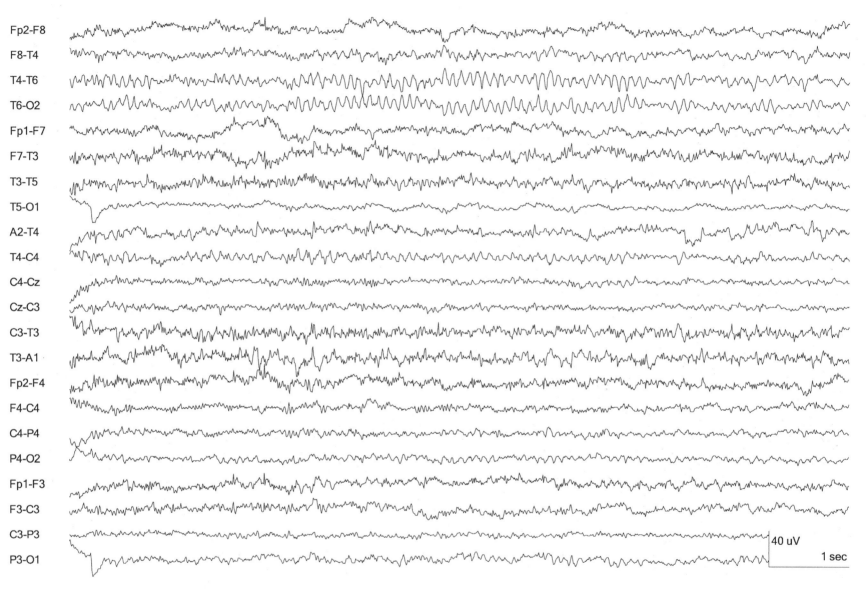

FIG. 3–9. Abnormal Alpha Rhythm Asymmetry. Even at a high gain, the left side's alpha rhythm is not present in this bipolar montage or in a referential montage. No other abnormality is evident, and this is evidence of dysfunction in the left thalamo-occipital system. (LFF 1 Hz, HFF 70 Hz)

OR T5 electrode is defective

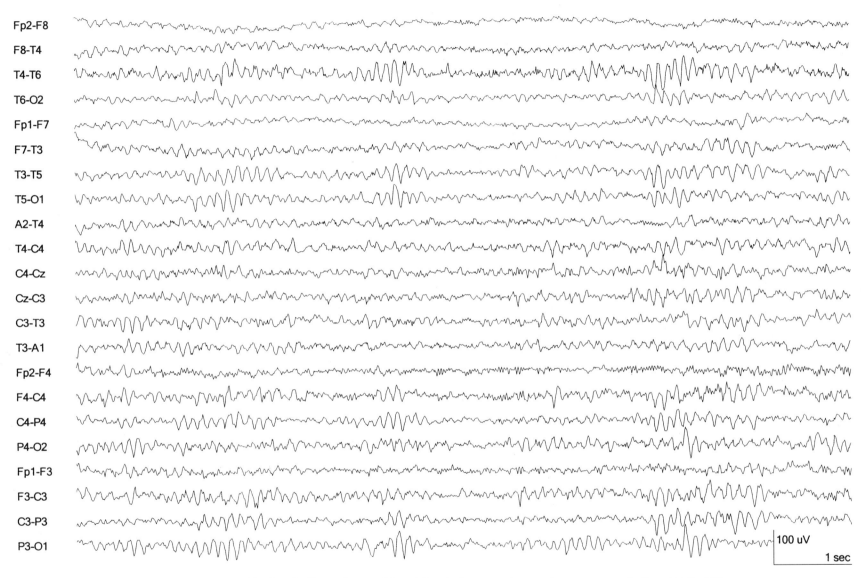

FIG. 3–10. Alpha Rhythm in Drowsiness. The alpha rhythm spontaneously appears and disappears with extension anteriorly and occasional replacement by theta frequency range activity. Increased frontal beta activity and slow roving eye movement artifact are other signs of drowsiness that are present. (LFF 1 Hz, HFF 70 Hz)

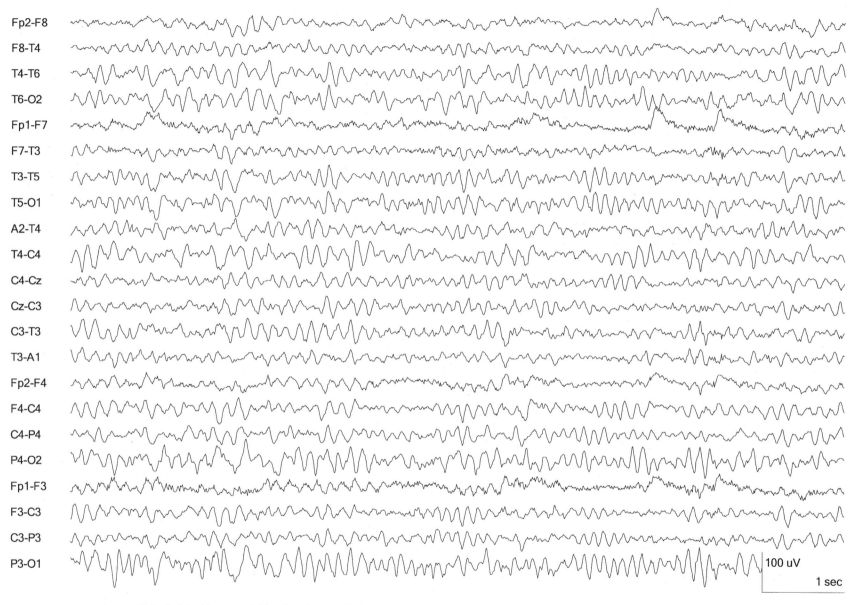

FIG. 3–11. Abnormal Slowing in the Alpha Rhythm. The alpha rhythm has normal posterior predominance and spindling and has the lower frequency activity and extension anteriorly that are compatible with drowsiness. However, other signs of drowsiness are minimal. Identifying this as abnormal depends on ascertaining that the EEG reflects the best awake state. (LFF 1 Hz, HFF 70 Hz)

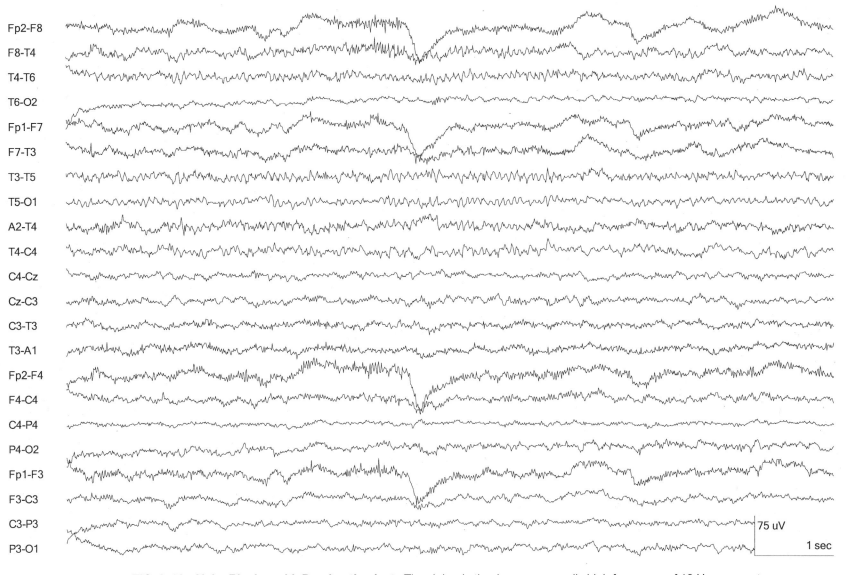

FIG. 3–12. Alpha Rhythm with Psychostimulant. The alpha rhythm has an unusually high frequency of 13 Hz but is otherwise normal. The unusual temporal distribution on the right is due to an asymmetric dipole. Eye-blink artifact in this segment does not correspond to alpha rhythm attenuation because of the lack of visual fixation with the brief opening and closing of the eyes. The EEG corresponds to a 14-year-old being treated with methylphenidate, which also produced the increased, generalized beta activity. (LFF 1 Hz, HFF 70 Hz)

GENERALIZED ALPHA ACTIVITY

Other Names
Alpha coma
Alpha-theta coma
Frontal arousal rhythm

Description
Alpha frequency range activity may occur with a generalized distribution. When it does, it is monotonous, monomorphic, symmetric, and most commonly anteriorly predominant (40) (Fig. 3–13). This is especially true for alpha bursts during normal non–rapid eye movement (NREM) sleep. Abnormal bursts of alpha into rapid eye movement (REM) and NREM sleep occur with a central predominance (26,41). In NREM sleep, these bursts occur in slow wave sleep stages and thereby have the name alpha-delta sleep. In both REM and NREM sleep, longer versions of such bursts represent microarousals and possibly sleep fragmentation. Generalized alpha due to coma or sedation has the most widespread distribution but still is best formed anteriorly (42). It is highly persistent and typically does not vary with stimulation but spontaneously increases or decreases slightly in frequency.

Frontally predominant alpha activity also occurs as an arousal response, especially in children. This pattern typically has a frequency between 7 and 10 Hz and lasts up to 20 seconds (43). The arousal alpha pattern also may occur as a harmonic of its typical frequency.

Distinguishing Features
Versus Alpha Rhythm

Generalized alpha activity may resemble the AR in drowsiness because of the AR's extension into the temporal and frontocentral regions. However, the AR remains distinguishable by its occipital predominance and reactivity to visual fixation and levels of alertness. Generalized alpha in the context of coma, regardless of its cause, does not respond to either condition.

Versus Mu Rhythm

The mu rhythm's frontocentral location overlaps with the predominant region of generalized alpha activity. However, a straightforward differentiation depends on the state in which it occurs and its morphology. Accompanying waveforms indicating wakefulness distinguish the mu rhythm from generalized alpha of any etiology. Furthermore, the mu rhythm's arciform morphology is not characteristic of generalized alpha.

Co-occurring Waves
Although generalized alpha activity in encephalopathy or coma often is the predominant wave present, it frequently is accompanied by other waves that typically occur with diffuse cerebral dysfunction. These include polymorphic delta activity, generalized theta activity, generalized beta activity, and spindles.

Clinical Significance
Generalized alpha activity is a nonspecific pattern that is most associated with coma, and when it occurs in the context of coma, it does not alter the medical prognosis (44). This is exemplified by generalized alpha having the same features when it accompanies coma due to reversible sedation and acute coma due to a major hypoxic-ischemic injury (42,45,46). Alpha coma due to brainstem infarction may differ by having a more posterior distribution and thus resemble a persistent AR (47). The disappearance of generalized alpha activity when a coma due to diffuse cerebral injury becomes prolonged also is not helpful in establishing a prognosis. Typically, generalized alpha is replaced within 10 days by generalized polymorphic delta activity, which also is nonspecific with regard to prognosis (48). However, an incomplete manifestation of the classic generalized alpha pattern through either the presence of reactivity or spontaneous variation may be an indicator of a greater chance for recovery (49).

Lissencephaly in infants also may produce generalized alpha activity (50). In such cases, the pattern often includes beta frequency activity, does not vary with behavioral state, and typically has a high amplitude that may reach amplitudes of 350 to 400 μV.

The most important aspect in interpreting the EEG as demonstrating generalized alpha is the consideration of whether it truly is demonstrating an AR. The presence of an AR when a patient appears comatose indicates that the patient is conscious and either feigning unresponsiveness or is in a de-efferented (locked-in) state due to a brainstem lesion (51,52). The alpha activity of the AR most likely has a different source than the alpha activity in generalized alpha with coma. This difference is demonstrated by the occurrence of alpha coma in children too young to generate an AR within the alpha frequency range (53).

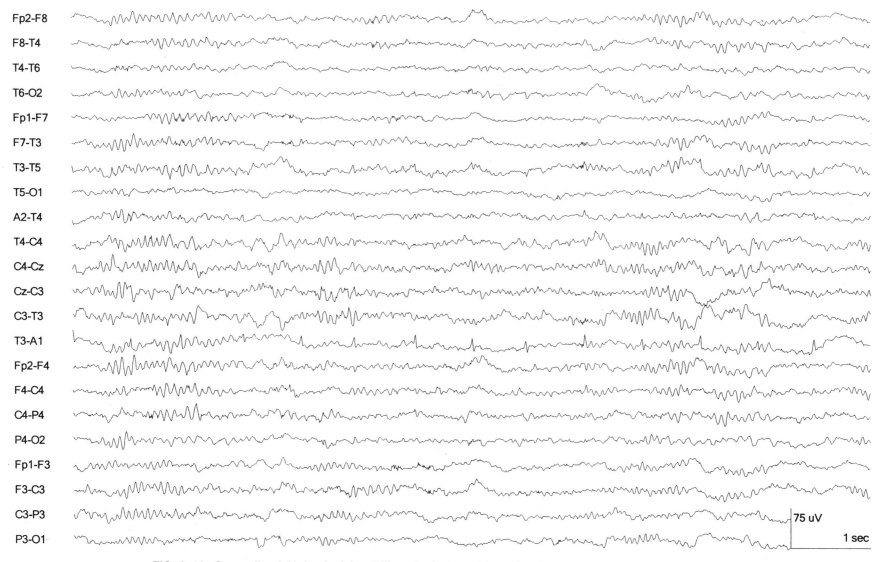

FIG. 3–13. Generalized Alpha Activity. Diffuse rhythmic activity with a frequency of about 10 Hz is present intermittently and amid diffuse lower amplitude polymorphic slowing. The EEG corresponds to medication-related encephalopathy, which was manifested by disoriented wandering. (LFF 1 Hz, HFF 70 Hz)

MU RHYTHM

Other Names
Rolandic mu rhythm
Central mu rhythm
Precentral alpha rhythm
Somatosensory alpha rhythm
Arceau rhythm (rythme rolandique en arceau)
Comb rhythm

Description
The mu rhythm takes its name from the morphology of its component waves and is distinct from other activity that happens to have the same morphology, which may be described with one of the synonymous terms mu, arciform, arceau, comb, wicket, and arcade. This morphology of regularly repeating waves that are sharply contoured in the direction of one polarity and rounded in the direction of the other may occur in many regions and with differing features and significances, as is evident with the wicket rhythm. For the mu rhythm, the rounded phase is positive and the sharply contoured one is negative (9) (Figs. 3–14, 3–15, and 3–16). This is opposite to the fourteen and six positive spike pattern. The mu rhythm has the medium amplitude of the AR and a frequency similar to the AR's typical 10 Hz (6). It usually is within 1 Hz of the AR in the same EEG but is more often 1 Hz slower than 1 Hz faster (7). Unlike the AR, a frequency of 8 Hz in an adult is not abnormal because 7-Hz mu rhythms commonly occur in otherwise normal EEGs. Overall, the mu rhythm's normal frequency range is from 7 to 11 Hz. The mu rhythm differs from the AR in its morphology and its central location. The mu rhythm is maximal at either C3 or C4, with Cz sometimes within the maximal field. More rarely, it is centered at P3 or P4 (9). It does not occur bilaterally symmetrically. Runs of the mu rhythm last one to several seconds and have a shifting asymmetry. A mu rhythm that is entirely unilateral is likely to be abnormal unless it is over a skull defect. The relevance of mu rhythm asymmetry has not been investigated as thoroughly as that of AR asymmetry.

The mu rhythm first appears as early as around age 2 years but commonly is not present until adolescence (13). It is most prevalent in young adulthood and is more likely to occur in females (14). Its prevalence declines after age 30 (10). Estimates of its overall prevalence vary but typically are in the range of 3% to 15%; thus, most normal EEGs do not demonstrate a mu rhythm (6,7). It is inconsistently present with repeated EEGs of the same patient. The most characteristic feature of the mu rhythm is its reactivity to motor activity or thoughts planning motor activity (54). The blocking that occurs with real or planned movements is bilateral but is maximal contralateral to the movement. Because it depends on conscious activity, the mu rhythm is present only in wakefulness and disappears with drowsiness and sleep (10). Similar to the AR, it also disappears with concentration. It is most evident with bipolar montages and with eyes opened because opened eyes block the AR, which may have a field that extends to the mu rhythm (9).

Distinguishing Features
Versus Cigánek Rhythm

The central location and occasional arciform morphology are the overlapping features of the mu and Cigánek rhythms. However, these two rhythms are easily distinguishable by frequency and field. The mu rhythm has frequency that more often is within the alpha frequency range and is usually asymmetrically placed with a parasagittally centered field. The Cigánek rhythm is midline in the central region. Attenuation with upper extremity movement is not always reliable as a distinguishing feature because such movement may be accompanied by arousal, which causes the Cigánek rhythm to attenuate (55). The mu rhythm attenuates in this circumstance as a result of the specific motor task.

Versus Rolandic Interictal Epileptiform Discharges

Mu fragments resemble interictal epileptiform discharges (IEDs) because of their sharp component followed by a rounded component. This appears similar to the morphology of a diphasic spike and slow wave complex. Distinguishing these fragments of normal activity from IEDs relies on identifying more sustained mu rhythms within the same portion of the EEG. Finding a rhythm of repeated waves with a morphology similar to the wave in question is strong evidence against the wave being an IED. Without the presence of a clear mu rhythm, a suspicious wave cannot be ascribed to be a fragment. Fragments rarely occur in the absence of longer duration waveforms.

Co-occurring Waves
Because the mu rhythm occurs in relaxed wakefulness, it often co-occurs with the AR. Other signs of wakefulness also occur, including blink and muscle artifacts.

Clinical Significance

The mu rhythm is the motor system's analogue to the visual system's AR and is a normal pattern. Like the AR, the mu rhythm's absence is not an abnormality. However, in contrast to the AR, the mu rhythm commonly is not present. The presence of a mu rhythm is genetic with possible autosomal dominant inheritance (56). According to magnetoencephalographic source analysis, the mu rhythm exists as a superimposition of two, independent, and adjacent signals. These are a 10-Hz signal, which originates from somatosensory cortex, and a 20-Hz signal, which is slightly anterior and originates from premotor cortex (57).

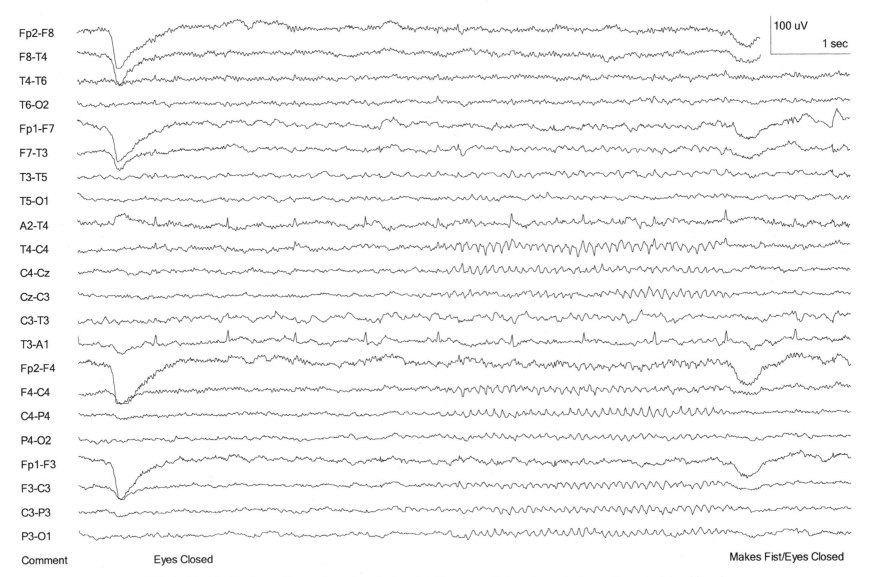

Fp2-F8
F8-T4
T4-T6
T6-O2
Fp1-F7
F7-T3
T3-T5
T5-O1
A2-T4
T4-C4
C4-Cz
Cz-C3
C3-T3
T3-A1
Fp2-F4
F4-C4
C4-P4
P4-O2
Fp1-F3
F3-C3
C3-P3
P3-O1

100 uV

1 sec

Comment   Eyes Closed   Makes Fist/Eyes Closed

FIG. 3–14. Mu Rhythm. Attenuation of central and right parasagittal arciform rhythm with contralateral hand movement demonstrates it to be a mu rhythm. Ocular artifact occurring with the mu rhythm attenuation corresponds to eye movement without opening, such as with eye flutter. (LFF 1 Hz, HFF 70 Hz)

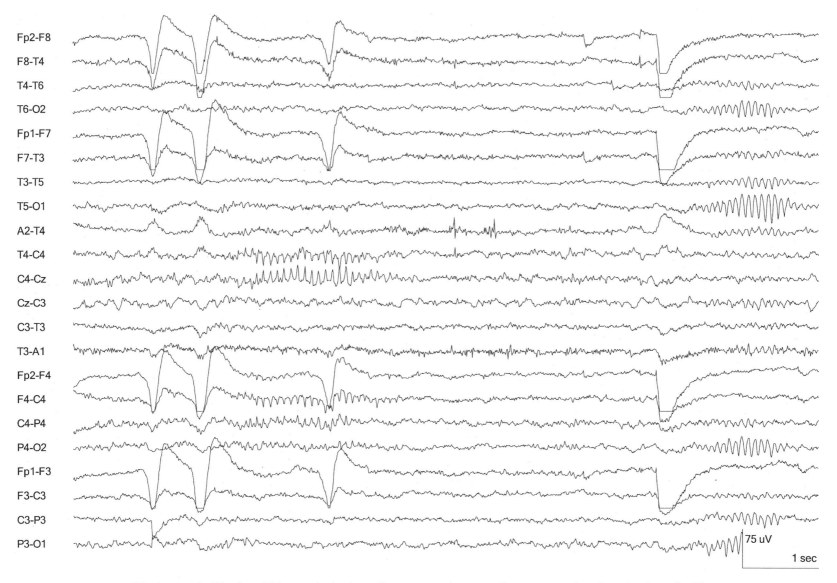

FIG. 3–15. Mu Rhythm. This mu rhythm's arciform pattern is unusually pronounced and contrasts well with the alpha rhythm present at the end of the segment. Unlike the alpha rhythm, it does not appear or block at the time of eye blink artifact. (LFF 1 Hz, HFF 70 Hz)

...but it is asymmetric!

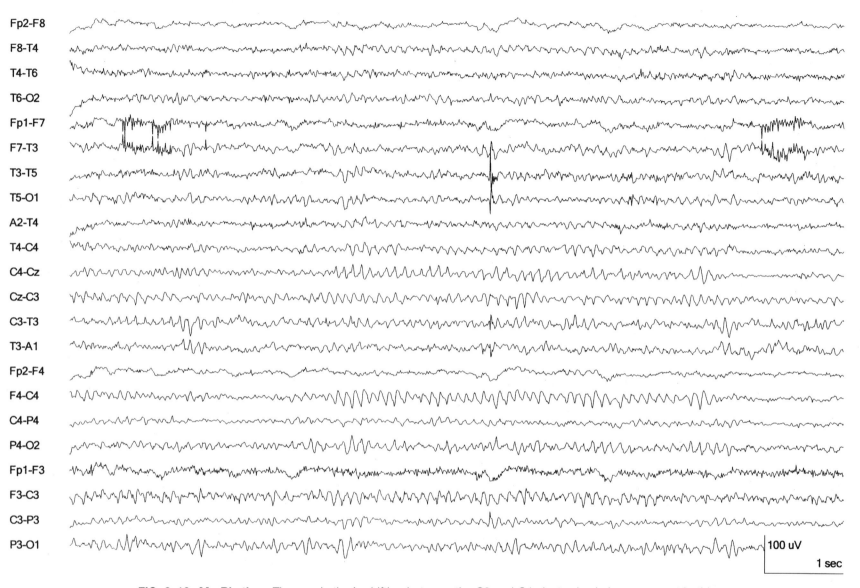

FIG. 3–16. Mu Rhythm. The mu rhythm's shifting between the C3 and C4 electrodes is less apparent in this figure than in Fig. 3–14 because this rhythm's frequency and amplitude are more similar to that of the surrounding activity. However, morphology and location distinguishes this as a mu rhythm. (LFF 1 Hz, HFF 70 Hz)

WICKET RHYTHM

Other Names
Third rhythm
Tau rhythm
Wicket fragment
Wicket spike
Wicket wave
Kappa rhythm

Description
The wicket rhythm constitutes a 6- to 11-Hz repetition of monophasic waves with alternating sharply contoured phases and rounded phases and, therefore, has an arceau appearance that is similar to the mu rhythm (58) (Figs. 3–17 and 3–18). Specifically, the frequency most commonly is within the alpha frequency range and the alternating waveform includes negative sharply contoured phases and rounded positive ones (9). The amplitude is in the medium range of other alpha frequency activity and typically between 60 and 200 μV. The wicket rhythm is maximal over the anterior or midtemporal region and occurs unilaterally with a shifting asymmetry that usually makes it bilaterally symmetric overall (7,43,59). Sometimes, the left temporal lobe is favored (58,60). Phase reversals sometimes are present within the rhythm or fragments of it. These phase reversals occur at F7, F8, T3, and T4 (9). Like the AR and the mu rhythm, the wicket rhythm is present in relaxed wakefulness, but unlike the other two, it is facilitated by drowsiness and even may occur in light sleep (43,61,62). Identification is easiest when the AR is absent, such as with the eyes opened or during drowsiness or sleep. The wicket rhythm is most commonly present in middle adulthood or older adults.

Distinguishing Features
Versus Interictal Epileptiform Discharges

Components of the wicket rhythm are termed wicket fragments or wicket spikes, and resemble IEDs because of their sharp component followed by a rounded component (Figs. 3–19 and 3–20). Morphologically, they are similar to a diphasic spike and slow wave complex. Furthermore, they occur over a temporal region, which is a common site for IEDs. Distinguishing these fragments of normal activity from IEDs relies on identifying either more sustained wicket rhythms within the same portion of the EEG or rhythmic trains of the fragments that have similarity to a wicket rhythm (63). Finding a rhythm of repeated waves with a morphology similar to the wave in question is strong evidence against the wave being an IED. Without the presence of a larger wicket rhythm, a suspicious wave cannot be ascribed to be a fragment. Fragments rarely occur in the absence of larger waveforms.

Versus Partial Seizure Ictal Rhythm

Like the ictal pattern for partial seizures, the wicket rhythm manifests as an abrupt replacement of the preceding background with rhythmic activity. Moreover, it occurs over the temporal lobe, which is a region that commonly produces ictal patterns within the theta frequency range. The key distinguishing feature is the wicket rhythm's lack of evolution in frequency, morphology, or distribution. Each of these features typically evolves during a focal seizure.

Versus Subclinical Rhythmic Electrographic Discharge of Adults

The wicket rhythm and the pattern called subclinical rhythmic electrographic discharge of adults (SREDA) are both rhythmic, temporal repetitions. However, SREDA has a much broader field with a center that is displaced from the center of the wicket rhythm's typical field. SREDA typically is posterior temporal and parietal. SREDA also differs by having a frequency that starts in the delta frequency range and evolves into the theta frequency range.

Versus Rhythmic Midtemporal Theta Activity

Rhythmic midtemporal theta (RMT) and wicket rhythms are similar in their location and occurrence in drowsiness. Furthermore, the wicket rhythm may occur in the theta frequency range, although it most commonly occurs in the alpha frequency range. The essential difference between the patterns is morphology. RMT does not have the wicket morphology, even when it is sharply contoured. RMT and wicket rhythms also differ in duration with wicket rhythms typically not lasting the typical minimum RMT duration of 5 or 10 seconds. However, these two patterns have overlapping features.

Co-occurring Waves

Because the wicket rhythm may occur in wakefulness and light sleep, all normal waveforms of these states may accompany it.

Clinical Significance

The wicket rhythm is a normal variant. Suspicion that it is more common in the presence of cerebral vascular disease requires validation with a control population (60,64). Wicket fragments also are a normal variant and, despite their similarity to IEDs, have no association with epilepsy (65). The wicket rhythm may be the auditory analogue of the AR, because it may decrease with auditory stimulation (66). Magnetoencephalographic source analysis localizes it to supratemporal auditory cortex (66).

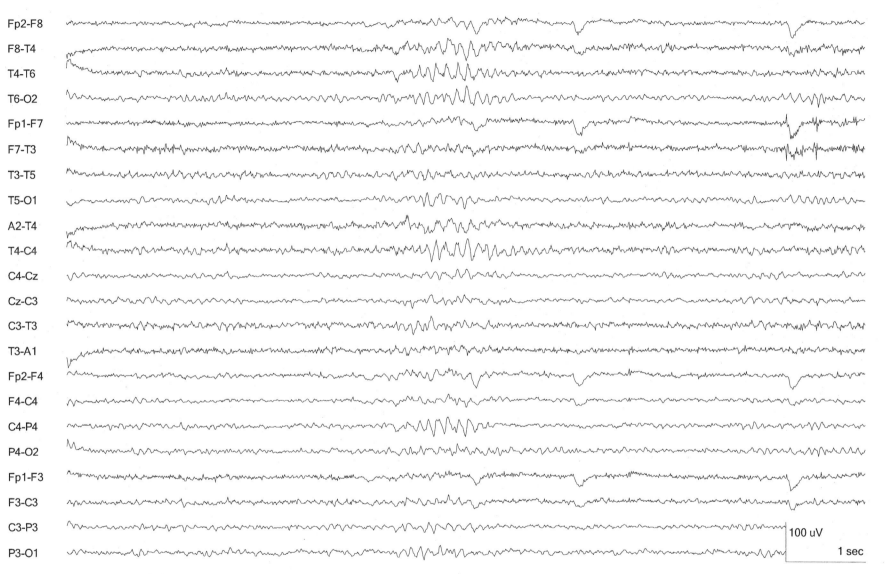

FIG. 3–17. Wicket Rhythm. An 8-Hz, right-sided wicket rhythm lasts slightly more than 1 second and occurs in drowsiness. The alpha rhythm is intermittent and poorly formed. (LFF 1 Hz, HFF 70 Hz)

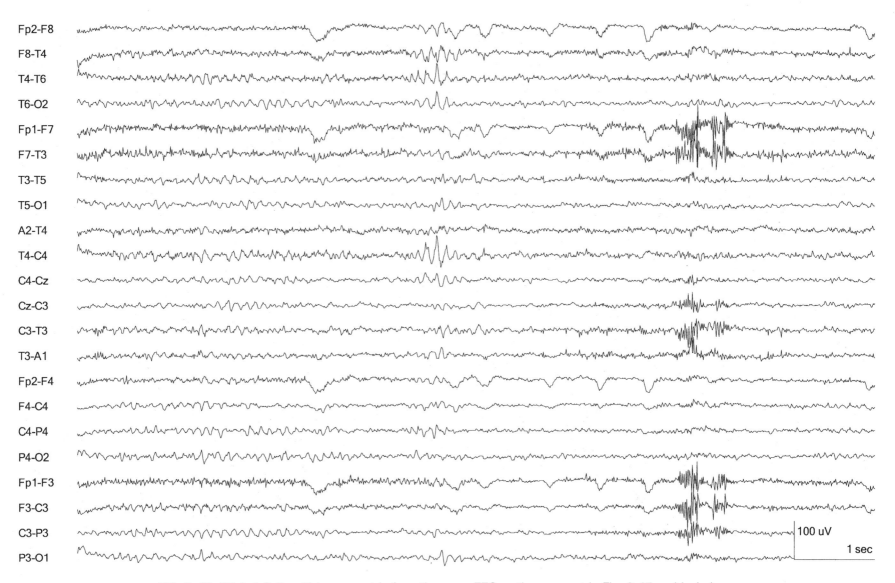

FIG. 3–18. Wicket Spike. This segment is from the same EEG as the segment in Fig. 3–17 and includes a fragment of a wicket rhythm with one component wave with greatest amplitude. If the fragment was shorter, the phase-reversing, high-amplitude component would appear similar to an interictal epileptiform discharge. Artifact from eye flutter and left-sided muscle activity also occurs. (LFF 1 Hz, HFF 70 Hz)

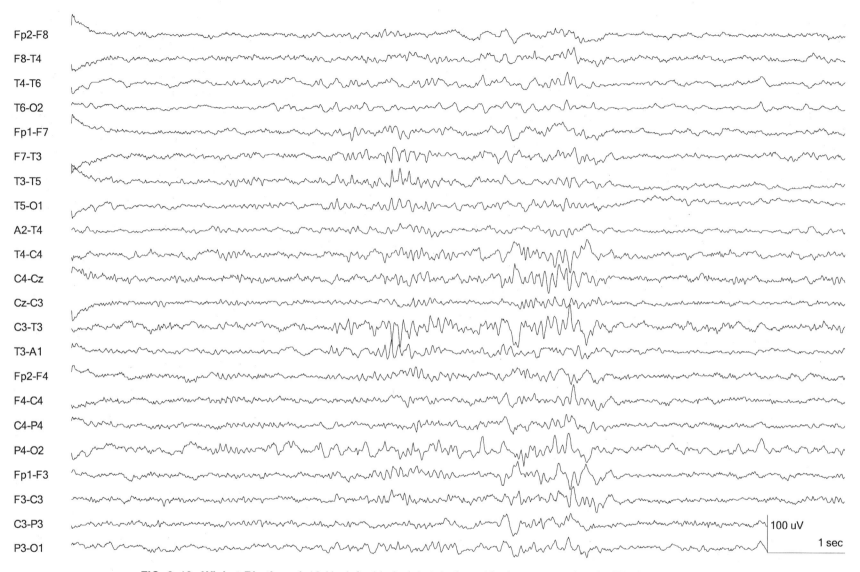

FIG. 3–19. Wicket Rhythm. A 10-Hz, left-sided wicket rhythm with phase reversal at the T3 electrode occurs for about a half second just before a sleep spindle. (LFF 1 Hz, HFF 70 Hz)

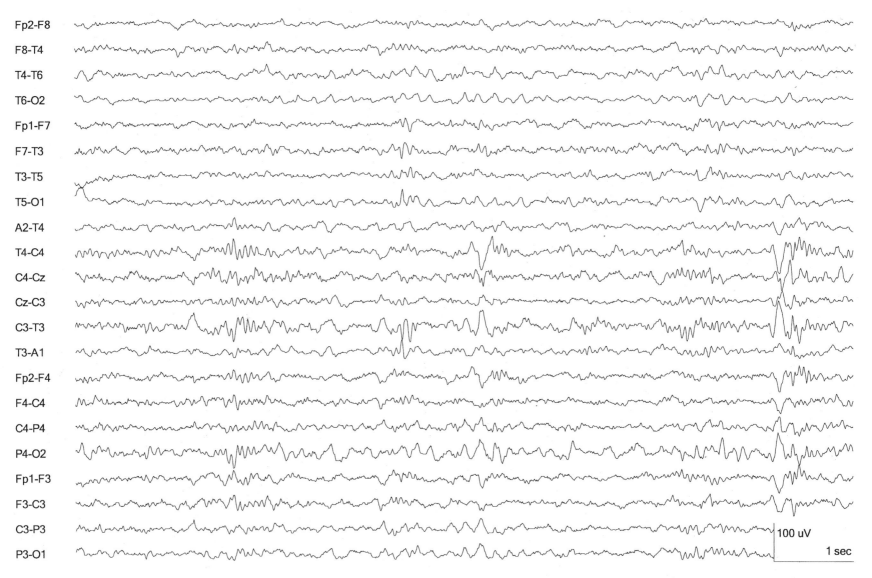

FIG. 3–20. Wicket Spike. This segment immediately follows the segment in Fig. 3–19 and includes a fragment of the wicket rhythm that is a phase-reversing spike at T3. A vertex sharp wave and K complex also occur. (LFF 1 Hz, HFF 70 Hz)

CHAPTER 4

Artifacts

CARDIAC ARTIFACTS

Types
Electrocardiographic (ECG)
Ballistocardiographic
Pacemaker
Pulse

Descriptions
The heart produces two types of electroencephalogram (EEG) artifact, electrical and mechanical. Both types are time-locked to cardiac contractions and are most easily identified by their synchronization with complexes in an electrocardiogram (ECG) channel.

The electrical artifact actually is the ECG, as recorded from head electrodes. Because of the distance from the heart and the suboptimal axis, the P wave and T wave usually are not visible. Essentially, the artifact is a poorly formed QRS complex (67) (Fig. 4–1). It is most prominent when the neck is short. The complex usually is diphasic, but some EEGs may depict it as either monophasic or triphasic. Overall, the artifact is best formed with referential montages because of their greater interelectrode distances and ECG field's approximately equal potential across the head. Because of the equipotential field, montages with an average reference have minimal ECG artifact (68). With bipolar montages, the artifact occurs with maximum amplitude and clearest QRS morphology over the temporal regions and often is better formed and larger on the left side (7). The R wave is most prominent in channels that include the ear electrodes and may demonstrate a dipole with A1 positive and A2 negative (9) (Fig. 4–2). ECG artifact may occur inconsistently by not being present with every contraction of the heart and may have an irregular interval when a cardiac arrhythmia is present. In either situation, it may be identified by its temporal association with the QRS complexes in an ECG channel. When its interval is regular, it still may be identified without an ECG channel by observing that the intervals between the artifacts occur in multiples of a time between cardiac contractions.

Cardiac pacemakers produce a different electrical artifact (Fig. 4–3). It is distinct from ECG artifact in both distribution and morphology. Pacemaker artifact is generalized across the scalp and comprises high-frequency, polyphasic potentials with a duration that is shorter than ECG artifact (7).

Mechanical artifact from the heart arises through the circulatory pulse and may be considered as a type of electrode artifact. It occurs when an electrode rests over a vessel manifesting the pulse and appears as a periodic slow wave with a regular interval that follows the ECG artifact's peak by about 200 msec (9,67) (Fig. 4–4). Sometimes it has a saw-tooth or sharply contoured morphology (68). It occurs most commonly over the frontal and temporal regions and less commonly over the occiput; however, it may be present anywhere (7). Pulse artifact is easily identified by touching the electrode producing it. This both confirms the movement of the electrode with the pulse and alters its appearance on the EEG as pressure is applied.

Ballistocardiographic artifact is another form of mechanical cardiac artifact. It results from the slight movements of the head or body that occur with cardiac contractions. This partly may be due to the pulsatile force on the aortic arch from the abrupt redirection of blood flow. Ballistocardiographic artifact is similar in morphology to pulse artifact but is more widespread. If it is due to electrode lead movement, it may involve one or a few electrodes. If it is due to movement of the head on a pillow, it involves a collection of posterior electrodes and is altered by repositioning the head or neck on a pillow. Occasionally, ballistocardiographic artifact is generalized.

Distinguishing Features
Versus Benign Epileptiform Transients of Sleep

Like benign epileptiform transients of sleep (BETS), ECG artifact typically comprises individual transients that are low amplitude, are morphologically conserved, and occur in the midtemporal regions. The temporal correspondence to simultaneously recorded ECG is the best means to differentiate these two waves. If an ECG channel is not present, identifying the wave in full wakefulness excludes BETS and identifying a regular interval between the waves supports ECG artifact. The interval between waves may vary but should be considered regular if it varies in multiples of a reasonable time interval between heart beats. Another distinguishing feature is the typical occurrence of ECG artifact bilaterally synchronously. This may occur with BETS but in a small minority of the occurrences.

Versus Focal Ictal and Interictal Epileptiform Discharges

ECG artifact may disrupt the EEG's background activity similarly to epileptiform discharges. Moreover, it usually is diphasic or triphasic with a fast component that has a duration within the spike range. When the artifact occurs either with a highly regular interval or can be compared to an ECG channel, differentiating it from interictal epileptiform discharges (IEDs) is straightforward. An episodic occurrence pattern requires careful scrutiny of the morphology and location. ECG artifact almost always occurs in channels that include electrodes that are low on the head, especially ear electrodes. When a wave only occurs in such channels and has a perfectly conserved morphology, it is likely to be ECG artifact. IEDs show greater variation between occurrences than ECG artifacts even when they recur as the same wave type, that is, they vary more in amplitude, duration, contour, and location than ECG artifact.

Paroxysmal tachycardia may produce ECG artifact that resembles an ictal pattern. Identifying it as artifact relies on the features that are used for distinguishing IEDs, including preservation in morphology and temporal association with the QRS complex in an ECG channel. The regular interval feature also is helpful because the artifact also will be present at times between the episodes of tachycardia.

Periodic Lateralized Epileptiform Discharges

The diphasic or triphasic morphology and periodic occurrence pattern are features that periodic lateralized epileptiform discharges (PLEDs) and ECG artifact share. Differentiating these waves is straightforward when comparison to an ECG channel is possible. When an ECG channel is not present, the regularity of the intervals between the transients is the key distinguishing feature. PLEDs usually are not nearly as regular in their interval as ECG artifact. This is especially true because the conditions for recording an EEG do not produce significant changes in heart rate. Other distinguishing features are distribution and frequency. Although ECG artifact may be unilateral, it often is bilateral, and PLEDs, by definition, are not bilaterally synchronous. Bilateral periodic epileptiform discharges (BiPEDs) are bilaterally synchronous, but BiPEDs usually have large, bifrontal fields. ECG artifact is usually maximal in the two temporal regions. The BiPEDs of Creutzfeldt-Jakob disease provide one exception to this distinguishing feature because they may be bilateral without a large field for a time during the course of the illness. Frequency is a less reliable means for differentiation. Most ECG artifact will be at 1 Hz or faster because a heart rate slower than 60 beats per minute is unusual. In contrast, PLEDs usually occur with intervals greater than 1 second. However, the interval between PLEDs varies, especially across different etiologies.

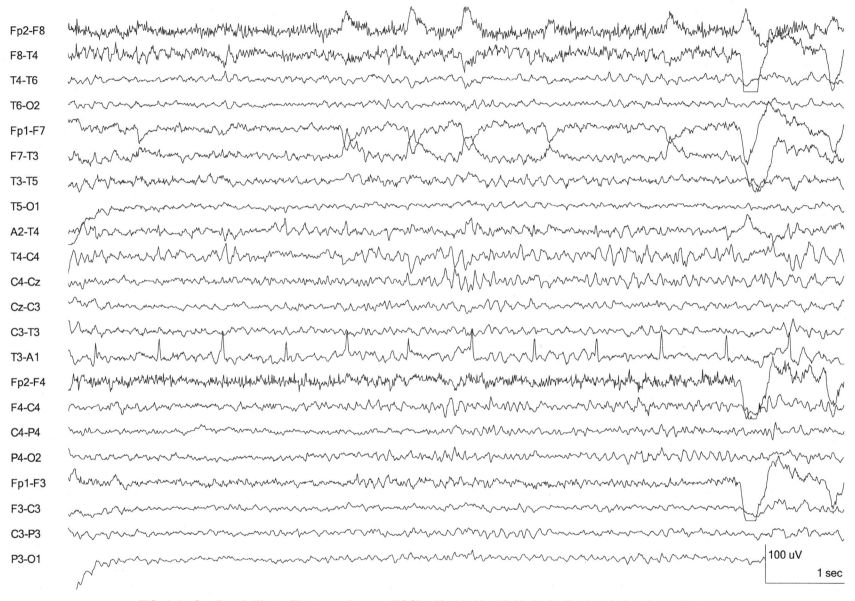

Fp2-F8
F8-T4
T4-T6
T6-O2
Fp1-F7
F7-T3
T3-T5
T5-O1
A2-T4
T4-C4
C4-Cz
Cz-C3
C3-T3
T3-A1
Fp2-F4
F4-C4
C4-P4
P4-O2
Fp1-F3
F3-C3
C3-P3
P3-O1

100 uV

1 sec

FIG. 4–1. Cardiac Artifact. Electrocardiogram (ECG) artifact is identifiable by its fixed period and morphology and is limited to T3-A1 channel in this bipolar montage. (LFF 1 Hz, HFF 70 Hz)

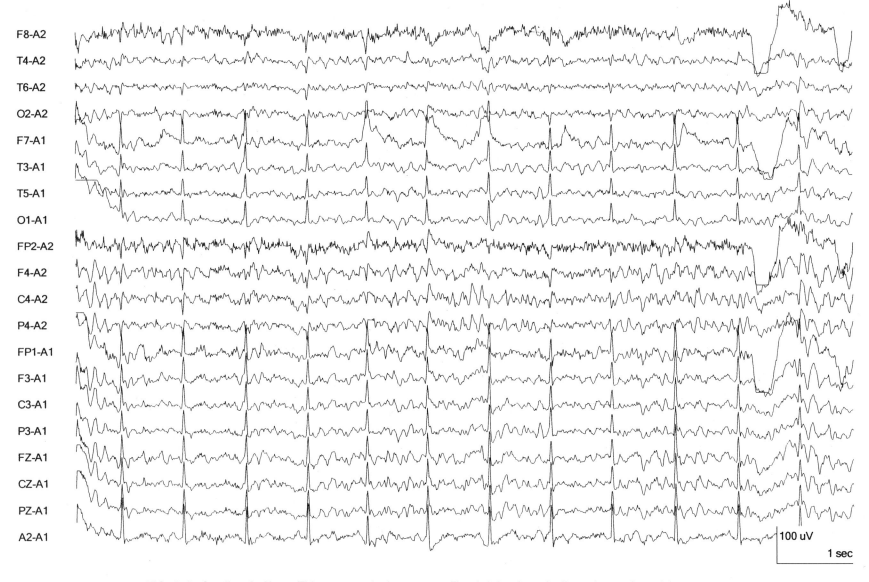

FIG. 4–2. Cardiac Artifact. This segment is the same as Fig. 4–1, but in an ipsilateral ear referential montage. The electrocardiogram (ECG) artifact remains predominant on the left side but now also is visible on the right in channels with greater interelectrode distances. The ear electrodes demonstrate the classical opposite polarity for the artifact. (LFF 1 Hz, HFF 70 Hz)

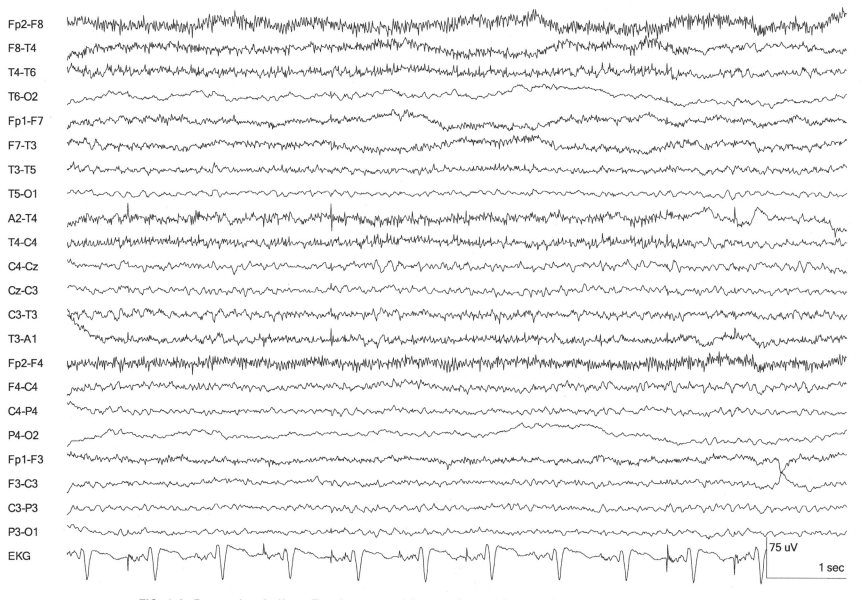

Fp2-F8
F8-T4
T4-T6
T6-O2
Fp1-F7
F7-T3
T3-T5
T5-O1
A2-T4
T4-C4
C4-Cz
Cz-C3
C3-T3
T3-A1
Fp2-F4
F4-C4
C4-P4
P4-O2
Fp1-F3
F3-C3
C3-P3
P3-O1
EKG

75 uV

1 sec

FIG. 4–3. Pacemaker Artifact. Transients comprising very fast activity recur in channels with the A1 and A2 electrodes. The transients are simultaneous to similar discharges in the electrocardiogram (ECG) channel and correspond to a permanent pacemaker's output. (LFF 1 Hz, HFF 70 Hz)

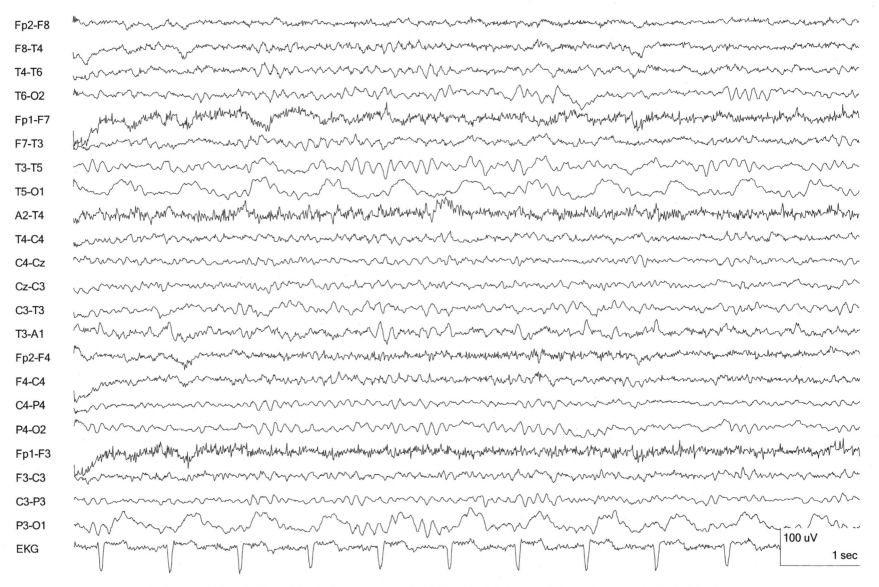

FIG. 4–4. Pulse Artifact. Focal slow waves at the left occiput follow each heart beat, as indicated in the electrocardiogram (ECG) channel. The slow waves are artifact due to electrode movement and were eliminated by repositioning the O1 electrode. (LFF 1 Hz, HFF 70 Hz)

ELECTRODE ARTIFACT

Types
Electrode pop
Electrode contact
Electrode/lead movement
Perspiration
Salt bridge
Movement artifact

Descriptions

Electrode artifacts usually manifest as one of two disparate waveforms, brief transients that are limited to one electrode and low-frequency rhythms across a scalp region. The brief transients are due to either spontaneous discharging of an electrical potential that was present between the electrode and the subjacent skin or due to mechanical disturbances to the electrode or its lead. The spontaneous discharges are called electrode pops, and they reflect the ability of the electrode and skin interface to function as a capacitor and store electrical charge across the electrolyte paste or gel that holds the electrode in place. With the release of the charge there is a change in impedance, and a sudden potential appears in all channels that include the electrode (Fig. 4–5). This potential may be superimposed on the background activity or replace it (9,69). Sometimes more than one pop occurs within a few seconds. Electrode pop has a characteristic morphology of a very steep rise and a more shallow fall. Essentially, it resembles the calibration pulses of analog EEG machines.

Poor electrode contact or lead movement produces artifact with a less conserved morphology than electrode pop. The poor contact produces instability in the impedance, which leads to sharp or slow waves of varying morphology and amplitude (Fig. 4–6). These waves may be rhythmic if the poor contact occurs in the context of rhythmic movement, such as from a tremor (7). Lead movement has a more disorganized morphology that does not resemble true EEG activity in any form and often includes double phase reversals, that is, phase reversals without the consistency in polarity that indicates a cerebrally generated electrical field (Fig. 4–7).

The smearing of the electrode paste between electrodes to form a salt bridge or the presence of perspiration across the scalp both produce artifacts due to an unwanted electrical connection between the electrodes forming a channel. Perspiration artifact is manifested as low-amplitude, undulating waves that typically have durations greater than 2 seconds; thus, they are beyond the frequency range of cerebrally generated EEG (7) (Fig. 4–8). It may appear as an unstable baseline for the cerebrally generated activity, sometimes causing adjacent channels to cross despite their low amplitude. This is due to shifts in the direct current (DC) offset potential from the unstable perspiration (68). The artifact typically includes several channels representing a region of scalp. Salt bridge artifact differs from perspiration artifact by being lower in amplitude, not wavering with low frequency oscillations, and typically including only one channel. It may appear flat and close to isoelectric (Fig. 4–9).

Distinguishing Features
Versus Ocular Artifact

Slow roving eye movements produce artifact that has a frequency and field similar to that perspiration artifact. The key distinguishing feature is the rhythmicity, phase reversal, and broad, bifrontal field of the eye movements. Roving eye movements occur with drowsiness and are an involuntary and repeated horizontal ocular movement (25). The movements have a relatively constant period and demonstrate a phase reversal because of the eyes' dipoles. With right gaze, the field around the right frontotemporal electrodes becomes more positive and the field around the left frontotemporal electrodes becomes more negative. This produces a phase reversal not seen with salt bridge artifact, even when the low-amplitude activity happens to be rhythmic.

Versus Interictal Epileptiform Discharges

Electrode pop resembles IEDs because both occur as paroxysmal, sharply contoured transients that interrupt the background activity. However, electrode pop involves only one electrode. Therefore, it does not have a field indicating more gradual decrease in the potential's amplitude across the scalp. The lack of a field including multiple electrodes is highly rare for IEDs except in young infants. The morphology of electrode pop also is different from spikes by having a much steeper rise and much slower fall.

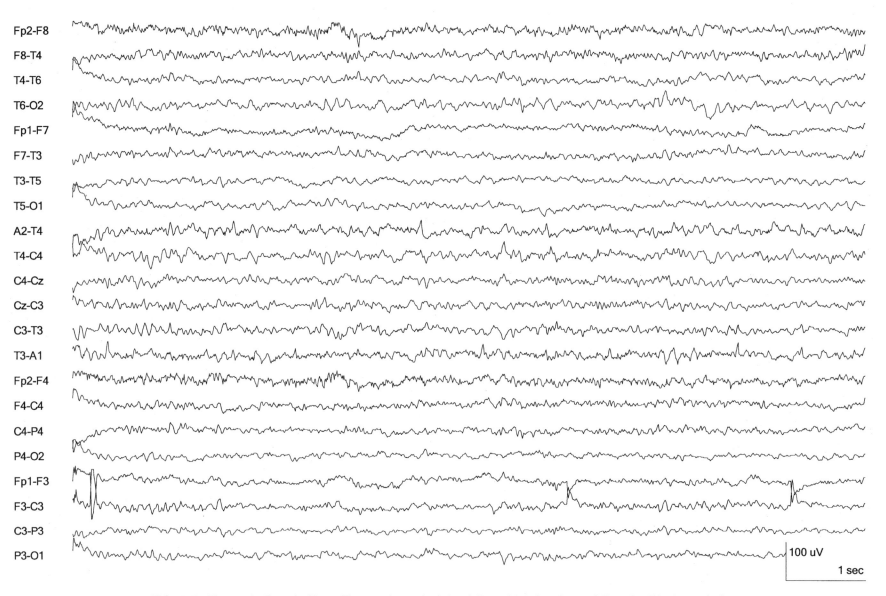

Fp2-F8

F8-T4

T4-T6

T6-O2

Fp1-F7

F7-T3

T3-T5

T5-O1

A2-T4

T4-C4

C4-Cz

Cz-C3

C3-T3

T3-A1

Fp2-F4

F4-C4

C4-P4

P4-O2

Fp1-F3

F3-C3

C3-P3

P3-O1

100 uV

1 sec

FIG. 4–5. Electrode Pop Artifact. The nearly vertical rise followed by the slower fall at the F3 electrode is typical of electrode pop artifact. Also typical is an amplitude that is much greater than the surrounding activity, a field that is limited to one electrode, and repeated recurrence within a short time. (LFF 1 Hz, HFF 70 Hz)

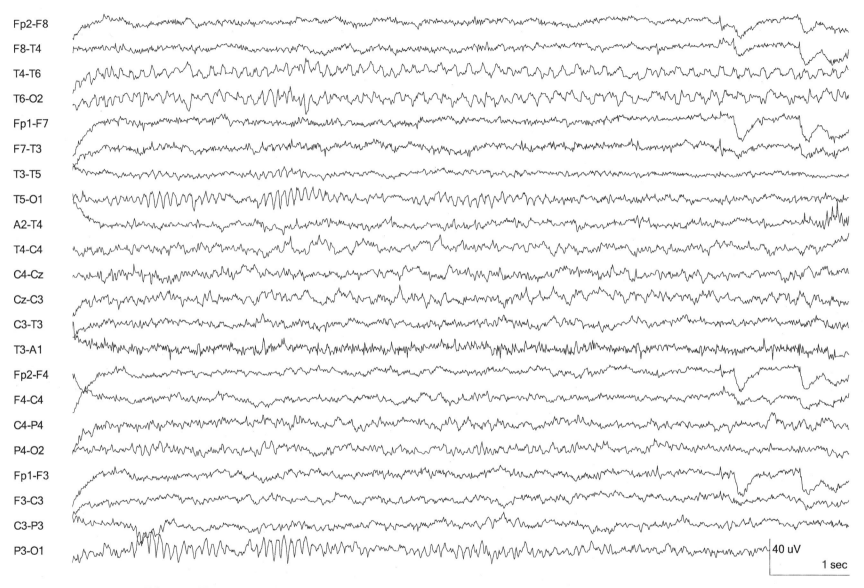

FIG. 4–6. Electrode Artifact. The focal slowing in the T4-T6 and T6-O2 channels has no field beyond the T6 electrode and has the oscillations typical of rhythmic electrode movement. (LFF 1 Hz, HFF 70 Hz)

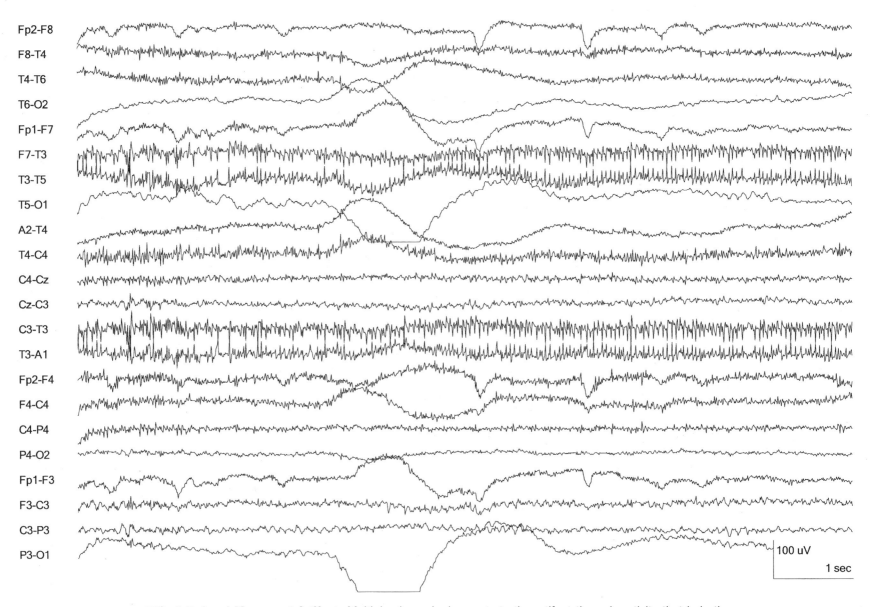

FIG. 4–7. Lead Movement Artifact. Multiple channels demonstrate the artifact through activity that is both unusually high amplitude and low frequency and also disorganized without a plausible field. (LFF 1 Hz, HFF 70 Hz)

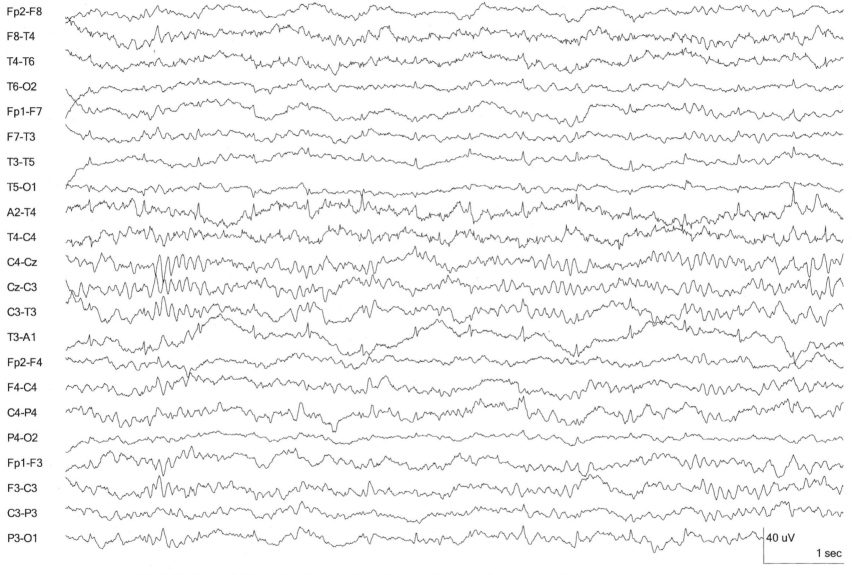

FIG. 4–8. Sweat Artifact. The decreased amplitude and very low frequency oscillations are present diffusely, which is consistent with the whole scalp's involvement. The recurring sharp waves across most channels are ECG artifact. (LFF 1 Hz, HFF 70 Hz)

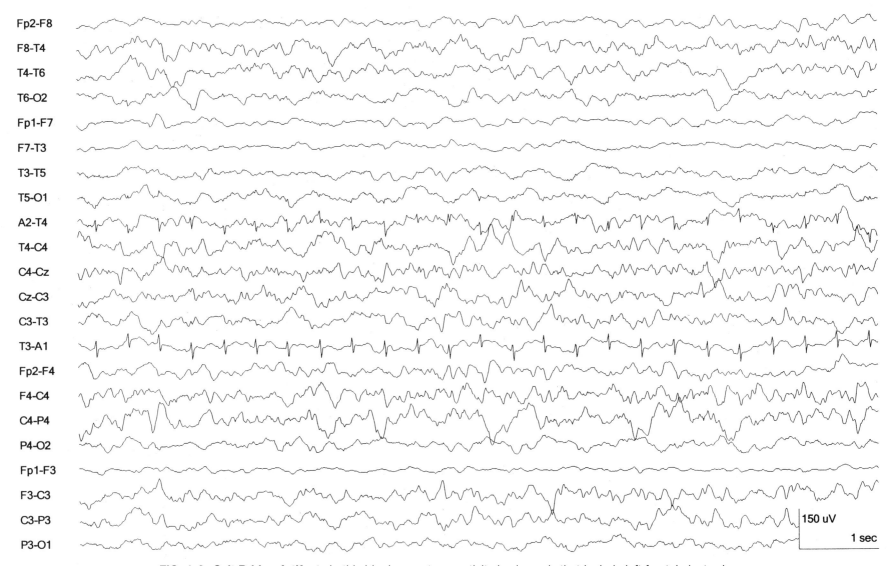

FIG. 4–9. Salt Bridge Artifact. In this bipolar montage, activity in channels that include left frontal electrodes is much lower in amplitude and frequency than the remaining background. The Fp1-F3 channel especially contrasts with the other channels. The lack of these findings when viewed in a referential montage confirms that an electrolyte bridge is present among the electrodes involved. (LFF 1 Hz, HFF 70 Hz)

EXTERNAL DEVICE ARTIFACT

Types
50/60 Hz ambient electrical noise
Intravenous drips
Electrical devices: intravenous pumps, telephone
Mechanical effects: ventilators, circulatory pumps

Descriptions
Numerous types of external devices produce EEG artifact and may do so through the electrical fields they generate or through mechanical effects on the body. The most common external artifact is due to the alternating current (AC) present in the electrical power supply. This noise is usually medium to low amplitude and has the monomorphic frequency of the current, which is 60 Hz in North America and 50 Hz in much of the rest of the world (Fig. 4–10). The artifact may be present in all channels or in isolated channels that include electrodes that have poorly matched impedances (9). Electrical noise may also result from falling electrostatically charged droplets in an intravenous drip. A spike-like EEG potential results, which has the regularity of the drip (69) (Fig. 4–11).

Electrical devices may produce other forms of noise. Anything with an electric motor may produce high-amplitude, irregular, polyspike-like, or spike-like artifact (Fig. 4–12). This is due to the switching magnetic fields within the motor. The artifact occurs with the motor's activity; thus, it may be constant or intermittent, as is the case with infusion pumps (71). Mechanical telephone bells are the classic source for a more sinusoidal form of this artifact but are increasingly a less common source of the intermittent form of this artifact.

Mechanical devices such as ventilators and circulatory pumps usually produce artifacts with slower components than other electrical devices. Their artifact may resemble ballistocardiographic or other electrode artifact in that the artifact is generated by movement of electrodes or leads as the body is moved by the device (Figs. 4–13 and 4–14). The artifact typically repeats with a fixed interval and is a slow wave or a complex including a mixture of frequencies superimposed on a slow wave. Two exceptions to this typical artifact pattern are the artifact resulting from ventilators that deliver air with an oscillating, high-pressure burst. This may produce rhythmic higher frequency artifact in channels that include electrodes either near the pharynx or in contact with a fixed surface, such as a pillow or bed. Thus, it may appear as intermittent, rhythmic activity and may be similar to alpha frequency activity when it is across the posterior head. Its highly monomorphic frequency and fixed repetition interval are its characteristic features.

Overall, the number of devices that may produce artifact and the variety of artifacts that each device may produce based on its settings greatly complicates the job of recognizing artifacts based on specific features. However, the challenge may be met by realizing that artifacts from external devices usually produce waveforms that are highly dissimilar to cerebrally generated waveforms. Because of this, highly unusual waveforms should always be suspected as artifact. Proving that the wave is artifact usually rests on the technologist recording the EEG. On seeing the unusual wave, the technologist should search the environment for possible causes and test the possibilities whenever possible by observing for a temporal association between the device's action and the artifact. When such information from the technologist is not present, the assumption that an unusual wave is artifact is preferred by convention over an assumption of abnormality.

Distinguishing Features
Versus Ictal Patterns

Because external device artifact may include fast components and demonstrate evolution within an occurrence, it may resemble ictal patterns. This artifact is most easily distinguished from ictal patterns by its short duration, regular repetition, and highly preserved morphology. Almost all sources for artifact produce either continuous artifact or artifacts that last less than several seconds and repeat as identical waves at least several times a minute. Such an occurrence pattern is very unusual for a seizure.

Versus Periodic Epileptiform Discharges

When an external device causes intermittent artifact, it often has a regular interval and may be similar to periodic epileptiform discharges (PEDs) in its periodicity. However, this type of artifact rarely has the diphasic or triphasic morphology of PEDs and usually has a distribution that is highly unusual for PEDs, such as the inclusion of electrodes that are not adjacent to one another. Also unusual for PEDs is a generalized occurrence, which is common for device artifact.

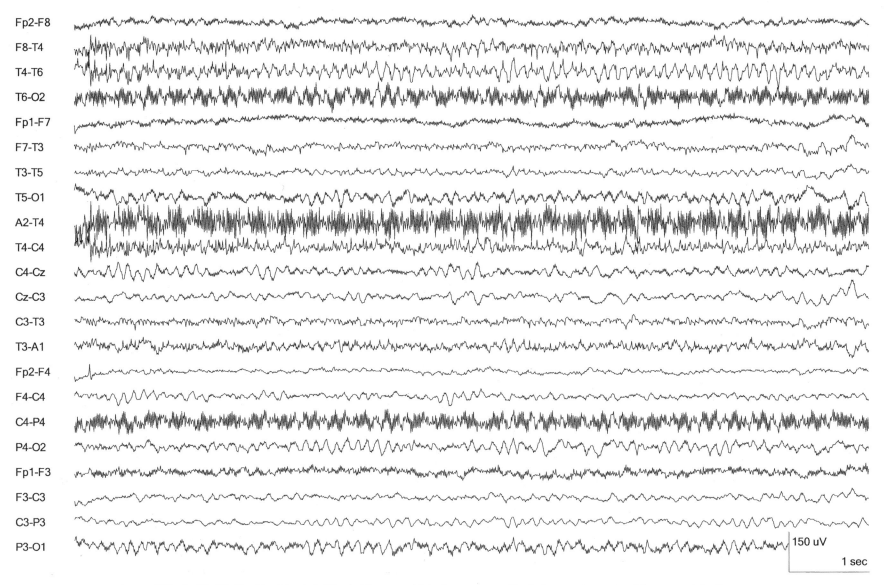

FIG. 4–10. 60-Hz Electrical Artifact. The very high frequency artifact does not vary and is present in the posterior central region, which does not typically manifest muscle artifact. This example was generated by eliminating the 60-Hz notch filter. (LFF 1 Hz, HFF 70 Hz)

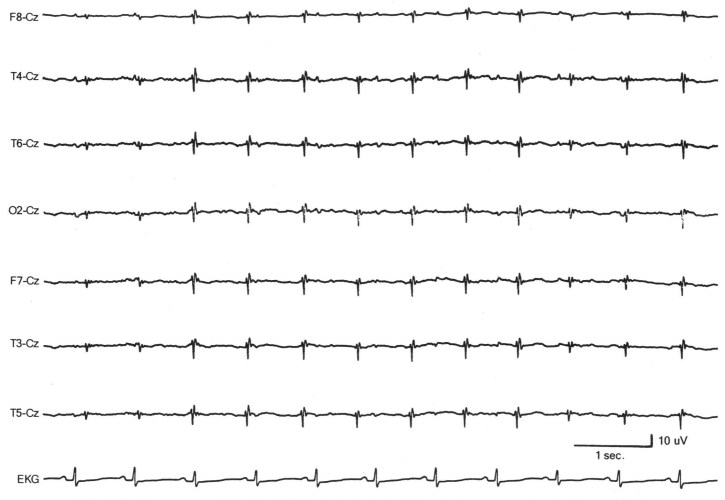

FIG. 4–11. Intravenous Drip Artifact. Triphasic and polyphasic transients are occurring simultaneous to the falling of drops in an intravenous infusion. Drip artifact differs from the artifact due to electrical infusion pumps, which is a low-amplitude form of the artifact in Fig. 4–12. This EEG corresponds to electrocerebral inactivity. (TC 0.12 sec, HFF 70 Hz). (From Bennett DR, et al. *Atlas of electroencephalography in coma and cerebral death.* New York: Raven Press, 1975:111.)

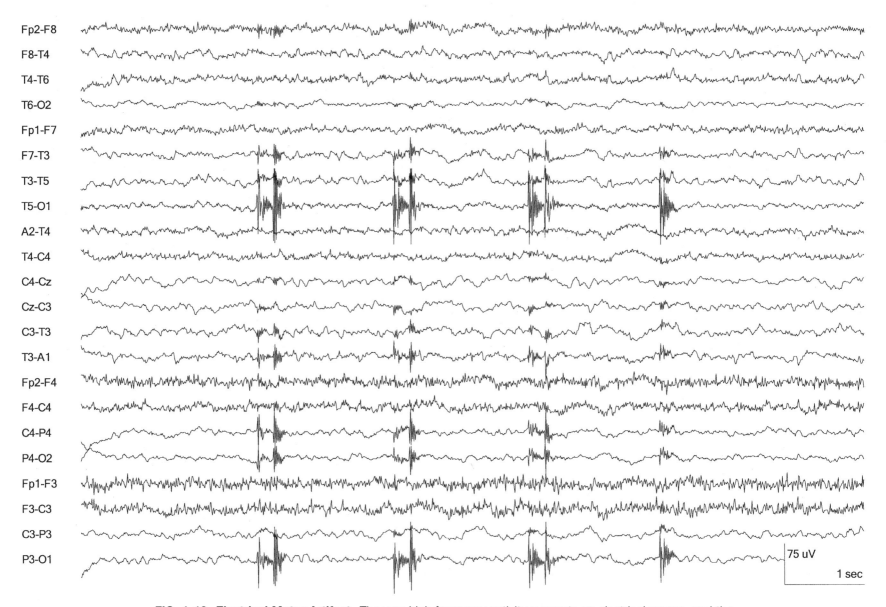

FIG. 4–12. Electrical Motor Artifact. The very high frequency activity suggests an electrical source, and the fixed morphology and repetition rate indicate an external device. This was caused by an electrical motor within a pump. (LFF 1 Hz, HFF 70 Hz)

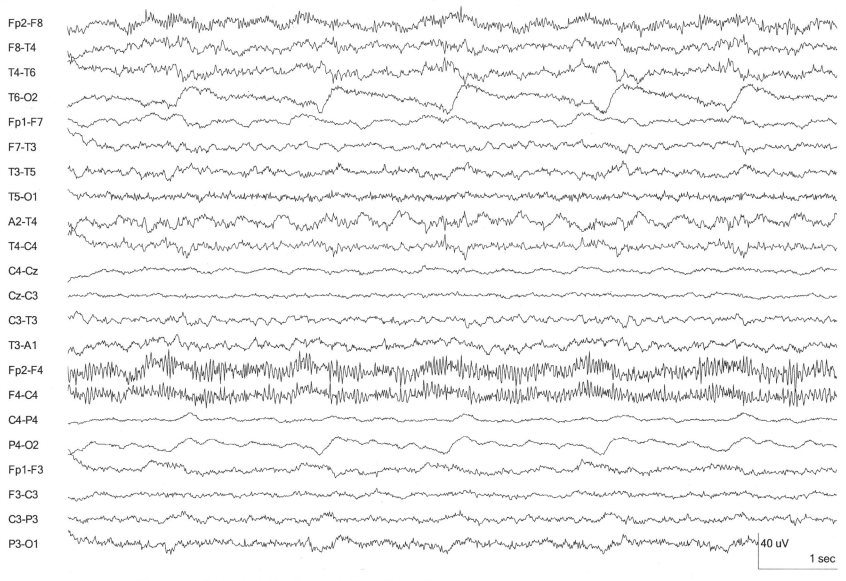

FIG. 4–13. Mechanical Ventilation Artifact. The artifact present across the right occiput has the fixed morphology and repetition rate of mechanical artifact. Its location relates to the head resting on the electrodes involved and moving at times of rapid airflow. The Fp2 and F4 electrodes generate artifact due to poor contact. (LFF 1 Hz, HFF 70 Hz)

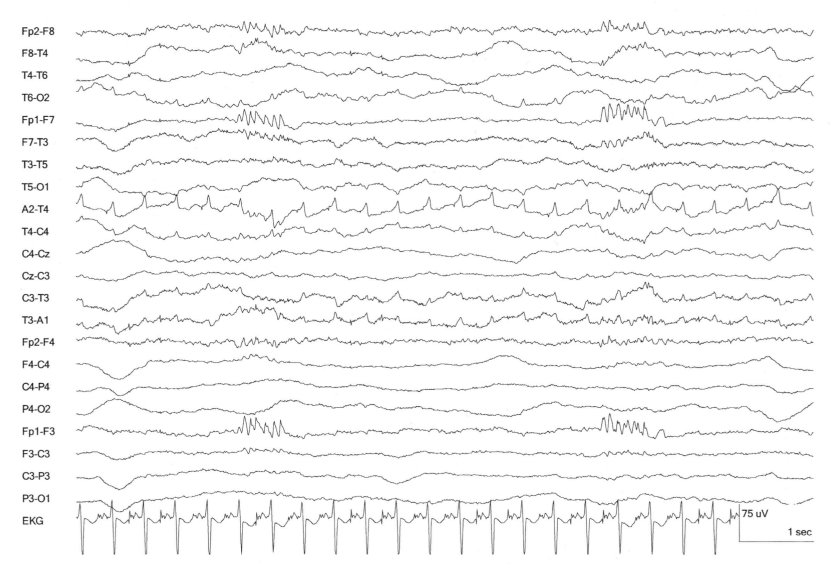

FIG. 4–14. Circulatory Pump Artifact. Sharply contoured, bilateral frontal repetitions occur with a fixed interval and are due to a pump providing circulatory support and extracorporeal membrane oxygenation. Pulse artifact is present in multiple channels and most apparent in the A2-T4 channel. (LFF 1 Hz, HFF 70 Hz)

MUSCLE ARTIFACT

Types
Glossokinetic (chew/swallow)
Photomyogenic (photomyoclonic)
Surface electromyography (scalp/facial muscle)

Descriptions
Movement during the recording of an EEG may produce artifact through both the electrical fields generated by muscle and through a movement effect on the electrode contacts and their leads. Although the muscle potential fields are the signals sought by electromyographers, they are noise to electroencephalographers. Indeed, electromyographic (EMG) activity is the most common and significant source of noise in EEG (72). EMG activity almost always obscures the concurrent EEG because of its higher amplitude and frequency (Figs. 4–15 and 4–16). Its frequency is higher than that of clinical EEG and too fast to be visually estimated. However, it may appear regular and in the beta frequency band or as repetitive spikes if the high-frequency filter (low-pass filter) is set at 35 Hz or less (9). Without this filtering, EMG artifact usually has a more disorganized appearance because the individual myogenic potentials overlap with each other. Occasionally, individual potentials are discernible (Fig. 4–17). This occurs with involuntary motor unit activity such as from fibrillations and has a classic EMG wave appearance. The duration of EMG artifact varies according to the duration of the muscle activity; thus, it ranges from less than a second to an entire EEG record. Similarly, the distribution varies; however, the artifact occurs most commonly in regions with underlying muscle, specifically the frontalis and masseters. Thus, EMG artifact most commonly occurs in channels including the frontal and temporal electrodes.

Repetitive EMG artifact may occur with photic stimulation as a time-locked facial muscle response to the flash of light. This is termed a photomyogenic or photomyoclonic response and occurs over the frontal and periorbital regions bilaterally (Fig. 4–18). It may extend to include a larger region when the myoclonus involves the neck or body. Larger regions of myoclonus commonly produce simultaneous electrode and movement artifact (7). The photomyogenic response has a 50-msec latency from the strobe's flash and, therefore, may occur synchronously with the occipital photic stimulation driving response (9). It may be present with eyes opened or closed but tends to occur more often with eyes closed. Its occurrence with eyes opened may be accompanied by ocular artifact. Obviously, it disappears immediately when photic stimulation is stopped.

Although the oropharyngeal muscles are not near EEG electrodes, swallowing and talking also produce artifact. This is partly EMG artifact from the pharyngeal muscles and partly due to the tongue's inherent dipole. The tongue's tip is electronegative compared to its base; thus, movement of the tongue toward or away from EEG electrodes alters the overall electrical field around them. This is termed glossokinetic artifact. The resulting artifact has a wide field with maximal amplitude frontally and comprises isolated slow waves, delta frequency range activity, or, more typically, slowing with superimposed faster frequencies (7). It often also includes simultaneous EMG artifact. Glossokinetic artifact is highly rhythmic when the tongue has a tremor or the patient is a nursing infant (69).

Distinguishing Features
Versus Beta Activity

Because the frontalis muscle runs over the frontal-central region, EMG artifact often co-localizes with the region of maximum beta activity and resembles it with its characteristic frequency greater than 25 Hz. Morphologic difference is the principal distinguishing feature. EMG artifact has a sharper contour and less rhythmicity when the high-frequency filter is set at more than 60 Hz. When it occurs as a rhythm within the beta frequency range, it does so as individual EMG potentials that have durations of less than 20 msec but are separated by an interval that gives it a beta frequency range appearance. The significant variation in this interval provides another distinguishing feature, especially when the interval becomes so brief that the potentials appear continuous. Such very fast activity is beyond the beta frequency range and almost always indicates muscle artifact.

Versus Paroxysmal Fast Activity

EMG artifact and paroxysmal fast activity (PFA) both develop abruptly and include high-amplitude, very fast activity. However, they differ in their frequency components. Muscle artifact contains a greater number of frequencies and, therefore, appears more disorganized. This basis in a superimposition of fast frequencies also makes muscle artifact appear slightly different with each occurrence. PFA has a more organized morphology that is stereotyped among occurrences.

Versus Photoparoxysmal Response

Because photoparoxysmal responses may have a maximal field frontally, their field may overlap with that of photomyogenic artifact. Furthermore, photomyogenic artifact has a spike-like morphology due to its basis as individual motor unit potentials. Differentiating the two patterns depends on morphologic differences and the degree of association between the transients and the flashing stimulation. Photomyogenic artifact is very sharply contoured and lacks after-going slow waves. Furthermore, it almost always occurs across a broad range of stimulation frequencies, occurs commonly at almost every stimulation frequency used, and does not persist beyond the period of stimulation. This contrasts with photoparoxysmal responses that typically occur at one or two stimulation frequencies, may not be time-locked with the stimulations, and may continue beyond the stimulation interval. Complicating the process of distinguishing these waveforms is the possibility of the two occurring simultaneously. Generalized seizures that follow photoparoxysmal responses also may follow brief bursts of myoclonus with myoclonus-associated photomyogenic artifact.

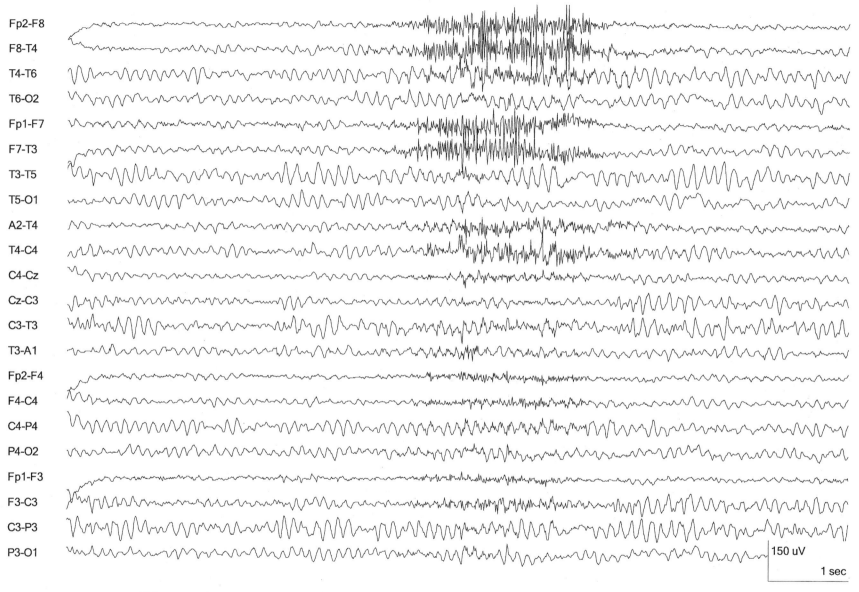

Fp2-F8
F8-T4
T4-T6
T6-O2
Fp1-F7
F7-T3
T3-T5
T5-O1
A2-T4
T4-C4
C4-Cz
Cz-C3
C3-T3
T3-A1
Fp2-F4
F4-C4
C4-P4
P4-O2
Fp1-F3
F3-C3
C3-P3
P3-O1

150 uV

1 sec

FIG. 4–15. Muscle Artifact. The high-amplitude, fast activity across the bilateral anterior region is due to facial muscle contraction and has a distribution that reflects the locations of the muscles generating it. Typical of muscle artifact, it begins and ends abruptly. (LFF 1 Hz, HFF 70 Hz)

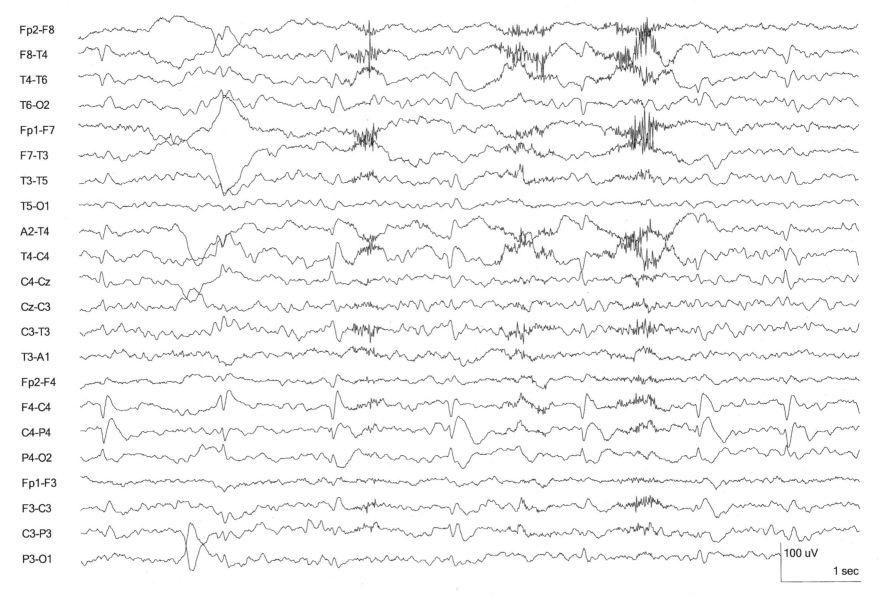

FIG. 4–16. Muscle and Movement Artifact. Three bursts of high frequency muscle artifact co-occur to more subtle low frequency movement artifact. These artifacts correspond to the periodic lateralized epileptiform discharges (PLEDs) that are broadly distributed across the right-side and recur about every 1½ seconds. (LFF 1 Hz, HFF 70 Hz)

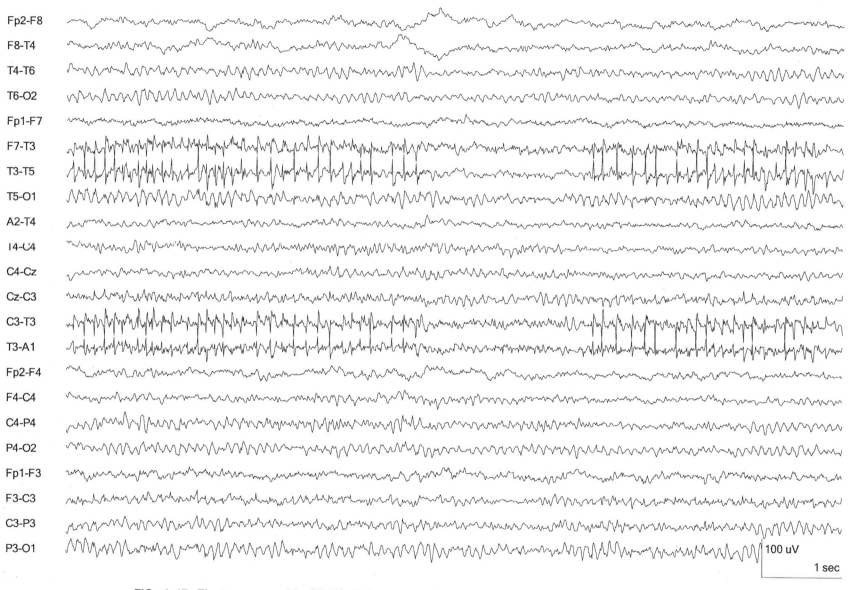

Fp2-F8
F8-T4
T4-T6
T6-O2
Fp1-F7
F7-T3
T3-T5
T5-O1
A2-T4
T4-C4
C4-Cz
Cz-C3
C3-T3
T3-A1
Fp2-F4
F4-C4
C4-P4
P4-O2
Fp1-F3
F3-C3
C3-P3
P3-O1

100 uV

1 sec

FIG. 4–17. Electromyographic (EMG) Artifact. The stereotyped potentials at the T3 electrode are EMG artifact. The potentials' durations are briefer than cerebrally generated spikes, and, unlike cerebrally generated activity, they have a field limited to one electrode. They also co-occur with more typical muscle artifact. (LFF 1 Hz, HFF 70 Hz)

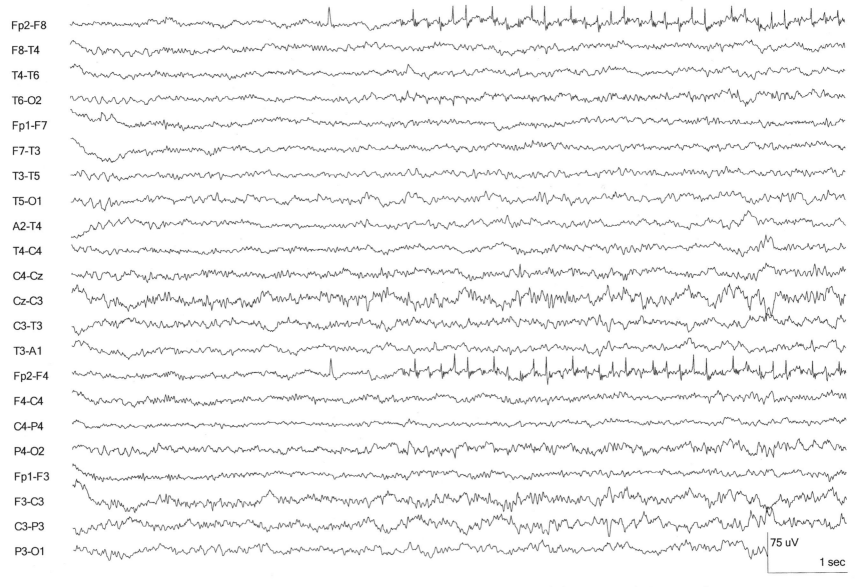

FIG. 4–18. Photomyogenic Artifact. Simultaneous to the 6-Hz strobe stimulations are transients across the frontal region that reflect an involuntary muscle contraction. At low stimulation frequencies, the transients more clearly resemble other electromyographic (EMG) potentials, such as in Fig. 4–17. (LFF 1 Hz, HFF 70 Hz)

OCULAR ARTIFACT

Types
Blink
Eye flutter
Lateral gaze
Slow/Roving eye movements
Lateral rectus spike
Rapid eye movements (REM) of REM sleep
Electroretinogram

Descriptions

Most ocular artifacts are due to each eye's inherent 100–mV electrical dipole (68). The dipole is oriented along the corneal-retinal axis and is positive in the direction of the cornea and negative in the direction of the retina. The dipole becomes relevant to the EEG recording when it becomes a moving electrical field, as occurs with changes in gaze and eye opening and closure. Vertical eye movements accompany eye opening and closure with deviation upward on closure. This is called Bell's phenomenon. Eyelid movement with its myogenic potentials also may contribute to ocular artifact with eye opening and closure (68). Blinking produces an ocular artifact because of the rapid movement of the eyes both up and down and appears on the EEG as a bifrontal, diphasic, synchronous slow wave with a field that does not extend beyond the frontal region (67) (Fig. 4–19). The amplitude of the artifact decreases quickly with greater distance from the orbits. The wave is maximum amplitude and surface positive at the frontal poles. Because the artifact is produced by deviation of the eyes upward, the negative end of the dipoles is not detectable with conventional montages.

Repetitive blinks usually appear as a sequence of the slow wave ocular artifacts and thus resemble rhythmic delta activity. However, blepharospasm may produce an artifact with a faster frequency. Although ocular flutter involves vertical eye movements, it differs from repetitive blinks by being more rapid and having lower amplitude. Because of this, its EEG artifact is more rhythmic and lower amplitude, which gives it a greater resemblance to rhythmic delta activity (Figs. 4–20 and 4–21). When periocular muscle contractions accompany the eye movements of ocular flutter, the resulting artifact may appear as a run of bifrontal spike and slow wave complexes (9). The spike arises from the brief EMG artifact related to the periocular contraction.

Both ends of the eyes' dipoles are detectable with lateral eye movements. This is observed with greater positivity on the side to which gaze is directed and greater negativity on the opposite side (9) (Fig. 4–22). With bipolar montages, positive and negative phase reversals are seen at the F7 and F8 electrodes. Ocular artifact from lateral gaze is most apparent during drowsiness, when the eyes demonstrate repeated, slow lateral movements. This produces rhythmic, slow artifact anteriorly with a field that is maximum at the frontal poles and temples and a frequency that is less than 1 Hz (Fig. 4–23). Because the amplitude is also low, the wave also resembles an unstable baseline for the superimposed EEG activity. The most characteristic feature of the low-amplitude slowing due to roving eye movements is the opposite polarity of the slowing in the left and right frontotemporal regions (7). This artifact typically occurs intermittently and is accompanied by slowing of the alpha rhythm.

The EEG during more rapid lateral eye movements sometimes includes a single motor unit potential from contraction of the lateral rectus muscle (69). This low-amplitude transient is termed a lateral rectus spike and usually is present at the F7 (left gaze) or F8 electrode (right gaze) (Fig. 4–24). The lateral rectus spike may be followed immediately by slower eye movement artifact in the same location and this may result in what appears as one wave with a morphology that resembles a focal IED (7).

Although they are lateral gaze movements, the rapid eye movements of REM stage sleep have a morphology that differs from lateral gaze during wakefulness. REM artifact appears as asymmetric waves with a quicker rise than fall (7). Of course, their location is the same as the other artifacts produced by lateral gaze.

Distinguishing Features
Versus Delta Activity

Isolated monomorphic frontal slow waves and frontal intermittent rhythmic delta activity (FIRDA) have the same wave duration and a similar field to ocular artifact from eye opening and closure. Blinks are more similar to isolated slow waves, and eye flutter is more similar to FIRDA. The field is the key distinguishing feature between ocular artifact and delta activity. Unlike delta activity, ocular artifact does not extend into the central region. However, a morphologic difference also exists due to ocular artifact's sharper contour. The two also may be distinguished based on recognized eye movements, as described in the technologist's notation. If notation is not present, then identification may be based on whether the wave is absent in drowsiness and sleep, states in which the eyes are closed. Using both supraorbital and infraorbital electrodes is the most definitive means for differentiation. Ocular artifact produces a phase reversal between infraorbital electrode and supraorbital electrode channels because the area of maximum potential exists between the electrodes. In contrast, the area of maximum potential for cerebrally generated slowing is above the orbits; thus, it does not produce a phase reversal between these channels.

Versus Interictal Epileptiform Discharges

When the slow wave artifact of ocular flutter occurs in combination with the faster frequency artifact from eyelid movement, a compound wave results that appears to be a bifrontal spike and slow wave complex. Although the frontal poles may be the center of a spike and slow wave complex's field, this is an unusual location. When the bilateral spike and slow wave of a generalized IED has a phase reversal, it usually is at F3 or F4. A focal spike and wave may occur at one frontal pole but it would not have bilateral symmetry. Spike morphology also may distinguish these waveforms. Because it is generated from muscle artifact, the spike of the simulated spike and wave complex is less stereotyped than the IED. Lastly, true IEDs usually occur in states beyond light drowsiness, which is the state for ocular flutter. Even when the IEDs occur only with drowsiness, they continue to occur into stage II non-REM sleep.

Another compound wave results from the combination of the brief myogenic potential from the lateral rectus and the slow wave artifact from lateral gaze. This appears especially similar to an IED because the lateral rectus spike results from a single motor unit potential and is, therefore, relatively stereotyped across occurrences like the spike of an IED. It also occurs in the anterior temporal region, which is a region that often produces focal IEDs. Distinguishing lateral rectus spikes from IEDs depends on the lateral rectus spike's consistent low amplitude, presence only at F7 and F8, and absence in some lateral eye movements that still demonstrate the slow wave artifact. IED spikes typically vary more in their amplitude and location, even if the variation is only minor and one interelectrode distance. They also sometimes occur without the aftergoing slow wave, which is the opposite of the lateral gaze artifact in which the slow wave may occur without the spike. A shifting asymmetry between F7 and F8 is not helpful because some individuals with temporal lobe epilepsy have bilateral independent temporal IEDs.

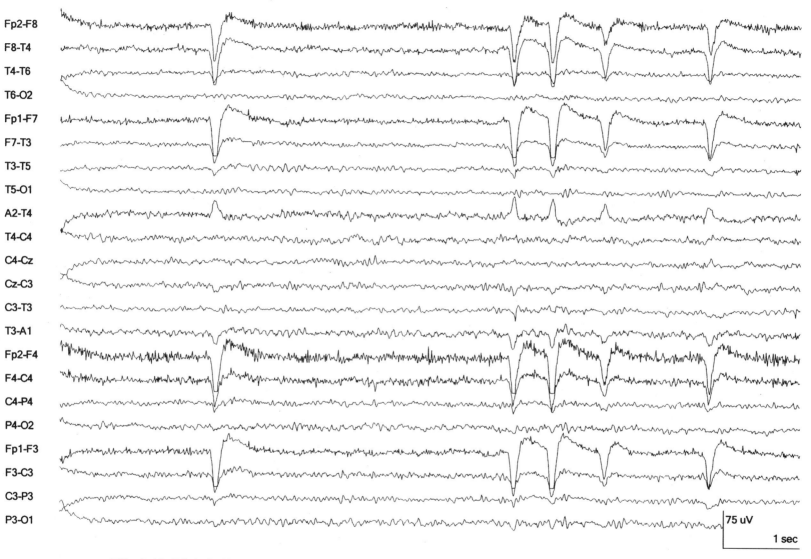

FIG. 4–19. Blink Artifact. Bifrontal, diphasic potentials with this morphology and field are reliably eye blink artifact. The amplitude often is less than what is depicted here but characteristically is greater than that of the surrounding activity. (LFF 1 Hz, HFF 70 Hz)

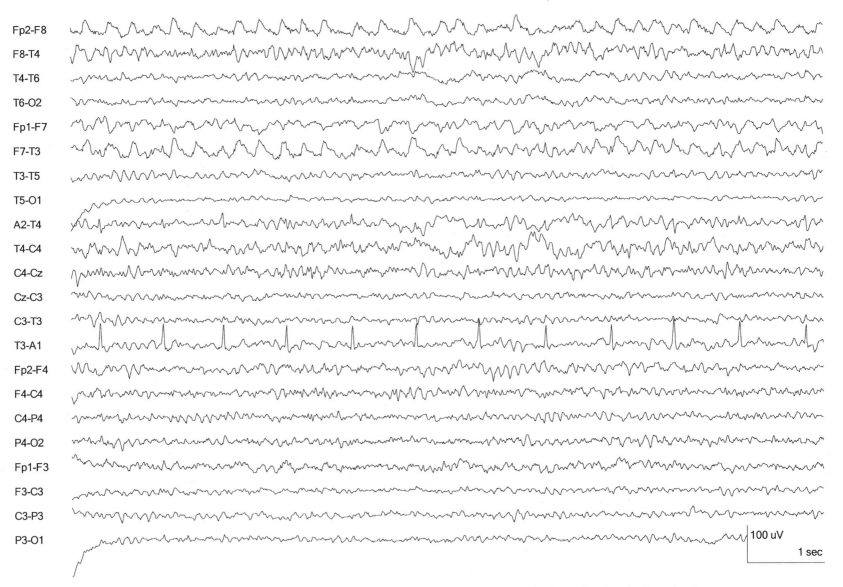

FIG. 4–20. Eye Flutter Artifact. Medium-amplitude, low-frequency activity that is confined to the frontal poles is identified as ocular artifact through its morphology. Compared to blink artifact, flutter artifact typically has a lower amplitude and a more rhythmic appearance. Electrocardiogram (ECG) artifact is produced by the A1 electrode. (LFF 1 Hz, HFF 70 Hz)

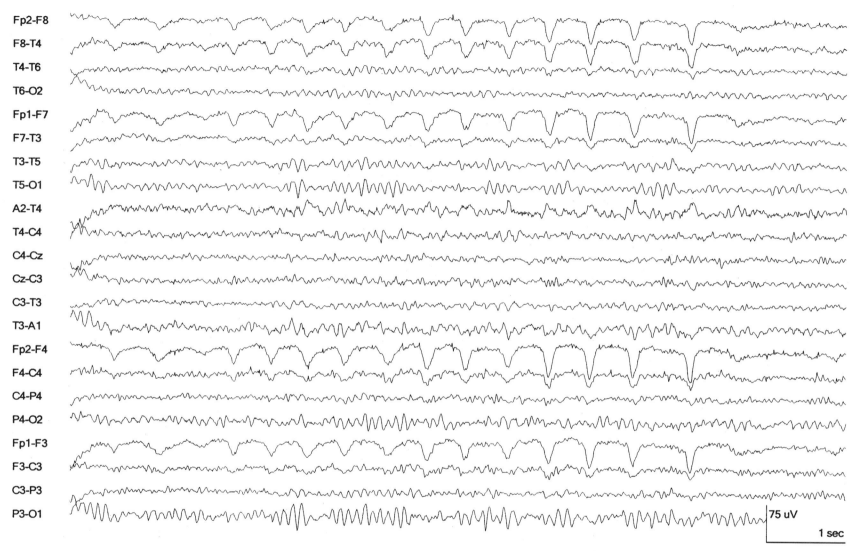

FIG. 4–21. Eye Flutter Artifact. Compared to Fig. 4–20, the eye flutter artifact in this example more closely resembles blink artifact. The rapid blinks of eye flutter may not allow fixation; therefore, the alpha rhythm may be sustained through the brief periods of eye opening. (LFF 1 Hz, HFF 70 Hz)

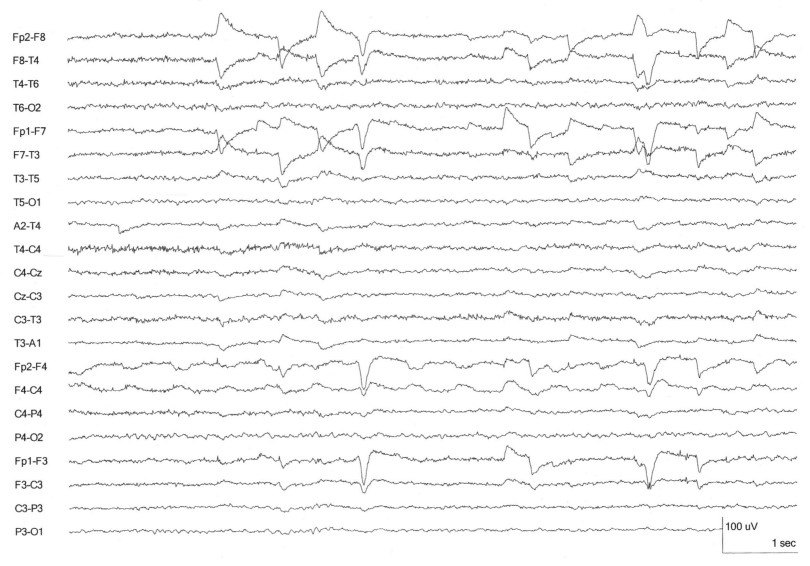

FIG. 4–22. Lateral Eye Movement Artifact. Although a horizontal, frontal dipole is the key finding with lateral eye movements, the artifact is also distinguished by its morphology, which has a more abrupt transition between the positive and negative slopes than blinks and most flutter. The initial gaze in this segment is to the right. (LFF 1 Hz, HFF 70 Hz)

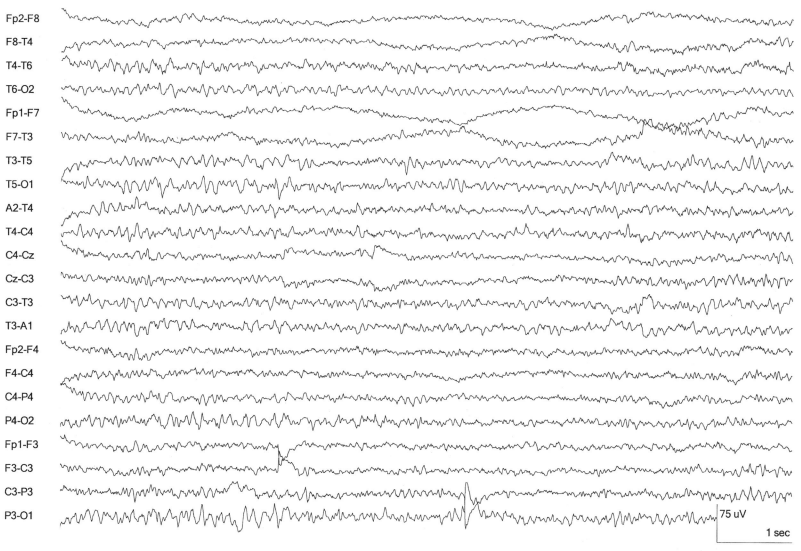

FIG. 4–23. Slow Roving Eye Movement Artifact. Unlike the saccades of the lateral gaze depicted in Fig. 4–22, slow roving movement artifact does not have abrupt changes. Instead, it reflects the smooth lateral movements with phase reversing slow activity. (LFF 1 Hz, HFF 70 Hz)

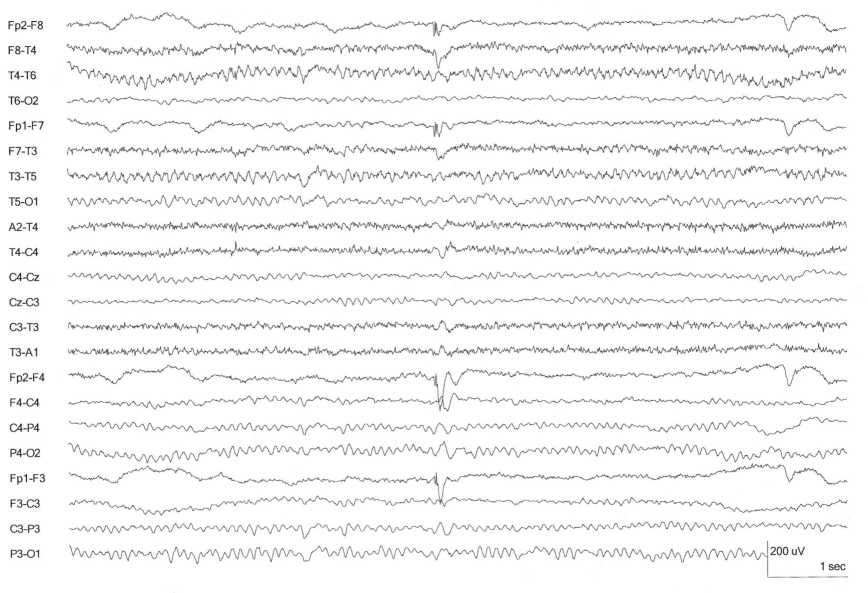

FIG. 4–24. Lateral Rectus Spike Artifact. The F7 or F8 location of lateral rectus spikes overlaps with the typical distribution for mesial temporal lobe interictal epileptiform discharges. The lateral rectus spikes differ by including very fast, myogenic activity and often is associated with artifact from the ocular dipoles. (LFF 1 Hz, HFF 70 Hz)

CHAPTER 5

Benign Epileptiform Transients of Sleep

BENIGN EPILEPTIFORM TRANSIENTS OF SLEEP

Other Names
BETS
Benign sporadic sleep spikes
Small sharp spikes

Description
BETS are low-amplitude, sharply contoured, monophasic or diphasic transients that occur in light sleep (Figs. 5–1, 5–2, and 5–3). They are most likely to occur in adults between 30 and 60 years and do not occur in children younger than 10 years (61). Stages I and II of non–rapid eye movement (NREM) sleep are the states in which they are most likely to occur, and they do not occur in wakefulness. Their waveform characteristically has one principal phase with an abrupt rise and a steeper fall (4). Forms with polyphasic potentials or after-going slow waves are less common. When an after-going slow wave is present, it has an amplitude that is less than the spike. BETS do not precede focal slowing but may precede a brief change in focal background activity with an increase in rhythmic theta or alpha frequency range activity.

With some exception, BETS are less than 90 μV in amplitude and 90 msec in duration and typically are about 60 μV in amplitude and 60 msec in duration. Their small size often results in the interpreter only noticing the largest of them, which hampers their identification because their morphologic consistency is an important feature in their identification. Multiple occurrences typically occur within a recording, and identifying several morphologically similar temporal spikes within only drowsiness or sleep supports the consideration of BETS. When multiple BETS occur within one recording, the discharges may have the same distribution, may be homotopically contralateral, and occasionally may occur synchronously over bilateral temporal regions (7). Overall, the shifting asymmetry should not demonstrate a significant majority of transients on one side. When they recur with the same distribution, they are almost always separated by more than 1 second and often by more than 10 seconds. Unlike other brief transients, they do not occasionally occur repetitively in a train (43).

BETS are usually centered in the midtemporal region and vary minimally in this localization. However, an exact localization may be difficult to identify because the center of the field is ambiguous. The field is typically broad and extends over the entire temporal lobe and may include the immediately adjacent frontal lobe. Because parts of the field may have equal potentials, cancellations may occur in bipolar channels, especially ones that include a posterior temporal electrode. For the same reason, BETS have an amplitude that is maximal in channels comprised of an electrode from each hemisphere. Montages with such channels sometimes also demonstrate a transverse dipole with a negative phase reversal over one temporal lobe and a positive one over the other.

Distinguishing Features
Versus Interictal Epileptiform Discharges

BETS are more likely to be mistaken for focal interictal epileptiform discharges (IEDs) than other transients because of their epileptiform morphology; occurrence over the temporal lobes; and occurrence during sleep, a state with greater IED frequency. Distinguishing them from IEDs is much easier when they recur. Compared to BETS, IEDs tend to vary more in their morphology with inconsistent amplitudes and durations. IEDs also are more likely to have a prominent after-going slow waves, with an amplitude equal to or greater than the spike or sharp wave. Furthermore, focal IEDs tend to have narrower fields, which usually are limited to an electrode and its nearest neighbors and also may have co-localized but independently occurring focal slowing. The presence of such slowing indicates the region is abnormal and, therefore, is consistent with IEDs and not consistent with BETS. The occurrence of the same transient during wakefulness also is a distinguishing feature by eliminating the possibility of BETS. When a discharge consistent with a BETS occurs only once during a recording and no other suspicious finding is present, determining whether the transient is a BETS may not be possible. In such instances, the interpreter may rely on the basic tenet of electroencephalogram (EEG) interpretation that undercalling abnormality is preferable to overcalling it. With this tenet, the interpreter may describe the transient within the report's body, state that the recording was normal, and state within the report's comment that the suspicious transient may have been a BETS.

Versus Cardiac Artifact, Electrocardiogram

Like BETS, electrocardiogram (ECG) artifacts typically are individual transients that are low amplitude, morphologically conserved, and occurring in the midtemporal regions recorded with ear electrodes. The temporal correspondence to simultaneously recorded ECG is the best means to differentiate these two waves. If an ECG channel is not present, identifying the wave in full wakefulness excludes BETS and identifying a regular interval between the waves supports ECG artifact. The interval between waves may vary but should be considered regular if it varies in multiples of a reasonable time interval between heart beats. Another distinguishing feature is the typical occurrence of ECG artifact bilaterally and synchronously. This may occur with BETS but in a small minority of the occurrences.

Versus Wicket Spikes

Wicket spikes have the same distribution as BETS but occur in wakefulness, have a larger amplitude, and have a more variable morphology. Furthermore, wicket spikes characteristically have a morphology that is similar to fragments of the background activity (wicket rhythm) in the same distribution. This morphology is more symmetric in the rise and fall with the peak of the spike being the sharply contoured side of an arciform wave.

Co-occurring Waves

Other evidence of drowsiness should accompany BETS. This may include an alpha rhythm that is slowed or poorly formed, slow roving eye movements, vertex sharp transients, rhythmic midtemporal theta activity, Cigánek rhythm, and positive occipital sharp transients of sleep.

Clinical Significance

BETS are commonly considered a normal phenomenon because the accumulating evidence regarding their epileptogenicity has gradually favored their classification as generally benign (73). The exceptions to this perspective tend to be from retrospective studies based in EEG laboratories that evaluate populations with high rates of epilepsy. Some of these studies find higher rates of BETS among individuals with epilepsy than among those without epilepsy, and others find higher likelihoods of EEGs demonstrating BETS at times when the patient has active epilepsy compared to being seizure free (74,75). The limitations of such studies are clear and include the issue of whether the EEGs were obtained in equivalent states of sleep deprivation. Sleep deprivation is more likely to be performed when an EEG is being obtained to evaluate for epileptiform abnormality, and it produces an increased frequency of BETS (76). In a study that compared patients with epilepsy to a control population that underwent the same sleep deprivation, the rates of BETS were without significant difference between the groups (77). BETS occurred in 24% of the control EEGs and 20% of those from the epilepsy patient population. Furthermore, depth electrode recordings of BETS demonstrate differences from the IEDs that occurred within the same recording (78).

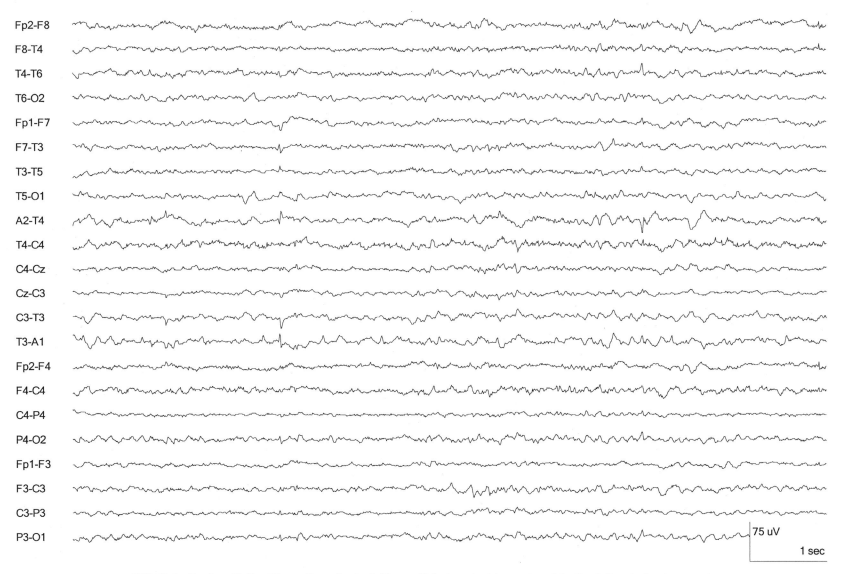

FIG. 5–1. Benign Epileptiform Transient of Sleep. This transient is centered in the left anterior temporal region and has a broad field that is also contralateral but with a lower amplitude. Brief rhythmic theta frequency range activity, another sign of drowsiness, follows the transient. (LFF 1 Hz, HFF 70 Hz)

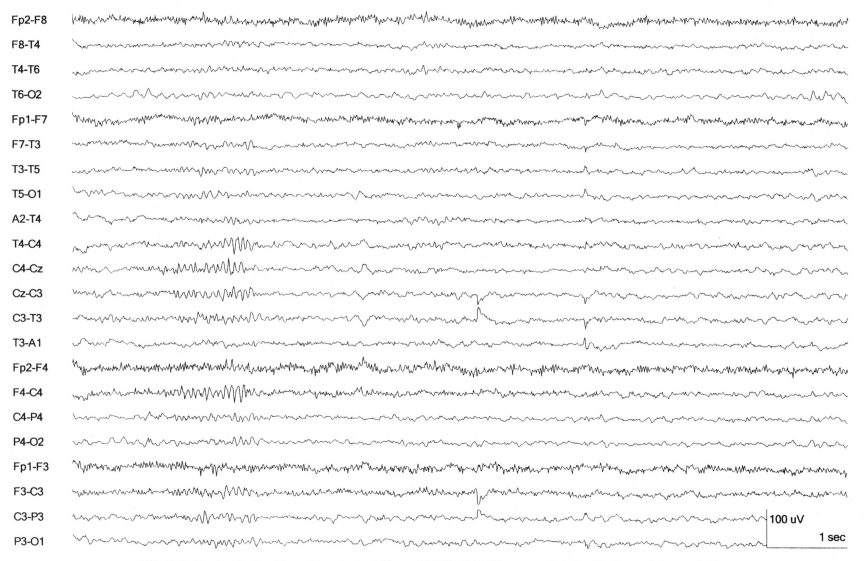

FIG. 5–2. Benign Epileptiform Transient of Sleep (BETS). A BETS centered at the T3 electrode has a field that includes the left central region and extends across the entire temporal region. On a Cz electrode referential montage, the field may be seen to involve the O1 electrode and have a transverse dipole with positivity at the T4 electrode. The C3 electrode pop preceding the BETS provides a morphologic comparison. A sleep spindle occurs earlier in the segment. (LFF 1 Hz, HFF 70 Hz)

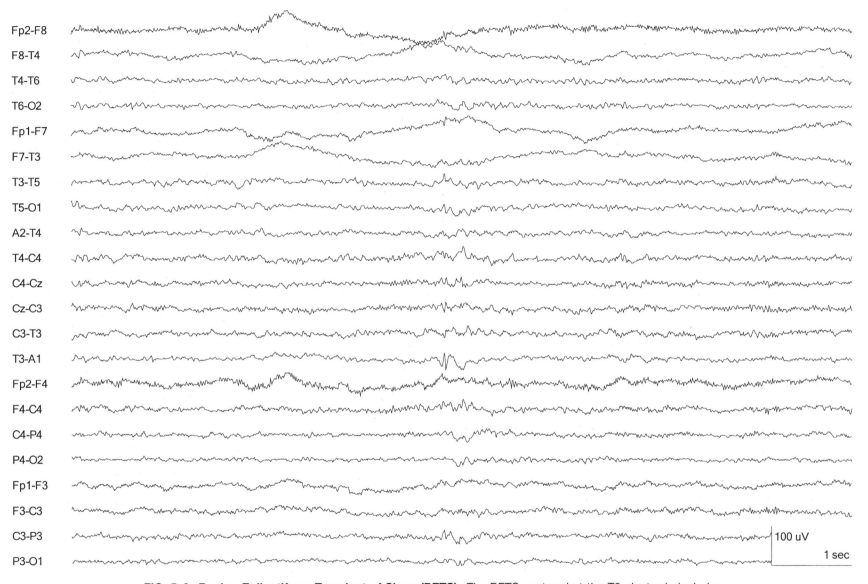

FIG. 5–3. Benign Epileptiform Transient of Sleep (BETS). The BETS centered at the T3 electrode includes an after-going slow wave of lower amplitude. Ocular artifact due to slow roving eye movements also is present and is another sign of drowsiness. (LFF 1 Hz, HFF 70 Hz)

CHAPTER 6

Beta Activity

FRONTOCENTRAL BETA ACTIVITY

Other Names
Fast activity
Sensory motor rhythm (SMR)

Description
As initially described and named by Hans Berger, beta activity constituted waves of 30 to 40 msec duration, which equates to rhythms of 25 to 33 Hz (79). However, this description was of beta activity in recordings that used only one channel and included subjects with skull defects. Beta activity now has a broader range of frequencies with a frequency definition of 13 Hz or greater. However, its occurrence within the frontal and central regions tends to have a frequency within the more narrow range of 20 to 30 Hz. Although frontocentral beta activity rarely has a frequency below 18 Hz or above 35 Hz, it may occur with frequencies anywhere from 14 to 40 Hz (6,14) (Figs. 6–1, 6–2, and 6–3). Frontocentral beta activity is state dependent, occurring with drowsiness and sometimes continuing through stage II of non–rapid eye movement (NREM) sleep. In drowsiness, it occurs as a burst, its amplitude may reach about 60 μV, and it may occur out of phase between the two hemispheres (25,54,80). Its distribution depends on age. When it first develops, which usually is between the ages of 6 months and 2 years, it is over the central and posterior head (7). During childhood, it gradually migrates anteriorly and is frontally predominant by early adulthood. Normal frontal-central beta activity is symmetric in its amplitude. An amplitude asymmetry greater than 35% is abnormal (7,14).

Distinguishing Features
Versus Muscle Artifact

Because the frontalis muscle runs over the frontal-central region, muscle artifact often co-localizes with the region of maximum beta activity. This artifact characteristically has a frequency greater than 25 Hz, and thus resembles frontal-central beta in this feature as well. Morphologic difference is the principal distinguishing feature. Electromyographic (EMG) artifact has a sharper contour with less rhythmicity when the high-frequency filter is set high. A high-frequency filter set to a frequency in the beta frequency range will give EMG artifact morphologic features of beta activity. When EMG artifact occurs as a rhythm within the beta frequency range, it does so as individual EMG potentials that have durations of less than 20 msec but are separated by an interval that gives it a beta frequency range appearance. The significant variation in this interval provides another distinguishing feature, especially when the interval becomes so brief that the potentials appear continuous. Such very fast activity is beyond the beta frequency range and usually indicates muscle artifact.

Versus Paroxysmal Fast Activity

Normal beta activity differs from paroxysmal fast activity (PFA) by typically beginning and ending gradually, even if only over a second. The abrupt change in amplitude and frequency components makes PFA more identifiable as a distinct pattern amid ongoing background activity.

Versus Sleep Spindles

Only beta activity that is localized to the vertex or midline frontal region appears similar to spindles, and this similarity is fostered by midline beta's association with drowsiness. However, midline beta differs from sleep spindles by not demonstrating abrupt beginning and ending. Such beta does not typically occur in bursts and instead usually builds up over seconds and persists for seconds before attenuating over seconds. Therefore, it does not have the characteristic spindle-like morphology. Furthermore, midline beta frequency activity usually has a predominant frequency greater than the 15 Hz that is typically the maximum frequency of sleep spindles.

Co-occurring Waves

Other signs of drowsiness always accompany frontal-central beta activity. These signs may include decreased muscle artifact, slow roving eye movements, intermittent alpha rhythm, slowed alpha rhythm, rhythmic temporal theta, and a Cigánek rhythm.

Clinical Significance

Frontocentral beta activity is a normal variant that most commonly is a sign of drowsiness or sleep onset but is present all of the time for some individuals. More rarely, it may accompany anxiety. Abnormally asymmetric frontal-central beta activity (greater than 35% between sides) may indicate cortical pathology beneath the region with the lower amplitude (7,14). However, artifactual low amplitude due to electrode positioning or function also must be considered. Rarely, cerebral pathology produces a focal increase in the amplitude of frontocentral beta activity; thus, the side of lower amplitude may be the normal side (9).

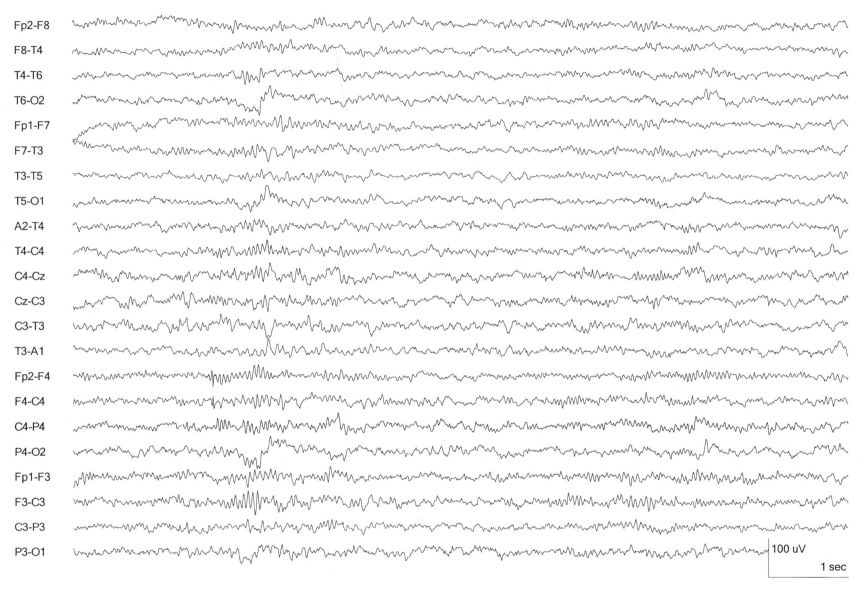

FIG. 6–1. Frontocentral Beta Activity. Increased beta activity is present diffusely but with paroxysmal greater activity in the frontocentral regions. Generalized theta activity also is present and is more visible at times when the beta activity declines. (LFF 1 Hz, HFF 70 Hz)

Fp2-F8

F8-T4

T4-T6

T6-O2

Fp1-F7

F7-T3

T3-T5

T5-O1

A2-T4

T4-C4

C4-Cz

Cz-C3

C3-T3

T3-A1

Fp2-F4

F4-C4

C4-P4

P4-O2

Fp1-F3

F3-C3

C3-P3

P3-O1

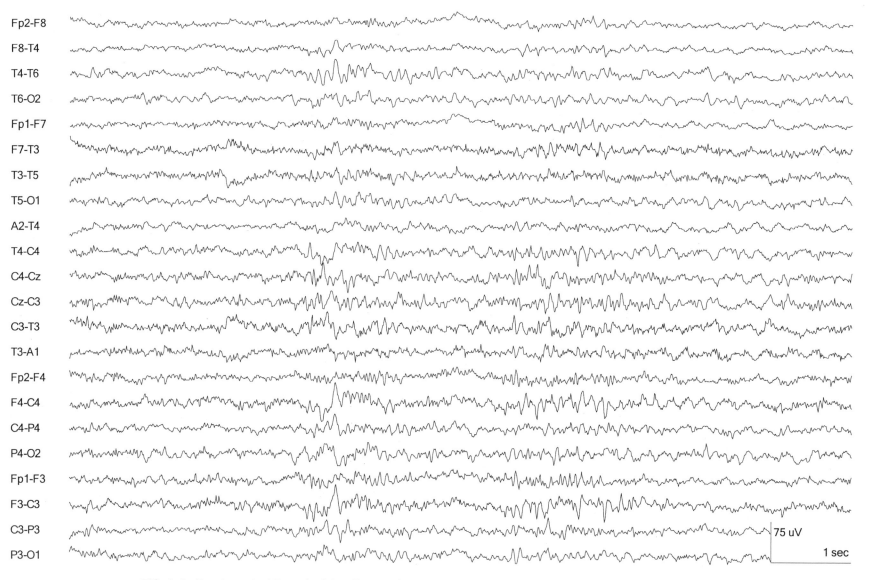

75 uV

1 sec

FIG. 6–2. Frontocentral Beta Activity. Bursts of beta activity occur in the central region within a background of generalized slowing. Both findings are consistent with drowsiness, which was behaviorally evident. (LFF 1 Hz, HFF 70 Hz)

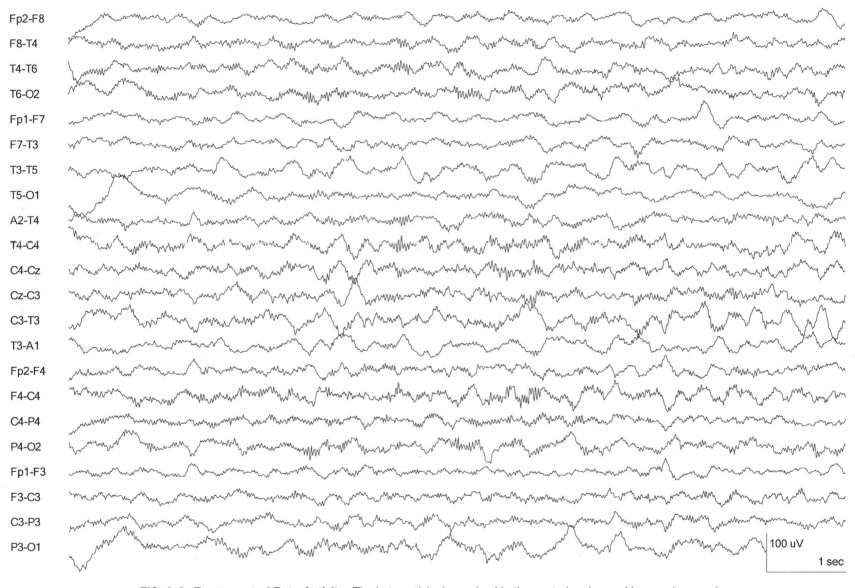

FIG. 6–3. Frontocentral Beta Activity. The beta activity is maximal in the central region and is superimposed on diffuse delta activity, indicating a deep stage of sleep. (LFF 1 Hz, HFF 70 Hz)

GENERALIZED BETA ACTIVITY

Other Names
Diffuse fast activity

Description
Although the electroencephalogram (EEG) of normal wakefulness includes a mixture of activities over most of the head, beta activity usually is low amplitude and not the predominant band (54). Beta activity is less than 20 μV in 98% of healthy awake subjects and less than 10 μV in 70%. When beta activity is predominant, the term generalized beta activity applies (Figs. 6–4 and 6–5). Beta activity comprises rhythms with frequencies within the beta range and individual waves with durations of the elements of beta frequency range rhythms. By definition, a beta rhythm has a frequency of 13.0 Hz or greater, and a beta wave has a duration of 77 msec or less. This definition is tempered by gamma activity, which is defined as activity with a frequency greater than 30 Hz but this is not as commonly used as a frequency term. Generalized beta activity usually is symmetric to within a 35% difference in amplitude (7). It also may have a frontal predominance, thereby overlapping with frontal-central beta activity (81). Although generalized beta activity may occur at any age, the amount of beta activity may change late in life (7). The direction of this change varies among published reports.

Distinguishing Features
Versus Generalized Paroxysmal Fast Activity

Generalized beta activity usually occurs over prolonged periods, with instances lasting less than 1 minute occurring rarely. It also tends to build and end gradually over several seconds. Both of the features distinguish it from generalized paroxysmal fast activity (GPFA), which characteristically has an abrupt beginning and end and a duration between 3 and 18 seconds (82). This abrupt change in amplitude and frequency components makes GPFA more identifiable as a distinct pattern amid ongoing background activity. Furthermore, GPFA typically has a maximum field over the frontal or frontal-central regions, whereas generalized beta activity is more evenly distributed. The occurrence of seizure-related artifact is another distinguishing feature; a seizure is likely to accompany GPFA lasting longer than 5 seconds (83).

Co-occurring Waves
Generalized beta may occur across all behavioral states and is not associated with another EEG wave specifically.

Clinical Significance
Generalized beta activity is most commonly a result of sedative medications; benzodiazepines and barbiturates are the most potent producers of such activity (7). Chloral hydrate, neuroleptics, phenytoin, cocaine, amphetamine, and meth-aqualone also may produce generalized beta activity, but they do so less readily and with less persistence than benzodiazepines and barbiturates (54,84,85). Beta activity is a common EEG accompaniment to coma due to sedation. Less commonly, anxiety and hyperthyroidism may produce generalized beta activity (7). Hypothyroidism may be accompanied by generalized beta activity, but this is in the context of decreased alpha activity (86). Generalized beta activity also may occur in the absence of any neurologic, psychiatric, or medical illness, but this is rare. Loss of beta activity may be the most sensitive EEG sign of cortical injury or fluid collection in either the subdural or epidural space, but this is most commonly a focal finding (14).

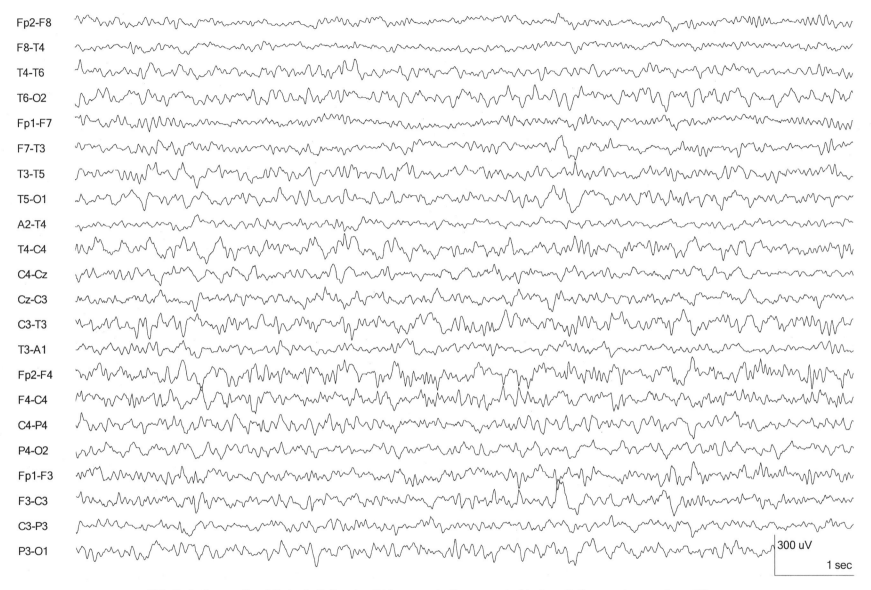

FIG. 6–4. Generalized Beta Activity. A mild increase in the amount of beta activity superimposed on diffuse slowing is consistent with sedation. Secobarbital was given for sedation. (LFF 1 Hz, HFF 70 Hz)

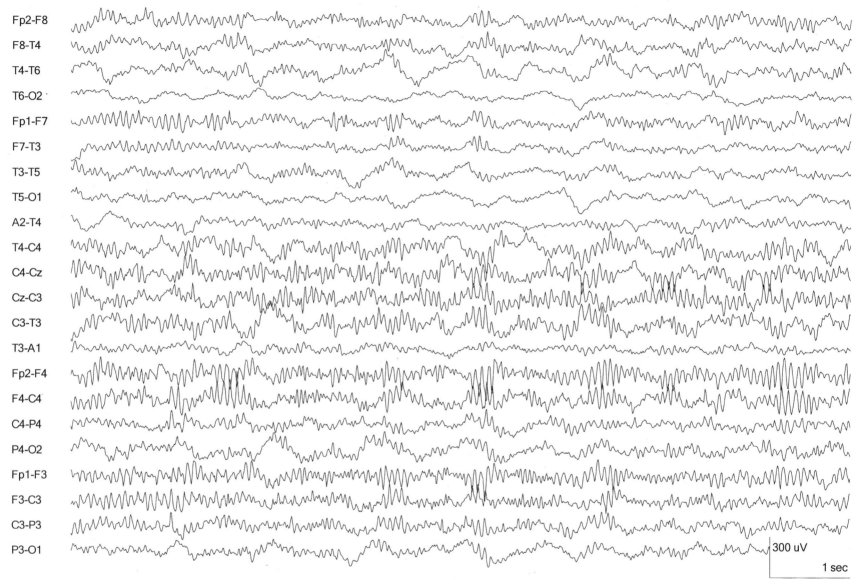

FIG. 6–5. Generalized Beta Activity. Abundant beta activity eclipses the other activity. Propofol was given for sedation. (LFF 1 Hz, HFF 70 Hz)

CHAPTER 7

Breach Effect

BREACH EFFECT

Other Names
Breach rhythm

Description

Because bone is a filter for electrical field activity that is biased toward the attenuation of higher frequencies, skull defects result in a change in the appearance of electroencephalogram (EEG) waves. This change is an overall increase in amplitude; a relative increase in the power of high-frequency rhythmic activity; and an increase in the sharpness of all other activity, including both transients and repetitions of all frequencies (Figs. 7–1 and 7–2). The amplitude increase usually is less than a factor of three times, but may be as much as five times the surrounding area (87,88). The sharpness may give sinusoidal activity an arciform morphology with the appearance of spikes at times when the rhythm demonstrates brief increases in amplitude.

Breach effects occur only over skull defects and abruptly diminish beyond the margins of the defect. Therefore, breach effects are best identified with bipolar montages with their better spatial resolution. Small skull defects, such as are produced by burr holes, do not produce a breach effect, presumably because the field that each electrode detects is larger than the hole. Specific questioning of the patient regarding head injuries and brain surgery is crucial in determining if a breach effect is likely to be present. Palpation of the scalp is not sufficient because the skull may have been replaced by an artificial material that does not have the filtering properties of bone.

Distinguishing Features
Versus Interictal Epileptiform Discharges

Interictal epileptiform discharges (IEDs) may occur within a region of breach effect as a consequence of the trauma that led to the skull defect. However, normal activity may have a spike-like appearance within a region of breach effect. This may occur when the background activity demonstrates increases in the amplitude that only last the duration of one wave and that wave appears abnormally sharp because of the breach effect. Determining whether the transient is an epileptic spike or background activity requires scrutinizing the surrounding background activity for wave elements that are similar in appearance to the transient. These surrounding elements may differ from the transient in their amplitudes or by occurring in a rhythmic train. The occurrence of several wave elements that are similar to the transient in question suggests that the transient truly is a component of the background and not an IED. Polyphasic IEDs are differentiated from breach effect activity through their occurrence as a complex with a slow wave or through their more characteristic morphology, which does not resemble the background activity.

Versus Beta Frequency Activity or Paroxysmal Fast Activity

Normal beta frequency activity is bilateral but may vary in distribution. Thus, it may be focal when it is at the midline. Therefore, focal fast activity within one hemisphere should raise suspicion for cerebral abnormality or a breach effect. The breach effect may be distinguished through its clearly circumscribed region of increased amplitude and its consistency. Paroxysmal fast activity (PFA) occurs in bursts with intervening return to a symmetric baseline or focal slowing within the region of the PFA.

Versus Electromyographic Artifact

Electromyographic (EMG) artifact tends to occur in skull regions with overlying muscle, that is, in the frontal and temporal regions, but it may be visible elsewhere. EMG artifact is easily distinguished by its inconsistent presence and its much higher frequency components. During sleep, the EMG artifact will disappear, but a breach effect becomes more apparent due to the generalized slowing. Although the frequencies within a breach effect are faster than the beta activity typically seen with the scalp EEG, they are slower than the predominant frequencies of EMG artifact. Breach effect frequencies are visible frequencies, and the frequencies within EMG artifact are so fast that they cease to appear as simple frequencies and demonstrate elements that appear as vertical lines.

Co-occurring Waves

The development with skull defects means breach effects may be associated with cerebral injury or pathology. If so, the background activity within, and sometimes beyond, the breach effect may be abnormally slowed or low in amplitude.

Clinical Significance

The breach effect is not due to a brain abnormality; it is a sign of a bone abnormality. Therefore, it is not an EEG abnormality. The presence of abnormal slowing or low amplitude within the breach effect's region is a separate matter and may indicate cerebral pathology (Fig. 7–3).

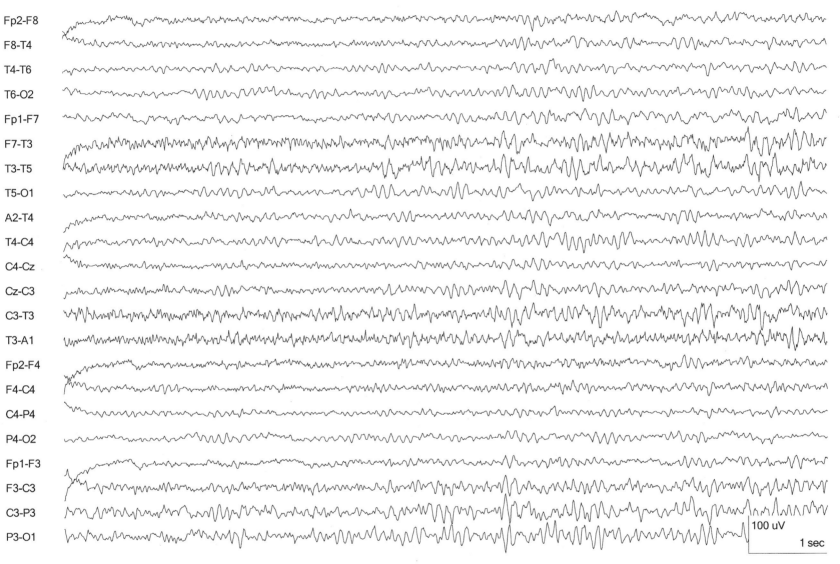

FIG. 7–1. Breach Effect. The increased beta activity and higher amplitude across the left temporal and parietal regions is consistent with the history of a similarly located craniotomy. (LFF 1 Hz, HFF 70 Hz)

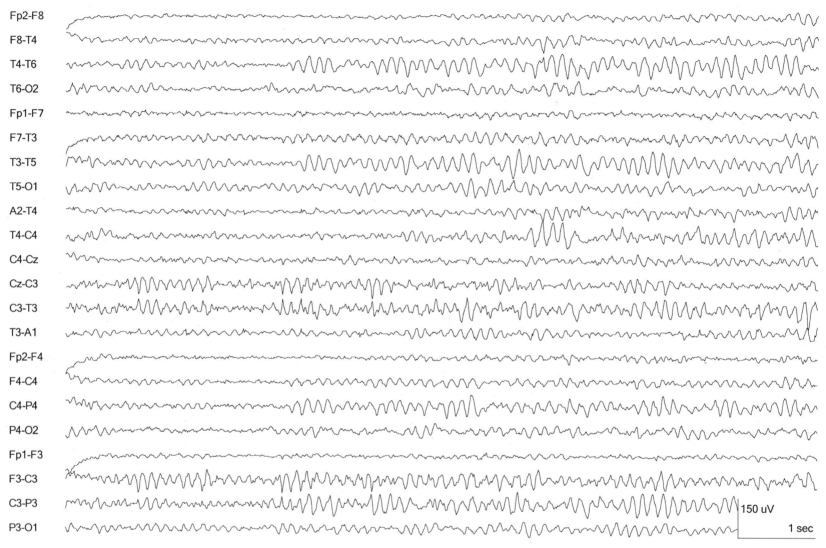

FIG. 7–2. Breach Effect. The left central bone defect gives the underlying activity a classic arciform morphology. (LFF 1 Hz, HFF 70 Hz)

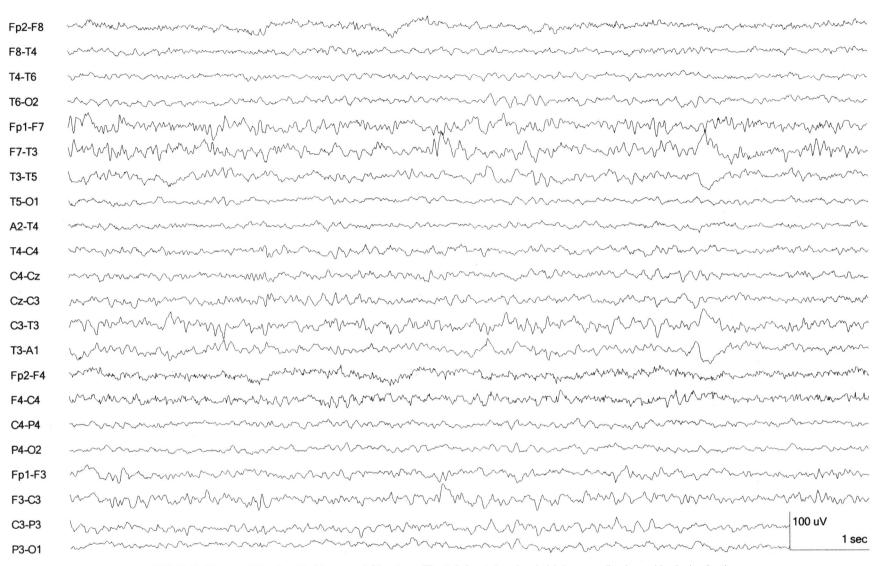

FIG. 7–3. Breach Effect with Abnormal Slowing. The left frontal region is higher amplitude and includes both slowing and a greater amount of fast activity. The EEG corresponds to a left frontal tumor that was partially resected. (LFF 1 Hz, HFF 70 Hz)

CHAPTER 8

Burst-Suppression Pattern

BURST-SUPPRESSION PATTERN

Other Names
Suppression-burst pattern (activity)

Description
The burst-suppression pattern (BSP) is characterized not so much by the features within the burst or the suppression but by their contrasting, adjacent amplitudes (Figs. 8–1, 8–2, and 8–3). The amplitudes of the bursts may vary from low (<20 µV) to high (>100 µV), but most often are between 20 and 100 µV. Similarly, suppressions may vary in amplitude but are almost always within the range of electrocerebral inactivity to medium amplitude (~50 µV). Because the abrupt change in amplitude defines this pattern, the amplitude difference must be clearly visible and usually greater than a 50% decrease. A threshold absolute amplitude decrease cannot be defined because BSPs may have amplitude differences as little as 10 µV if the bursts are 15 µV, but a 10-µV decrease is not significant if the higher amplitude activity is 60 µV.

The temporal relationships between the bursts and suppressions vary considerably with the possibility of either the bursts or the suppressions being longer in duration. Some definitions specify that the term burst-suppression indicates that the bursts are longer than the suppressions and suppression-burst indicates that the suppressions are longer (7). However, BSP commonly is used without such specificity. Individual bursts typically have a duration of 1 to 3 seconds and, regardless of the duration, often recur quasi-periodically (7,89).

Bursts usually are bilaterally synchronous and commonly are generalized but may be unilateral. They may comprise multiple and intermingled sharps and spikes or occur as rhythmic activity. The rhythmic activity may be regular or irregular and have a predominant frequency anywhere in the spectrum from the delta through the beta ranges, and bursts of delta frequency range activity usually have superimposed faster frequencies. Regardless of whether the bursts are rhythmic or not, burst morphology usually is not conserved among occurrences within an electroencephalogram (EEG) with rhythmic bursts having conserved regularity and frequency. When activity is present during suppressions, it typically is in the delta frequency range. In general, suppressions with less of an amplitude decrease include activity closer to the normal background frequencies than lower amplitude suppressions; thus, they may be as fast as the alpha frequency range (89).

Distinguishing Features
Versus Periodic Epileptiform Discharges

Similar to BSPs, periodic epileptiform discharges (PEDs) constitute an abruptly recurring pattern that includes spikes or sharps, which often are bilateral (bilateral periodic epileptiform discharges [BiPEDs]) and of higher amplitude than the background. Furthermore, many clinical situations that produce BSPs instead may be accompanied by PEDs, especially BiPEDs. Differentiating these two patterns depends mostly on morphology. Unlike the bursts of BSP, PEDs typically are briefer and have a more conserved morphology that also includes a recurring temporal relationship between sharply contoured transients (spikes or sharp waves) and slow waves. Moreover, the relationship among the wave elements is epileptiform with the slow wave following a sharp wave or one or more spikes. Occasionally, bursts are morphologically conserved, but they comprise multiple sharply contoured waves and slow waves without the epileptiform pattern (90). Bursts also are usually longer in duration than PEDs and, unlike PEDs, commonly have durations longer than 1 second.

Co-occurring Waves

BSP always occurs in the context of diffuse cerebral dysfunction; thus, it is accompanied by other EEG features of such states, especially generalized polymorphic delta activity. Some clinical situations that lead to BSP also produce myoclonus, and the myoclonus of such states accompanies the bursts. Tonus, ocular movements, or orofacial movements also may accompany the bursts of BSP, each of which has their own characteristic muscle or movement artifact (7,91). Therefore, muscle artifact may be superimposed on the bursts with a slight lag from the burst's beginning. Rarely, the muscle artifact accompanies the suppressions (92).

Clinical Significance

The BSP occurs in the context of diffuse cerebral dysfunction with coma and indicates a clinical severity that is greater than generalized rhythmic activity but less than electrocerebral inactivity. Such situations include cerebral anoxia (generalized ischemic encephalopathy), hypothermia, end-stage status epilepticus, and high levels of sedation (93). Hypothermia typically is accompanied by BSP between body temperatures of 18°C and 24°C, but BSP is not uncommon within the broader range of 14°C to 28°C (94). The levels of sedation that produce BSP also suppress the respiratory drive and other brainstem reflexes; thus, intact brainstem reflexes in the context of BSP and sedation suggests that the sedation is not the only cause for the BSP (95). The bursts when sedation is responsible tend to comprise more regular rhythmic activity. Anoxia tends to produce irregular polymorphic bursts comprising delta activity and spikes (96). BSP also may follow head trauma, but only when the trauma produces cerebral anoxia. Unilateral bursts in a BSP indicate that the hemisphere contralateral to the bursts is more dysfunctional, as most commonly occurs with a large infarction. However, a large resection or large tumor are other possible causes for unilateral bursts. Clinical worsening may be apparent in BSP with shortening of the burst durations, simplification of the burst morphology, and decreasing amplitude of the suppressions (7). Overall, BSP is nonspecific for prognosis because reversible sedation may produce it. However, it is a sign of poor prognosis for cerebral recovery when its cause is known to be an irreversible process (97).

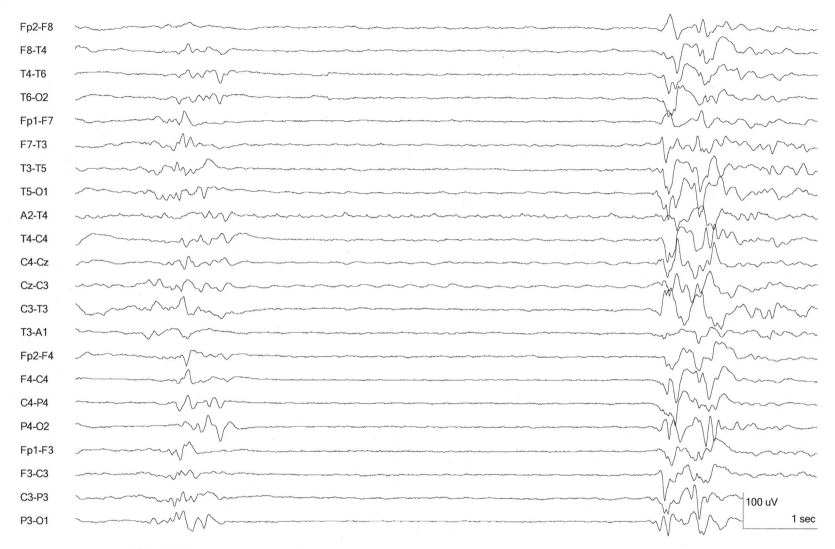

FIG. 8–1. Burst-suppression Pattern. Bursts of irregular, predominantly slow wave activity occur without consistent morphology or periodicity. The bursts last 1 to 2 seconds and are separated by suppressions lasting 2 to 6 seconds. The EEG corresponds to coma following a period of severe hypoxia-ischemia. (LFF 1 Hz, HFF 70 Hz)

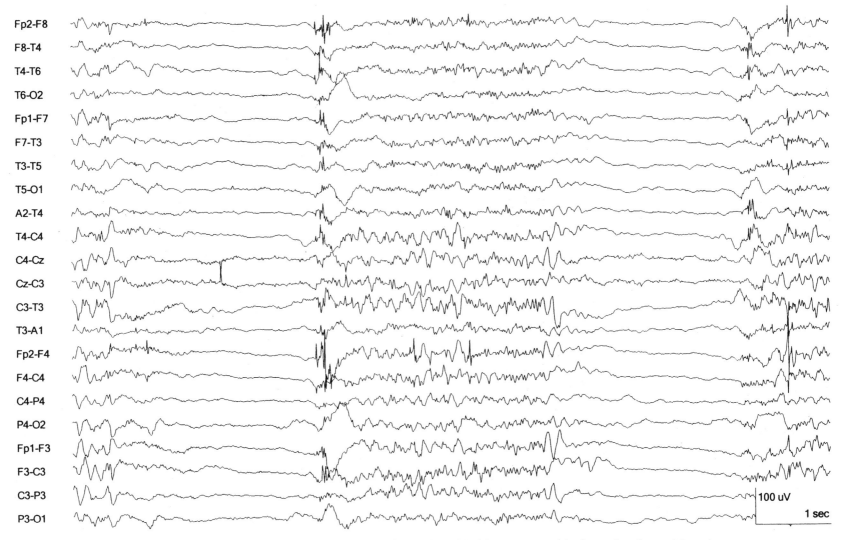

FIG. 8–2. Burst-suppression Pattern. Bursts of irregular, mixed frequency activity have durations of 3 to 4 seconds and are separated by suppressions lasting 2 to 3 seconds. Brief muscle artifact is superimposed on both the bursts and suppressions with the most significant artifact occurring at the beginning of the second burst. The EEG corresponds to anoxic encephalopathy. (LFF 1 Hz, HFF 70 Hz)

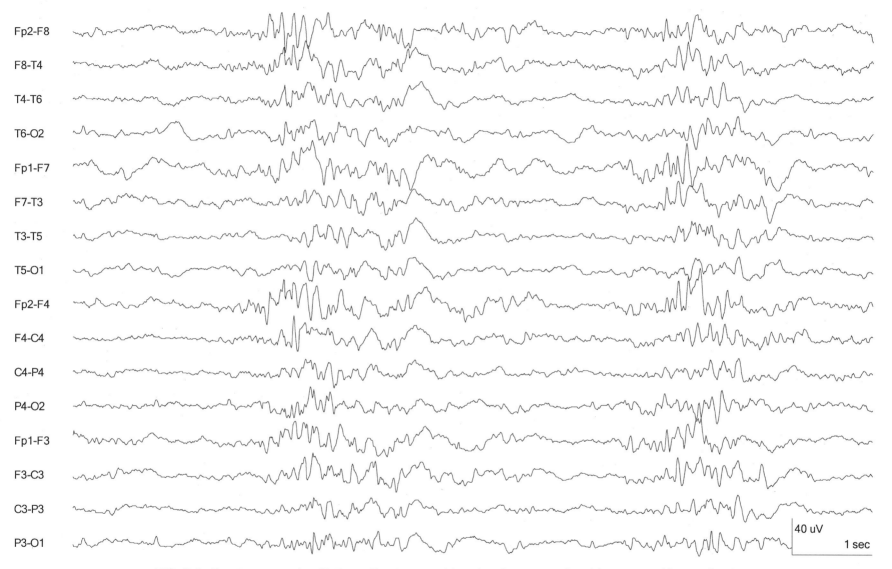

FIG. 8–3. Burst-suppression Pattern. Bursts comprising sharply contoured activity repeat without a fixed interval. The EEG corresponds to anesthesia with desflurane and was normal at other times. (LFF 1 Hz, HFF 70 Hz)

CHAPTER 9

Cone Waves

CONE WAVES

Other Names
Occipital wave
O wave

Description
Cone waves are isolated slow waves that occur over the occiput with a monophasic and triangular morphology (Fig. 9–1). They have medium to high amplitudes and durations that typically are greater than 250 msec. They occur only from infancy through mid childhood and are state dependent with occurrence only in non–rapid eye movement (NREM) sleep (7).

Distinguishing Features
Versus Polymorphic Delta Activity

By definition, cone waves are in the delta frequency range; thus, they resemble the slow waves of polymorphic delta activity (PDA) in their duration. Their occurrence only in NREM sleep is only somewhat helpful in distinguishing them from PDA because the background activity of stages III and IV NREM sleep includes much PDA. Occurrences in stages I and II NREM sleep are more distinguishing because PDA is rare in these stages. Cone waves' characteristic and stereotyped morphology is more helpful in distinguishing them from PDA. PDA, by definition, varies in morphology and typically is not triangular.

Versus Positive Occipital Sharp Transients of Sleep

Positive occipital sharp transients of sleep (POSTS) are similar to cone waves in their triangular morphology, occipital distribution, and occurrence in NREM sleep. However, POSTS differ by having a shorter duration, which is typically less than 200 msec, and a positivity at the center of the field, which is evident through a phase reversal. Cone waves also occur in younger individuals than POSTS, which are rare before 3 years and most common after childhood. Unlike cone waves, POSTS also may be diphasic.

Co-occurring Waves
Cone waves occur only during NREM sleep and, thus, are accompanied by the electrographic features of this state. This includes diffuse, polymorphic theta or delta background activity, vertex sharp transients, sleep spindles, and K complexes. Cone waves are not accompanied by evidence of wakefulness, such as the alpha rhythm.

Clinical Significance
Cone waves are a normal variant and have no clinical significance either through their presence or their absence.

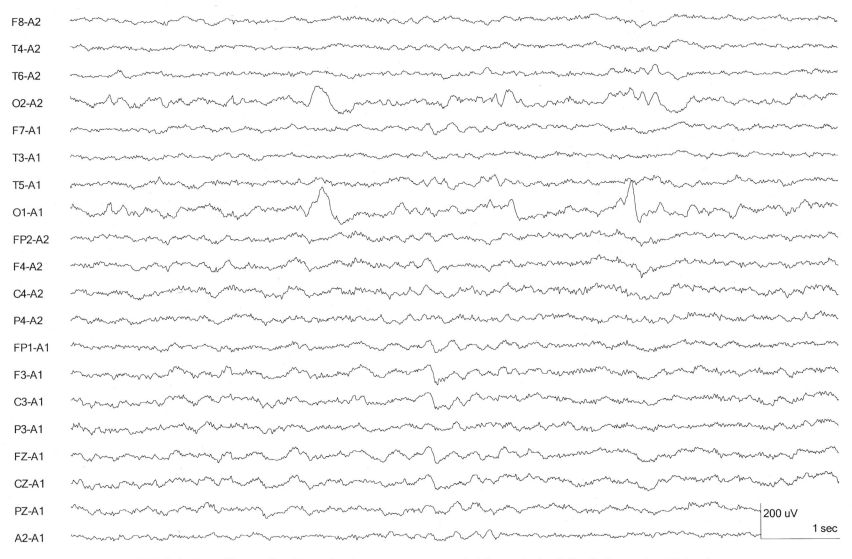

FIG. 9–1. Cone Waves. Two triangular slow waves are present at the occiput with the first occurring bilaterally and lasting 400 msec and the second occurring unilaterally and lasting 250 msec. The amplitude, shape, and duration of the slow waves contrasts the surrounding generalized theta frequency activity of non–rapid eye movement (NREM) sleep. (LFF 1 Hz, HFF 70 Hz)

CHAPTER 10

Delta Activity

POLYMORPHIC DELTA ACTIVITY

Other Names
Abnormal slowing
Anterior bradyrhythmia (if frontal bilateral)
Arrhythmic delta activity
Zeta waves

Description
Delta activity comprises both rhythmic activity with a frequency less than 4 Hz and individual waves that would produce a rhythm of less than 4 Hz if they occurred in succession. Therefore, intermittent waves with durations greater than 250 msec are included under the heading of delta activity (Figs. 10–1, 10–2, 10–3, 10–4). This differs from the original definition of delta activity, introduced by Grey Walter in 1936 and defined as all activity below the alpha frequency range (6). Walter later modified the definition with the insertion of the theta range between alpha and delta. Polymorphic delta activity (PDA) is a common finding on electroencephalograms (EEGs) that may be distinguished as either normal or abnormal based on features and circumstances. However, abnormal PDA may have several features of normal PDA, including bilateral symmetry in frequency and amplitude, superimposed faster frequencies, and an increase in frequency with alerting stimulation such as noise or touch. Nevertheless, abnormal PDA commonly and characteristically has consistent asymmetry, asymmetrically superimposed faster frequencies, and lack of change with alerting stimulation. Focal PDA that has a region of maximum slowing and minimal faster frequencies is especially abnormal and indicates a focal lesion in the white matter that is deep to the most abnormal region within the focal

slowing (9). Although PDA is the characteristic finding of non–rapid eye movement (NREM) sleep and it disappears with greater alertness, it still may occur in full wakefulness as specific patterns described here under different headings, including posterior slow waves of youth (PSWY), cone waves, and others.

Zeta waves are a delta wave with a distinctive sharply diphasic morphology (Fig. 10–5). They have a "Z" or saw-toothed shape that includes a rise followed by an overshooting fall and ending with a minor rise. This morphology varies somewhat between waves, even within a run of several individual waves. They usually occur in runs lasting 1.5 to 3 seconds and including two or three waves (98). Their amplitude usually is greater than 100 μV and may reach 400 μV. Although they most commonly have a focal frontal field, they may occur over any region of the scalp and also may occur bisynchronously.

Distinguishing Features
Versus Intermittent Rhythmic Delta Activity

Beyond containing waves of similar durations, intermittent rhythmic delta activity (IRDA) and PDA may occur in similar clinical circumstances and may occur independently within the same EEG. However, they have clear distinguishing features with differences in rhythmicity, persistence, and distribution. As its name indicates, PDA is not regular and does not occur with the rhythm characteristic of IRDA. Furthermore, IRDA's rhythms are intermittent, brief, monomorphic bursts that stand apart from the more normal background. This differs from PDA with its persistence as an ongoing background pattern and varying frequency and morphology. Bilateral PDA is also more likely to be generalized.

Versus Polymorphic Theta Activity

Irregular slowing may occur across a spectrum of frequencies and includes both the theta and delta frequency ranges. The division between these two ranges is arbitrary but useful for quickly communicating an EEG's general appearance. Nevertheless, the duration of the individual waves is the essential distinguishing feature, with waves of longer than 250 msec indicating delta activity.

Co-occurring Waves

The normal PDA of NREM sleep is accompanied by vertex sharp transients, sleep spindles, K complexes, and positive occipital sharp transients of sleep (POSTS); however, these other signs of NREM sleep occur more in stages I and II than in III and IV. Indeed stages III and IV may include only PDA and have no electrographic features that would distinguish it as normal sleep and not severe encephalopathy. Conversely, encephalopathy may be distinguished through the occurrence of focal findings such as epileptiform discharges, greater slowing, superimposed faster activity, and attenuations or electrodecrements.

Clinical Significance

Generalized PDA indicates either encephalopathy or sleep, and encephalopathy in this context is a nonspecific state of diffuse neuronal dysfunction that may be as severe as coma. PDA is so intrinsic to NREM sleep that the amount of PDA is the defining factor for stages III and IV, which, collectively, also are called slow wave sleep. An epoch is determined to be stage III NREM sleep when delta frequency activity composes at least 20% and not more than 50% of its activity. Stage IV is defined by the occurrence of delta frequency range activity over more than 50% of the epoch.

The encephalopathy producing generalized PDA may be a reversible state due to transient physiologic abnormality or due to endogenous or exogenous sedatives. Physiologic abnormalities may occur during migraine, syncope, and ischemia and after a seizure (99–102). Metabolic dysfunction is the principal source for endogenous sedation and may be produced by hepatic and renal disease. Exogenous sedatives are specific toxins and pharmaceuticals, such as narcotics (103). Generalized PDA also may be irreversible as from a diffuse cerebral insult such as anoxia, infection, hypoglycemia, and inflammation; developmental abnormality usually with global cognitive impairment; or certain degenerative or dementing illnesses such as stroke, advanced Alzheimer's disease, and sometimes schizophrenia (104–110). Specifically, PDA occurs when serum glucose is less than 35 mg/100 ml, and all other frequencies are absent when the glucose drops below 18 mg/100 ml (104). Lower serum glucose concentrations will produce generalized attenuation. Inflammatory causes of PDA include encephalitis, purulent meningitis, and some autoimmune diseases such as Sydenham's disease and Behcet's disease (111).

Regardless of its cause, generalized PDA is similar to focal PDA as a sign of cerebral white matter abnormality (42,112). This abnormality must be significant and include either cellular toxicity or mechanical compression. Interstitial edema alone does not appear to produce abnormal slowing (113). Often the pathology is accompanied by cerebral cortical abnormality, but abnormality limited to the cerebral cortex does not produce slowing. It produces attenuation and loss of the faster frequencies (114). PDA with a more paroxysmal pattern typically is more deeply situated (89). With clinical worsening, frontal IRDA (FIRDA) and occipital IRDA (OIRDA) may progress to PDA (42).

Compared to generalized PDA, focal PDA typically is more persistent, more polymorphic, and less reactive to stimulation or behavioral state (42). Furthermore, it is more clinically specific by usually indicating a similarly localized structural or functional abnormality (115). However, it also may occur with diffuse abnormalities or from a lesion in the distant site of the posterior fossa (116,117). Structural abnormalities usually have more continuous PDA. Among such lesions, abscesses typically have a larger field and higher amplitude than similarly sized tumors (118). In addition to seizures, transient and fluctuating PDA may indicate migraine, mild trauma, and a transient ischemic attack (7).

Zeta waves most commonly occur in the context of acute cerebral lesions, usually disappear with recovery, but may persist for years. In one series, 87% of patients whose EEG demonstrated zeta waves had a structural lesion on neuroimaging and the positive predictive value of zeta waves for a lesion was found to be 96% (119). They are more likely to occur with trauma, a hematoma, or a tumor than with infarction (27).

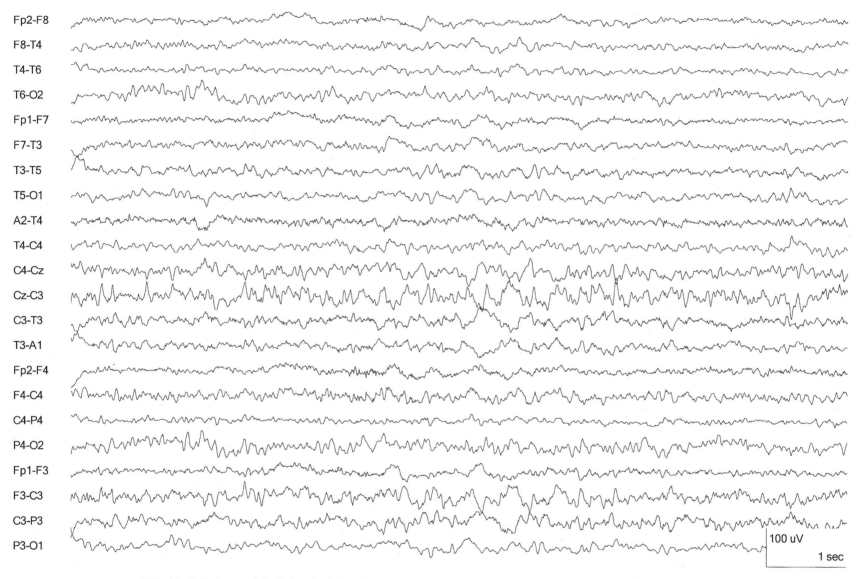

FIG. 10–1. Polymorphic Delta Activity. Slowing is present in the left posterior region and co-localizes with a left parieto-occipital meningioma. The asymmetric slowing exceeds the generalized slowing that corresponds to an encephalopathy. (LFF 1 Hz, HFF 70 Hz)

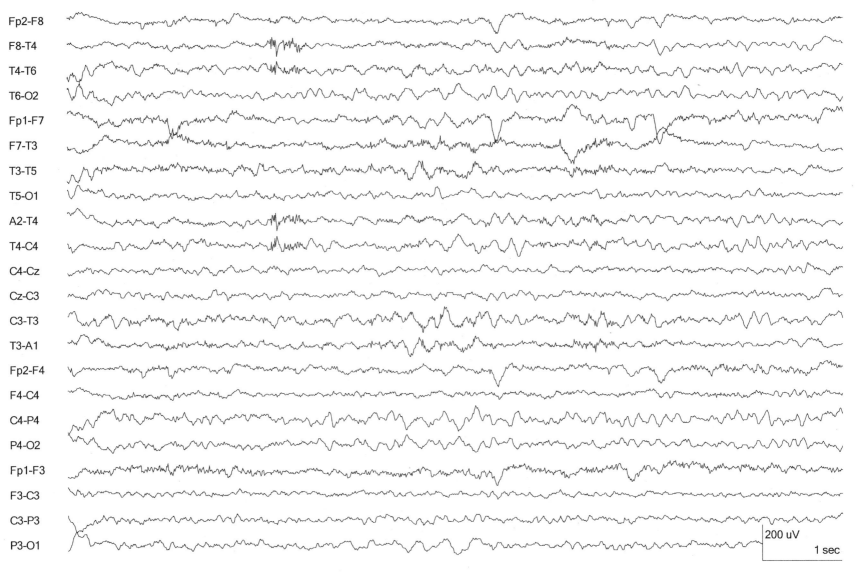

FIG. 10–2. Polymorphic Delta Activity. Intermittent and generalized delta activity interrupts the poorly formed posterior dominant rhythm, which is in theta frequency range and normal for this 1-year-old. The slowing corresponds to drowsiness. (LFF 1 Hz, HFF 70 Hz)

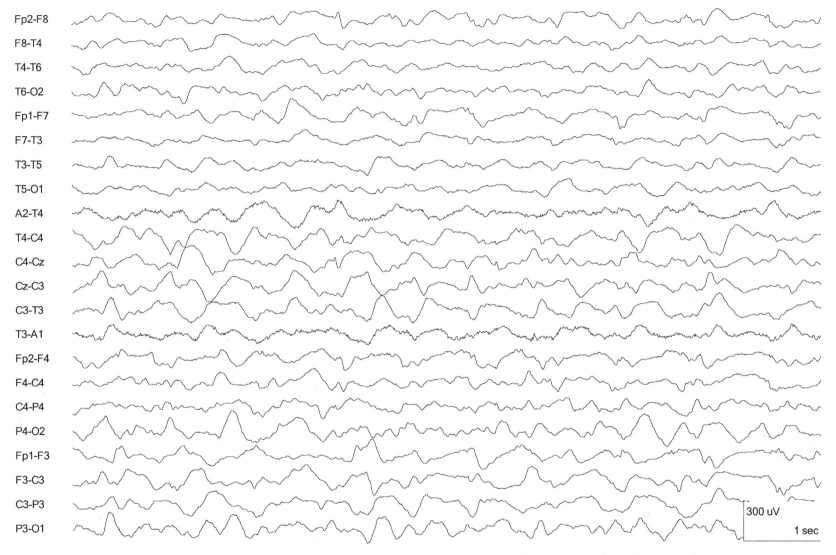

FIG. 10–3. Polymorphic Delta Activity. Abnormal generalized slowing that corresponds to the vegetative state of late-stage subacute sclerosing panencephalitis. (LFF 1 Hz, HFF 70 Hz)

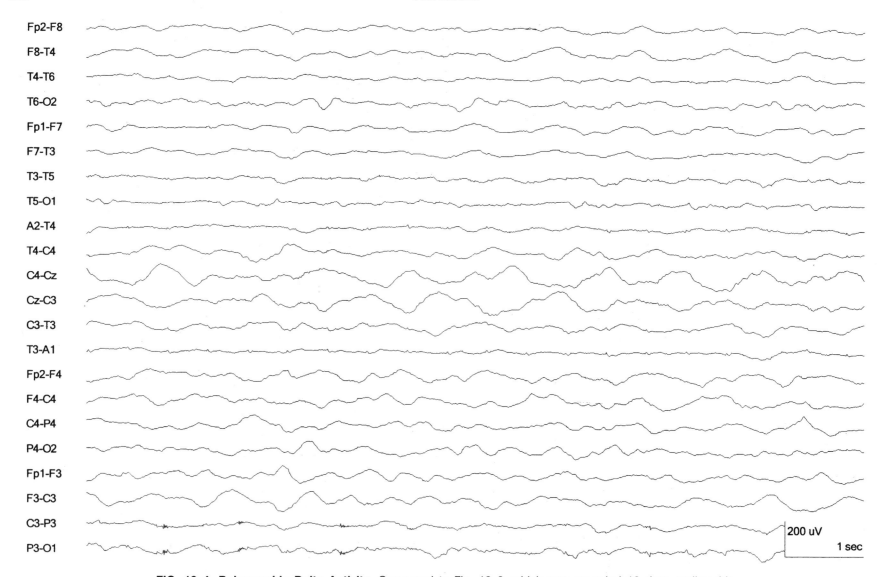

FIG. 10–4. Polymorphic Delta Activity. Compared to Fig. 10–3, which was recorded 10 days earlier, this segment has greater generalized slowing and lower amplitude. Medical deterioration had occurred. (LFF 1 Hz, HFF 70 Hz)

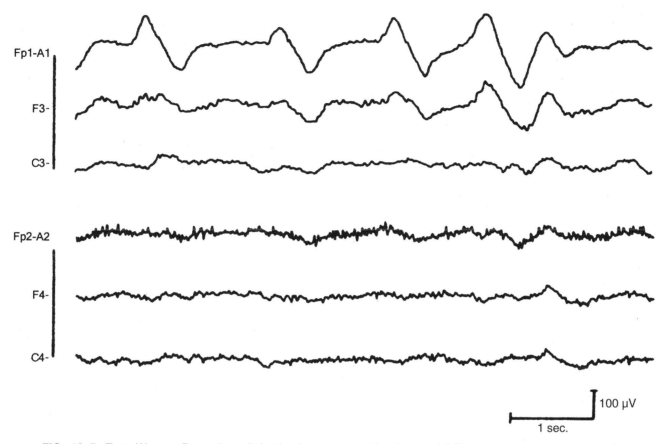

FIG. 10–5. Zeta Waves. Repeating, diphasic slow waves with minor variability are present across the left frontal region. The waves resemble the letter "Z" when the page is turned 45 degrees clockwise. The EEG corresponds to a left frontal cerebral tumor. (From Westmoreland BF, Klass DW. Unusual EEG patterns. *J Clin Neurophysiol* 1990;7:224, with permission.)

RHYTHMIC DELTA ACTIVITY

Other Names
Intermittent rhythmic delta activity (IRDA)
Frontal IRDA (FIRDA)
Occipital IRDA (OIRDA)
Temporal IRDA (TIRDA)
Monorhythmic delta
Projected slow waves
Parenrhythmia (German)
Rythmes a distance (French)
Phi rhythm

Description

The name IRDA suitably describes this pattern of brief runs of monomorphic activity within the delta frequency range (less than 4 Hz). The waves constituting the runs are regular and may be sinusoidal or saw-toothed with phases that rise more rapidly than they fall. They occur as a burst, that is, a sudden change to the background, and continue for periods often between 2 and 6 seconds with a frequency typically close to 2.5 Hz and an amplitude typically between 50 and 100 μV (42). Their field is typically is large and most commonly has a frontal focus, which is termed FIRDA (Figs. 10–6 and 10–7). However, the focus in children may be occipital instead, termed OIRDA (Fig. 10–8). Unilateral FIRDA and OIRDA also occur, but the more common form of unilateral IRDA is centered in the temporal region (Figs. 10–9 and 10–10). This is termed TIRDA. Regardless of its location, IRDA typically attenuates with alerting behavior as identified by spontaneous eye opening or the delivery of exogenous stimuli (42,89).

The phi rhythm is a brief, paroxysmal, bisynchronous, occipital delta rhythm that is defined as including at least three monomorphic delta waves within 2 seconds of eye closure. It usually has a latency of less than 0.5 seconds after eye closure, a frequency of 2 to 4 Hz, an amplitude of 100 to 250 μV, and a duration of 1 to 3 seconds (28). Thus, its waveform has features resembling OIRDA, but it differs most importantly by being triggered by decreased visual attention and not co-existing with electrographic evidence of cerebral dysfunction. OIRDA often has superimposed generalized slowing (6,13). Although it typically is symmetric, it may have a shifting asymmetry (27).

Distinguishing Features
Versus Ocular Artifact

Isolated monomorphic slow waves and FIRDA have the same wave duration and a similar field to ocular artifact from eye opening and closure. Blinks are more similar to isolated slow waves, and eye flutter is more similar to FIRDA. The field is the key distinguishing feature between ocular artifact and delta activity. Unlike delta activity, ocular artifact does not extend into the central region. However, a morphologic difference also exists due to ocular artifact's sharper contour. The two also may be distinguished based on recognized eye movements. Notation by the technologist is helpful for this. If notation is not present, then identification may be based on whether the wave is absent in drowsiness and sleep, states in which the eyes are closed. The use of both supraorbital and infraorbital electrodes is the most definitive means for differentiation. Ocular artifact produces a phase reversal between infraorbital electrode and superorbital electrode channels because the area of maximum potential exists between the electrodes. In contrast, the are of maximum potential for cerebrally generated slowing is above the orbits; thus, it does not produce a phase reversal between these channels.

Versus Hypersynchrony

There is no distinguishing morphologic or distribution difference between IRDA and hypersynchrony of any cause. Differentiating these waveforms depends on knowing the behavioral correlate to the EEG pattern.

Versus Posterior Slow Waves of Youth

PSWY and OIRDA have similar distributions and wave durations, and both occur in childhood. The waves constituting IRDA and PSWY both typically have durations of 0.35 to 0.5 seconds. However, PSWY occur individually and with varying morphology; they do not have the essential regular, rhythmic features of OIRDA. Furthermore, PSWY interrupt the alpha rhythm; thus, they are not accompanied by the diffuse slowing that typically is OIRDA's background activity.

Versus Polymorphic Delta Activity

Beyond containing waves of similar durations, IRDA and PDA may occur in similar clinical circumstances, and they may occur independently within the same EEG. However, they have clear distinguishing features with differences in rhythmicity, persistence, and distribution. As its name indicates, PDA is not regular and does not occur as the rhythm characteristic of IRDA. Furthermore, IRDA's rhythms are intermittent, brief, monomorphic bursts that stand apart from the usually normal background, which differs from PDA with its persistence and varying frequencies. Bilateral PDA also is more likely to be generalized.

Versus Triphasic Waves

FIRDA and triphasic waves (TW) have similar distributions and recurrence patterns. Both recur in repetitions that typically last several seconds. Differentiation between the patterns rests essentially on morphology. FIRDA is comprised of monophasic slow waves and TW clearly include multiple phases. The distinction may be more difficult if FIRDA has superimposed faster frequencies that give the appearance of notched slow waves suggestive of subtle initiating spikes or sharps. Distinguishing notched FIRDA due to a mixture of frequencies from TW relies on identifying a consistent location of the notch along the slow wave's slope. A mixture of frequencies will produce notching that is more random. A subtle spike or sharp wave always will be present at the same location with regard to the slow wave's apex. More rarely, FIRDA will have a subtle spike or sharp wave that is intrinsic to the wave and not due to superimposed faster frequencies. This is termed epileptic FIRDA and should be considered as an interictal epileptiform pattern.

Co-occurring Waves

Because IRDA, polymorphic delta activity, and polymorphic theta activity may be produced by the same clinical conditions, they may occur within the same record (9). This is true both for FIRDA and OIRDA with diffuse abnormal slowing to the delta or theta frequency ranges and for TIRDA with focal abnormal slowing present over a temporal lobe.

Clinical Significance

IRDA is a highly nonspecific pattern that may indicate either focal pathology or diffuse abnormality and may be a sign of epilepsy (120). Furthermore, the focal pathology may be supratentorial or infratentorial (40,42); the diffuse abnormality may be due to toxic, metabolic, anoxic, congenital, degenerative, or endogenous dysfunction such as from epilepsy or confusional or basilar migraine (121–125); the pattern does not differ based on whether or not the underlying abnormality is focal (126,339,340). IRDA also may precede or co-exist with other electrographic signs of diffuse cerebral dysfunction. It is an early sign of Creutzfeldt-Jakob disease that may last for several weeks before being replaced by the more characteristic periodic complexes (127). FIRDA may co-exist with and separate the periodic complexes of subacute sclerosing panencephalitis (SSPE) in about half of cases and usually does so in more than one EEG (128).

FIRDA and OIRDA are more likely to occur as an abnormality is developing or resolving than in the context of chronic and stable pathology (42). As such it may be an early sign of neuronal dysfunction and typically accompanies metabolic deterioration in the context of cerebrovascular disease (129). Uremia and hyperglycemia are among the most common metabolic abnormalities. FIRDA and OIRDA also may accompany increasing intracranial pressure, even as a sign of incipient herniation (89). However, its occurrence as a sign of progression, such as increasing intracranial pressure, is with co-existing abnormal slowing, which indicates the underlying pathology. As signs of focal pathology, FIRDA and OIRDA are nonlocalizing, and the difference in location is due only to brain development (9,42). FIRDA most commonly occurs in mid adulthood and OIRDA in mid childhood (129,130). The same pathology with the same location may produce either pattern, depending only on the age of the patient. However, OIRDA is much more often associated with epilepsy and much less likely to be accompanied by encephalopathy. Among seizure types, absence and generalized tonic-clonic seizures most commonly occur in patients with OIRDA. Although it resembles OIRDA, the phi rhythm is not associated with epilepsy and is a normal variant.

Unilateral FIRDA and OIRDA more often indicate focal pathology than diffuse neuronal dysfunction and sometimes are present contralateral to the pathology. However, contralateral occurrence also is possible. When bilaterally symmetric FIRDA and OIRDA are due to a focal lesion, this lesion classically is near the third ventricle, diencephalic or mesencephalic midline, brainstem, or cerebellum.

TIRDA is even more specific for focal pathology and, also in contrast to FIRDA and OIRDA, is highly indicative of ipsilateral pathology. Moreover, TIRDA has a greater diagnostic specificity because it is closely associated with mesial temporal lobe epilepsy and hippocampal sclerosis (131–133). Essentially, it has the same clinical significance as temporal interictal epileptiform discharges (7).

The phi rhythm also is a nonspecific abnormal pattern. It has been associated with encephalopathies, migraine, and focal pathology in the posterior fossa (27).

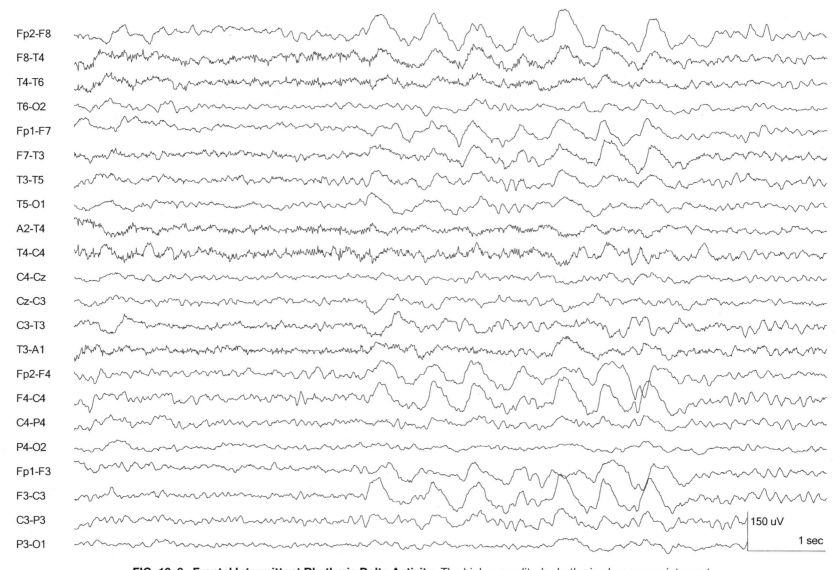

Fp2-F8

F8-T4

T4-T6

T6-O2

Fp1-F7

F7-T3

T3-T5

T5-O1

A2-T4

T4-C4

C4-Cz

Cz-C3

C3-T3

T3-A1

Fp2-F4

F4-C4

C4-P4

P4-O2

Fp1-F3

F3-C3

C3-P3

P3-O1

150 uV

1 sec

FIG. 10–6. Frontal Intermittent Rhythmic Delta Activity. The higher amplitude rhythmic slow waves interrupt more normal activity and correspond to acute encephalopathy following hemodialysis for chronic renal failure. (LFF 1 Hz, HFF 70 Hz)

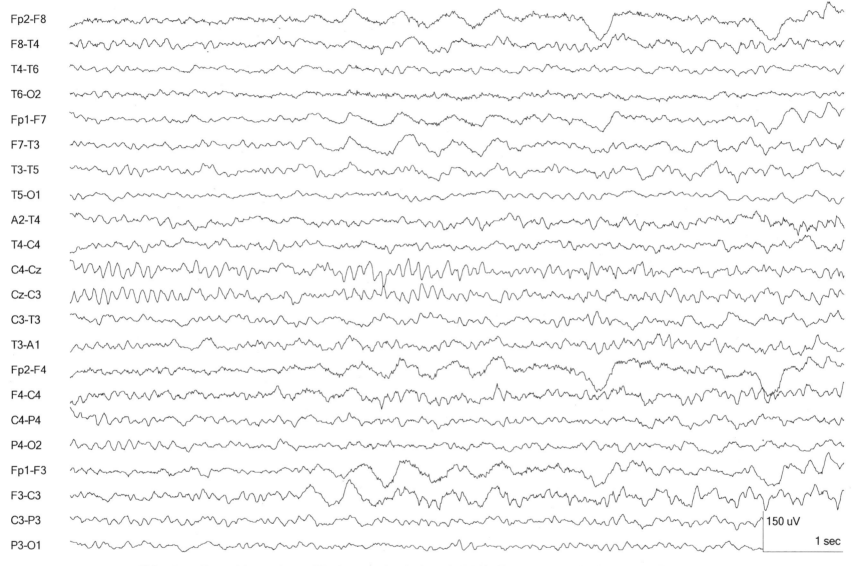

FIG. 10–7. Frontal Intermittent Rhythmic Delta Activity (FIRDA). The lower amplitude makes FIRDA in this figure less obvious than in Fig. 10–6, although it also corresponds to acute encephalopathy related to medical complications of chronic renal failure. A blink artifact slow wave follows the FIRDA and is distinguished by a field that does not extend as far posteriorly. (LFF 1 Hz, HFF 70 Hz)

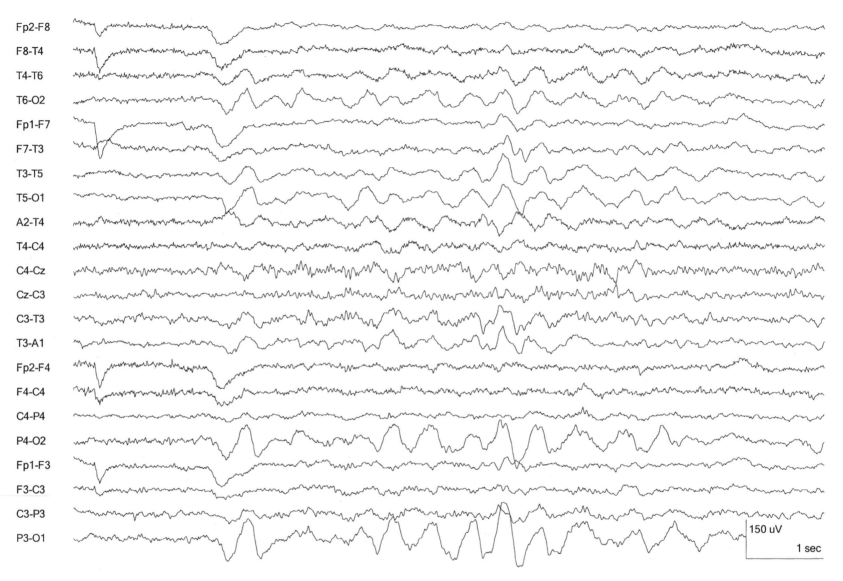

FIG. 10–8. Occipital Intermittent Rhythmic Delta Activity. The 2-Hz activity is bilaterally symmetric with a posterior field that extends into the temporal regions. The EEG corresponds to a 15-year-old with hypertensive encephalopathy related to chronic renal failure. Low-amplitude ocular artifacts are present frontally. (LFF 1 Hz, HFF 70 Hz)

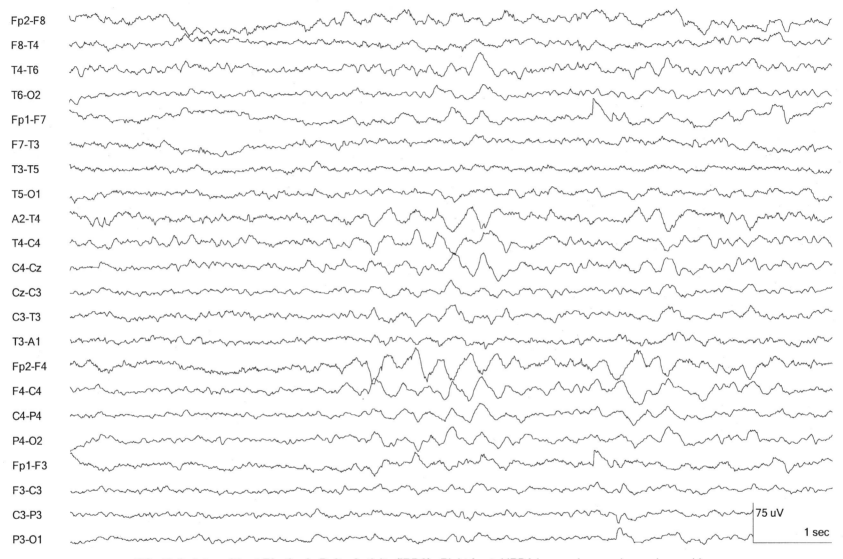

FIG. 10–9. Intermittent Rhythmic Delta Activity (IRDA). Right frontal IRDA is superimposed on polymorphic, mixed background and occurs in the context of severe, diffuse traumatic brain injury with the most significant edema within the right basal ganglia. (LFF 1 Hz, HFF 70 Hz)

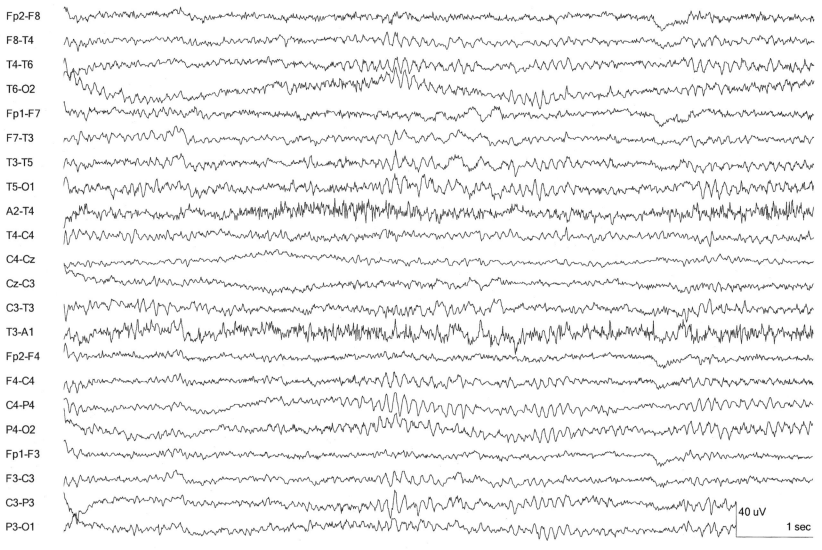

FIG. 10–10. Temporal Intermittent Rhythmic Delta Activity. Brief and poorly formed rhythmic slow waves are present across the left temporal region. The EEG was obtained following the development of complex partial seizures in the context of hypertensive encephalopathy. Magnetic resonance imaging (MRI) scan was normal. (LFF 1 Hz, HFF 70 Hz)

CHAPTER 11

Fourteen and Six Per Second Positive Bursts

FOURTEEN AND SIX PER SECOND POSITIVE BURSTS

Other Names
14 and 6 per second positive spikes
Ctenoids

Description
Fourteen and six positive bursts (14&6) are regular repetitions with an arciform morphology that are centered in the posterior temporal region and occur with a broad distribution across the adjacent regions (Figs. 11–1 and 11–2). The distribution may be unilateral, bisynchronous, or bilateral asynchronous. When they occur unilaterally, they may occur in greater number on the right side. The pattern is common between the ages of 8 and 14 years and rare in early childhood. After adolescence, it declines in incidence (13). Drowsiness and light sleep are the states most likely to demonstrate 14&6. It is not present in full wakefulness or deep sleep (134).

The terms positive and spike in the wave's name refer to its arciform morphology and not to surface polarity. The sharply contoured component of each arciform element is oriented downward in commonly used montages, that is, in the positive direction according to convention. Although 14 Hz and 6 Hz are the two most common frequencies for the burst, a range of frequencies may be manifested. Typically, the wave's repetitions occur at between 13 and 17 Hz or 5 and 7 Hz, with the faster frequencies occurring in late childhood and adolescence and the slower frequencies in middle childhood. Occasionally, the frequency evolves from the faster to the slower within one repetition. Alternatively, a manifestation of the faster frequency form may end with a single, diphasic, high-amplitude, N-shaped potential (135).

The repetitions usually last less than 2 seconds in total and with an amplitude that rarely is greater than 150 µV. More commonly, the duration is 0.5 to 1 second and the amplitude is about 75 µV. Because 14&6 have broad, uniform fields, they are best recorded with long interelectrode distances. A contralateral ear reference montage provides maximal amplitude waves. An ipsilateral ear reference montage may misrepresent the localization as frontal because the ear region and much of the posterior scalp may be within an isoelectric field. Posterior skull defects increase the likelihood of observing a 14&6 because of the breach effect (136).

Distinguishing Features
Versus Ictal Patterns for Partial Seizures

Ictal patterns for partial seizures and some occurrence of 14&6 are similar—both may demonstrate an evolving and focal pattern. However, the two patterns are distinguishable through their duration and distribution. The 14&6 usually lasts less than 1 second and rarely lasts more than 2 seconds. Ictal patterns for partial seizures usually last at least several seconds. More distinguishing is the occurrence of 14&6 bilaterally, either synchronously or, more importantly, asynchronously. Partial seizures do not have two fields. Even if a 14&6 pattern during one occurrence appears suggestive of an ictal pattern, other occurrences during the same electroencephalogram (EEG) are likely to be present and often manifest in another of 14&6's variations.

Versus Rhythmic Midtemporal Theta

The 14&6 has a much broader distribution than rhythmic midtemporal theta (RMTT). RMTT rarely extends beyond the temporal lobe and the immediately adjacent frontal lobe, whereas 14&6 commonly includes the occiput and parietal regions. Any occurrence of beta frequency range activity provides an even more clear distinction. The duration is somewhat differentiating, but less so than the distribution and frequency. RMTT more commonly lasts more than 2 seconds, but it may be as brief as 1 to 2 seconds.

Versus Sleep Spindles

When 14&6 manifests as 14-Hz parietal activity, it is similar to sleep spindles. However, its broad distribution across the posterior scalp differentiates it from sleep spindles. Although sleep spindles may occur displaced from the midline and with a shifting asymmetry, they remain confined to the central regions.

Versus Phantom Spike and Wave

When 14&6 occurs bisynchronously at 6 Hz, it is similar to the phantom spike and wave (PhSW) posterior variant (137). Both patterns occur in children during drowsiness and have durations typically less than 2 seconds. The distribution of the field is the key distinguishing feature; PhSW is maximal along the midline and 14&6 is more lateral. Other differentiating features are the PhSW's diphasic morphology and low-amplitude spike. The 14&6 pattern is monophasic.

Versus Subclinical Rhythmic Electrographic Discharge in Adults

Both subclinical rhythmic electrographic discharge in adults (SREDA) and 14&6 may manifest as paroxysmal rhythmic theta frequency activity with a broad field across the posterior scalp during drowsiness. Furthermore, 14&6 sometimes demonstrates frequency evolution, a characteristic of SREDA. The two patterns may be differentiated by the frequencies within the evolving pattern. SREDA progresses from theta to delta, and 14&6 progresses from beta to theta. The duration of the pattern also differentiates them. SREDA lasts as short as 10 seconds, and 14&6 lasts as long as 2 seconds. The age of the EEG's subject may be helpful, because SREDA is most common in the elderly and 14&6 is most common in children.

Co-occurring Waves

The EEG patterns of drowsiness or early sleep accompany 14&6. These include an attenuated or slowed alpha rhythm, vertex sharp transients, and ocular artifact indicating slow roving eye movements. When the subject is a child, hypnogogic hypersynchrony and posterior slow waves of youth also may be seen.

Clinical Significance

Initially believed to be an epileptiform abnormality, 14&6 are now known to be a normal variant (61,138,139). The only exception to this is when they are present in great abundance. In such instances, they may be a sign of metabolic encephalopathy, especially hepatic, and are accompanied by diffuse slowing and triphasic waves consistent with the type and degree of encephalopathy (61,140,141). The 14&6 also may be elicited by diphenhydramine (142).

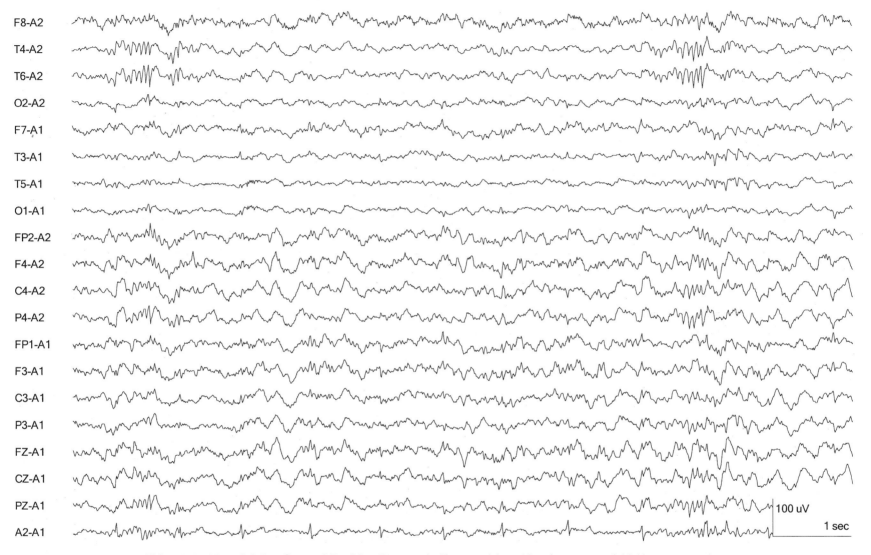

FIG. 11–1. 14 and 6 Per Second Positive Bursts. Arciform activity with a frequency of 15 Hz occurs twice across the right mid and posterior temporal region. The 6 per second form does not occur, but the first burst is interrupted by a slower wave, which forms the diphasic N-shaped potential. The EEG was normal and corresponded to a 13-year-old with a remote history of seizures and who was otherwise healthy. (LFF 1 Hz, HFF 70 Hz)

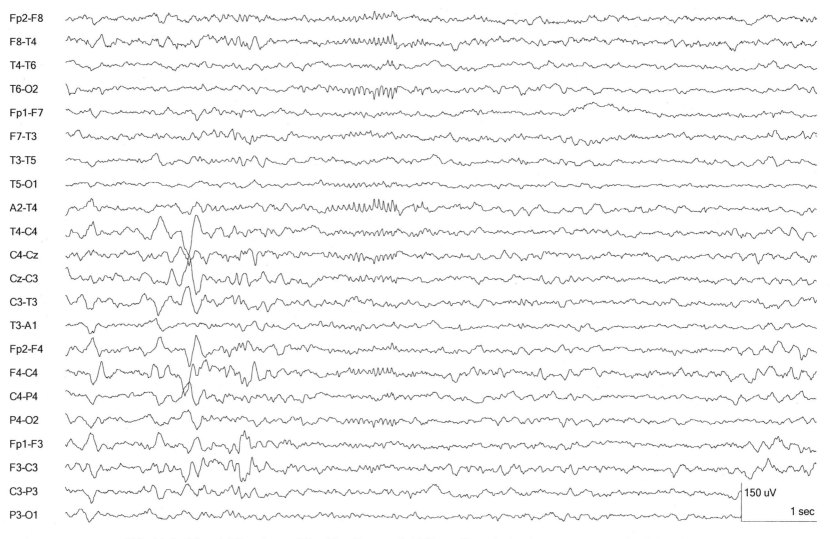

FIG. 11–2. 14 and 6 Per Second Positive Bursts. A 15-Hz arciform rhythm is present across the right mid to posterior temporal region with a duration of about 1 second. The direction of the arciform rhythm's sharply contoured components differs between the channels of this bipolar montage; thus, the components are negative in some channels. (LFF 1 Hz, HFF 70 Hz)

CHAPTER 12

Hypersynchrony and Hypersynchronous Slowing

HYPERVENTILATION HYPERSYNCHRONOUS SLOWING

Other Names
None

Description
Hyperventilation may produce bilateral, rhythmic, in-phase, low-frequency activity, which is termed hypersynchronous slowing (Figs. 12–1, 12–2, and 12–3). The timing and duration of hyperventilation hypersynchronous slowing (HVHS), when it occurs, is highly variable, and it may quickly follow the beginning of hyperventilation and continue beyond hyperventilation's end or it may be present for only a few seconds at the end of hyperventilation. Furthermore, it may appear and disappear during hyperventilation. Overall, it is more likely to occur in the context of hypoglycemia (52). When HVHS continues beyond the hyperventilation, it usually resolves within 1 minute of hyperventilation's discontinuation. Persistence for longer than 90 seconds beyond hyperventilation is abnormal. Regardless of its duration beyond the end of hyperventilation, HVHS should not return after its resolution. This is termed the "re-build up" phenomenon.

HVHS's frequency and paroxysmal onset are its more conserved features (13). Often, the onset is not a run of rhythmic activity; instead it occurs as individual, bilateral, sometimes sharply contoured, slow waves that meld together with continued hyperventilation. HVHS's frequency at onset may be in either the theta or delta frequency ranges, and it slows with continued hyperventilation. The final frequency usually is between 1.5 and 4 Hz, with lower frequencies occurring more commonly in children. Children and young adults are much more likely to manifest hyperventilation hypersynchrony, and the age range with maximum prevalence is 8 to 12 years (143). HVHS in children and

adults differ with a posteriorly maximum field in children and an anteriorly maximum one in adults (7). Also, amplitudes are higher in children and may reach 500 µV (10). HVHS may demonstrate a shifting asymmetry with an overall distribution that does not show lateralization (9).

HVHS results from hypocapnic cerebral vasoconstriction with decreased cerebral blood flow (144,145). It is independent of oxygenation and is facilitated by cerebral ischemia and hypoglycemia (7). Serum glucose concentrations less than 80 mg/dl facilitate HVHS, whereas concentrations greater than 120 mg/dl hamper it (143).

Distinguishing Features
Versus Intermittent Rhythmic Delta Activity

There is no morphologic or distribution difference between HVHS and intermittent rhythmic delta activity that is independent to hyperventilation. The occurrence during hyperventilation is the key distinguishing feature.

Versus Generalized Interictal Epileptiform Discharges

Generalized interictal epileptiform discharges (IEDs) that are provoked by hyperventilation are similar to HVHS in frequency, maximal field, and the sudden development and disappearance during hyperventilation. Furthermore, the common occurrence of impaired verbal recall and motor responsiveness during HVHS in children without epilepsy complicates the differentiation issue (146). When clearly visible spikes are present in association with slow waves, differentiation is straightforward. However, differentiation is more difficult when the spike is low amplitude and gives the slow wave only a notched appearance because notching may occur during HVHS as a manifestation of superimposed faster frequencies. The key distinguishing feature is HVHS's lacking of a time-locked location for the sharply contoured wave with regard to the slow wave's peak. Although the sharply contoured wave occurs along the slope of the slow wave, its location along that slope is fixed with regard to the overall slow wave morphology for generalized IEDs. HVHS's notching occurs with a random, less stereotyped, relationship to the slow wave's slope.

Co-occurring Waves
Glossokinetic muscle artifact from the swallowing of accumulated saliva commonly occurs at the end of hyperventilation.

Clinical Significance
HVHS with an overall symmetry is normal regardless of age. Its greater prevalence and greater hypersynchrony in children and young adults likely reflects a vascular reactivity that diminishes with aging; thus, occurrence in later adulthood is not an abnormality. Asymmetric HVHS indicates either cerebral ischemia on the side with greater slowing or impaired vascular reactivity on the side with lesser slowing; thus, it must be interpreted in the context of the baseline electroencephalogram (EEG). Therefore, evidence of baseline slowing ipsilateral to the side of greater HVHS slowing supports the presence of ipsilateral cerebral hypoperfusion. In this instance, HVHS becomes additional evidence for already identified abnormality. Asymmetric HVHS without any other EEG asymmetry should be interpreted with caution because of the unclear lateralization of the abnormality.

The re-build up phenomenon is characteristic of moyamoya disease, especially if the maximal delta hypersynchrony occurs 5 minutes after hyperventilation ends (143,147,148). Re-build up reflects impairments in vascular reactivity, and this sign should not be pursued in suspected moyamoya disease because of the risk for hyperventilation-related cerebral ischemia (149).

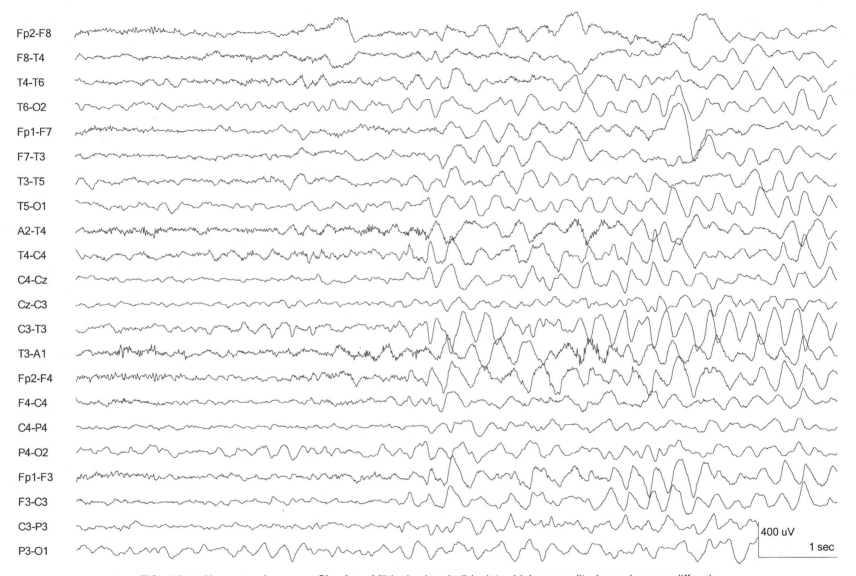

FIG. 12–1. Hypersynchronous Slowing. Mild slowing builds into higher amplitude and more diffusely synchronized activity without the abruptness of a paroxysmal change. This segment occurred 160 seconds into hyperventilation. (LFF 1 Hz, HFF 70 Hz)

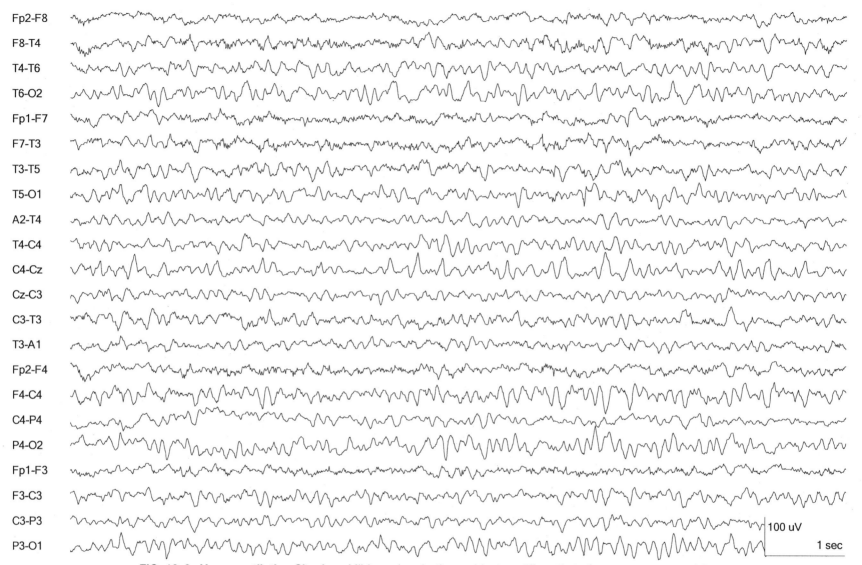

FIG. 12–2. Hyperventilation Slowing. Mild synchronization, evident as diffuse theta frequency range activity, is present in this EEG only during hyperventilation. An abrupt transition into hypersynchronous slowing is not present. (LFF 1 Hz, HFF 70 Hz)

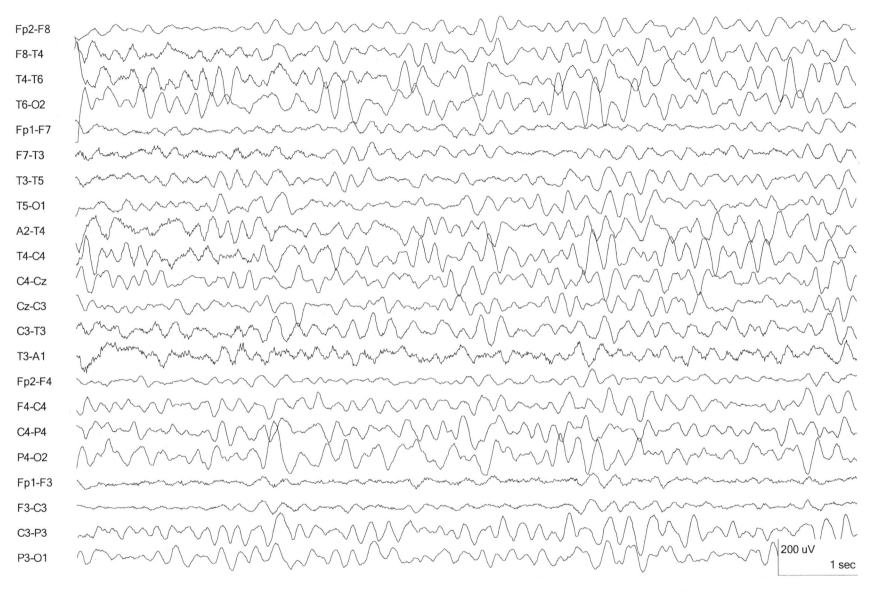

FIG. 12–3. Hypersynchronous Slowing. Because infants hyperventilate when they cry, hypersynchronous slowing may accompany the movement and muscle artifact related to crying. The slowing continues temporarily for this 9-month-old after he quiets. (LIFF 1 Hz, HFF 70 Hz)

HYPNOPOMPIC, HYPNAGOGIC, AND HEDONIC HYPERSYNCHRONY

Other Names
Paroxysmal hypnagogic hypersynchrony
Paradoxical arousal response

Description
In children, the transition between wakefulness and sleep may be accompanied by paroxysmal changes to the background activity during which there is bilateral, rhythmic, regular, in-phase activity (Figs. 12–4 and 12–5). When such activity occurs with drowsiness, it is called hypnagogic hypersynchrony, and when it occurs on arousal from sleep, it is called hypnopompic hypersynchrony. However, the two forms have no other relevant differences. The field of either hypersynchrony may range from just the bifrontal region to include all channels and commonly is maximum in the midfrontal region (13). The frequency typically is 3 to 5 Hz and the amplitude varies from lower than the surrounding background to high voltage and up to 300 μV (13,14). Occasionally, the superimposition of lower amplitude faster frequencies gives the slow waves a notched appearance that suggests the presence of a spike element (7). Both types of hypersynchrony first develop around the age of 6 months and are most prevalent before 2 years with about half of children manifesting it (7). It begins to become less prevalent around 3 years, uncommon by 6 years, and highly unusual by 12 years.

Hypersynchrony also may occur in infants while feeding (Fig. 12–6). Such hypersynchrony is termed hedonic hypersynchrony and typically has a longer duration than hypersynchrony related to transitions between sleep and wakefulness but has no other significance morphologic differences.

Distinguishing Features
Versus Cigánek Rhythm

Occurrence in a drowsy state, building amplitude of theta frequency range activity, and duration are similarities between hypnagogic hypersynchrony and the Cigánek rhythm; however, the two are most easily differentiated by distribution. Hypnagogic hypersynchrony is a more generalized phenomenon.

Versus Generalized Interictal Epileptiform Discharges

Hypnopompic, hypnagogic, and hedonic hypersynchrony (collectively, HH) and generalized IEDs share a typical frequency, maximal field, and a sudden occurrence and disappearance. When an IED's spike is low amplitude compared to the slow wave, the wave may be notched and appear similar to HH. The key distinguishing features are HH's lack of fixed location for the spike along the slow wave's slope and tendency for the slow waves to have a rising and falling amplitude during a burst. Generalized IEDs tend to have more uniform slow wave amplitudes.

Co-occurring Waves
Other signs of drowsiness usually accompany hypnopompic and hypnagogic hypersynchrony. These include slowing of the alpha rhythm into the theta frequency range, attenuation of the alpha rhythm, slow roving eye movements, central beta frequency activity, and generalized theta activity. Occasionally, hypersynchrony occurs in wakefulness and without other signs of drowsiness; thus, it may occur independent to other signs of the wake-sleep transition.

Hedonic hypersynchrony may occur in the context of movement and muscle artifact, which is manifested by either a rhythmic or periodic pattern with the frequency of the oral activity.

Clinical Significance
HH is a normal pediatric phenomenon when it occurs at times consistent with sleep-wake transitions. Its presence or absence does not carry any clinical relevance (7).

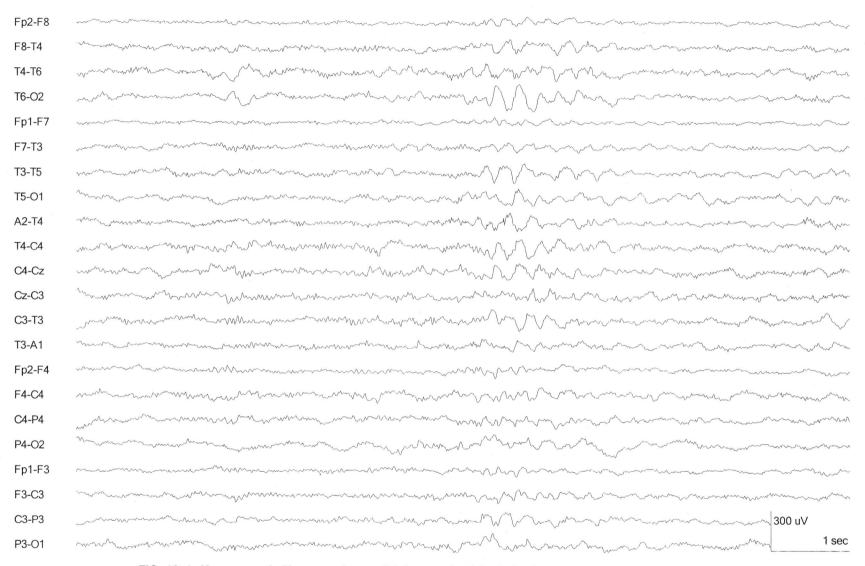

FIG. 12–4. Hypnopompic Hypersynchrony. Brief, generalized rhythmic slowing accompanies stimulation to awaken the patient. With arousal, the activity becomes more persisting. (LFF 1 Hz, HFF 70 Hz)

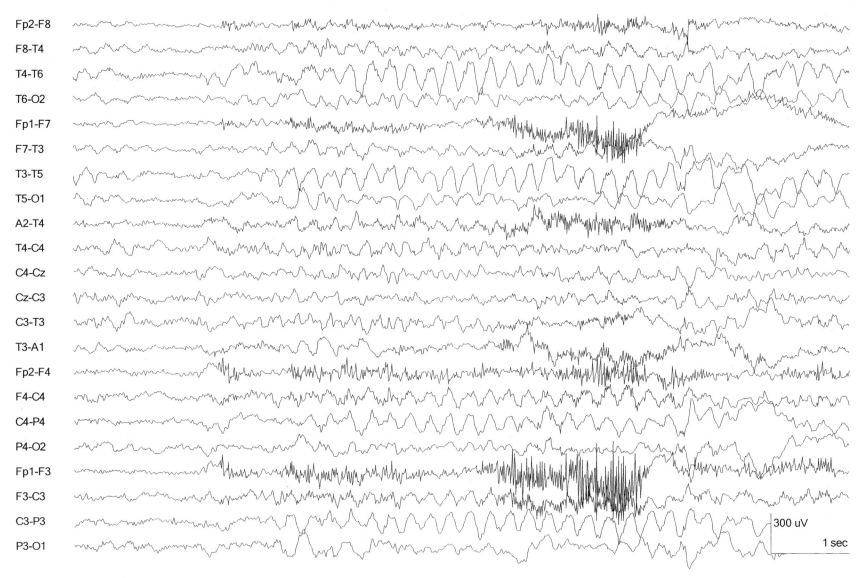

FIG. 12–4 *(continued).* (LFF 1 Hz, HFF 70 Hz)

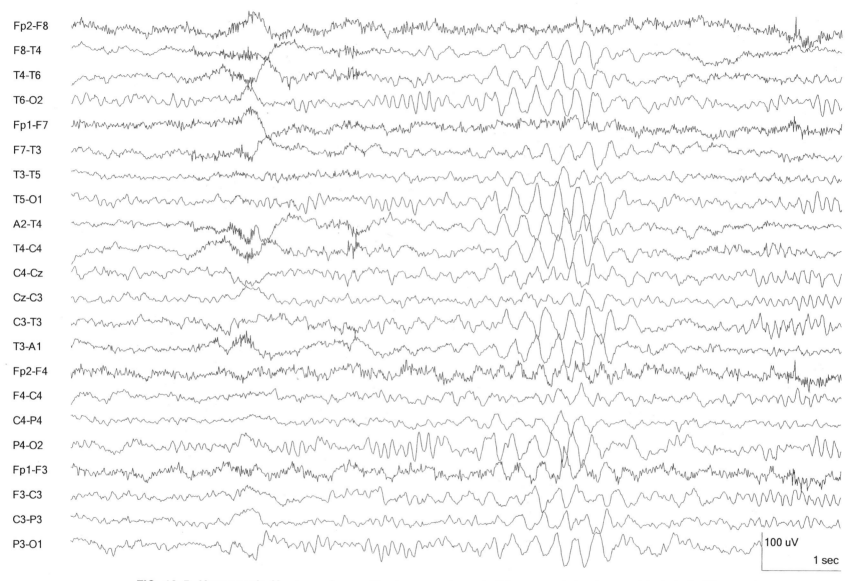

FIG. 12–5. Hypnagogic Hypersynchrony. The hypersynchrony in this segment develops suddenly but still demonstrates some transition in its buildup and resolution. Slow roving eye movement artifact and an intermittent alpha rhythm are accompanying signs of drowsiness. (LFF 1 Hz, HFF 70 Hz)

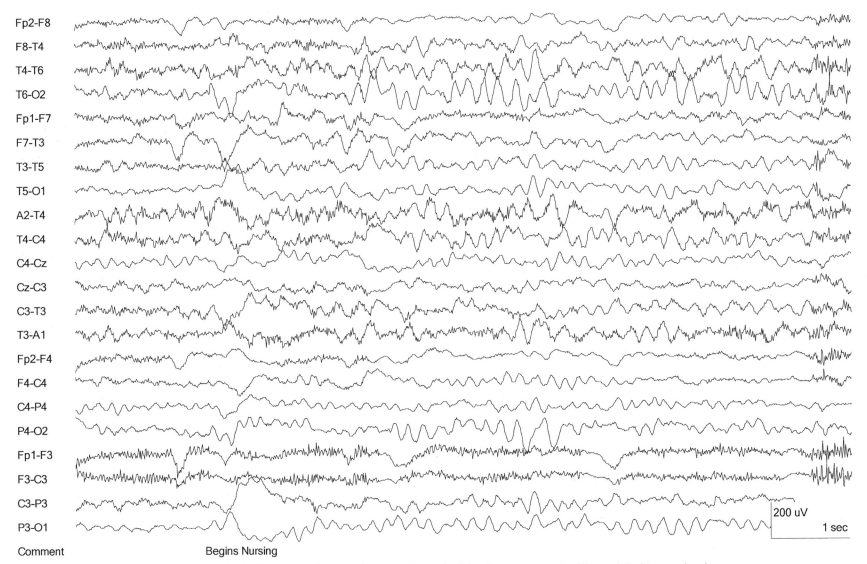

FIG. 12–6. Hedonic Hypersynchrony. Hypersynchrony builds after movement artifact related to nursing in a 9-month-old. Oropharyngeal movement artifact would be lower frequency, less monomorphic, and less persistent. (LFF 1 Hz, HFF 70 Hz)

CHAPTER 13

Ictal Epileptiform Patterns

ICTAL EPILEPTIFORM PATTERNS FOR FOCAL SEIZURES

Other Names
Electrographic seizure
Subclinical seizure
Partial seizure

Description
Unlike the ictal patterns for generalized seizures, the ictal patterns for focal seizures usually are dissimilar to the interictal pattern and cannot be predicted based on the particular type of seizure (61). However, they have several key features that are commonly present. The ictal pattern for focal seizures almost always is stereotyped for the person and usually includes evolving, repetitive sharp waves (9) (Figs. 13–1, 13–2, and 13–3). Infrequently, they do not include evolution and instead are regular repetitive spikes, desynchronization, or regular rhythmic slowing (7,150). The repetitive spike and desynchronization patterns most commonly accompany focal motor seizures.

The evolution that more commonly occurs classically involves one or more of the following sharp wave features: frequency, amplitude, topography, and morphology. Frequency evolution may begin in any of the normal encephalogram (EEG) frequency bands and may manifest as either an increase or decrease in frequency (7). The change usually is several Hertz with a crossing from one frequency band to another. Amplitude evolution usually is an increase in amplitude, often following an attenuation at the beginning of the seizure. The attenuation may be either generalized or focal at the region of ictal onset (150). At maximum amplitude after an evolving increase in amplitude, the amplitude of a focal seizure rarely is much beyond the range of the background EEG activity, that is, an abnormally high amplitude is unusual. The topographic

evolution reflects the anatomic spread of the seizure. Although focal seizures may have brief generalized changes at their onset, such as slowing, attenuation, or one or more high-amplitude sharp waves graphic evolution usually begins early in the seizure and is manifested as an increase in the distribution of the rhythmic activity from the region of ictal onset to a larger region containing the original region. Occasionally, propagation produces evolution in which the onset region is not included in the eventual region of ictal activity. The generalized activity at the onset lasts less than a few seconds and is replaced by the better formed and evolving focal rhythmic activity. Morphologic evolution is almost always present and is manifested by a gradual decrease in the complexity of the overall EEG activity. The decrease is due to the replacement of the background activity, which comprises multiple and independent frequencies, with the ictal rhythm (which is simpler due to a tightly interconnected system).

The evolution of the focal seizure's ictal rhythm may lead to a generalized pattern. This is expected as a partial seizure secondarily generalizes. A generalized ictal rhythm that develops from a focal one is not secondary bilateral synchrony. Secondary bilateral synchrony is an interictal pattern and does not demonstrate the obvious evolution of partial seizure ictal pattern. The ictal pattern of a secondarily generalized focal seizure typically shares the generalized paroxysmal fast activity (GPFA) features of a seizure that is generalized at its onset.

The electrographic resolution of focal seizures usually is either evolution into the background activity or a replacement of the evolving pattern by repetitive epileptiform bursts (7). The bursts are then followed by either slowing or suppression, with the maximum expression of the slowing or suppression often occurring in the ictal onset zone. Increased focal interictal epileptiform discharge frequency also may occur postictally in the ictal onset zone with gradual resolution (9).

Distinguishing Features
Versus Focal Alpha, Beta, Delta, or Theta Activity

Because the ictal patterns of focal seizure typically include focal, monomorphic activity, it must be distinguished from a burst of normal activity within one frequency band. Most ictal patterns are most easily distinguished through attention to whether evolution is present. Other than the fixed rhythmic delta activity of some seizures, most focal seizures with rhythmic activity demonstrate clear evolution. Stereotypy is another distinguishing feature, and one that applies to delta activity without evolution. However, normal bursts of rhythmic activity may be like ictal patterns by being relatively stereotyped. Association with changes in the surrounding area is another distinguishing feature. Ictal patterns often follow or precede either runs of co-localized focal interictal epileptiform discharges or periods of attenuation. They also may be followed by broad and abnormal slowing. Of course, the most important distinguishing feature is whether the pattern is associated with a behavioral change. This test is the most important because ultimately any electrographic pattern could be considered an ictal pattern if it reliably corresponds to an individual's seizure.

Versus Fourteen and Six Per Second Positive Spikes

Ictal patterns for focal seizures and some occurrences of fourteen and six positive bursts (14&6) are similar by both demonstrating an evolving and focal pattern. However, the two patterns are distinguishable through their duration and distribution. The 14&6 usually lasts less than 1 second and rarely lasts more than 2 seconds. Ictal patterns for focal seizures usually last at least several seconds. More distinguishing is the occurrence of 14&6 bilaterally, either synchronously or, more importantly, asynchronously. Focal seizures do not have two fields, especially bilateral fields that are independent but otherwise similar. Even if a 14&6 pattern during one occurrence appears suggestive of an ictal pattern, other occurrences during the same EEG are likely to be present and often manifest in another of 14&6's variations.

Versus Rhythmic Midtemporal Theta Activity and Wicket Rhythm

Like the ictal pattern for focal seizures, rhythmic midtemporal theta (RMT) activity and the wicket rhythm manifest as an abrupt replacement of the preceding background with rhythmic activity. Moreover, they occur over the temporal lobe, which is a region that commonly produces ictal patterns. The key distinguishing feature is the lack of evolution in frequency or distribution. Each occurrence begins and ends without a significant change in frequency or localization.

Versus Subclinical Rhythmic Electrographic Discharge of Adults

Unlike typical focal seizure ictal patterns, subclinical rhythmic electrographic discharge of adults (SREDA) does not demonstrate evolution in its distribution across the scalp or in its wave morphology and does not lead to slowing following its resolution. Furthermore, the alpha rhythm usually is unaffected by SREDA, and it rarely is present during bilateral ictal patterns. Most importantly, SREDA is not associated with any alteration in awareness or any behavioral change.

Co-occurring Waves
Focal seizures do not have the bilateral and forceful movements of generalized seizures, but they still commonly produce significant artifact. This may be electromyographic (EMG) artifact from repetitive facial movements, ocular artifact from repetitive blinking, or glossokinetic artifact from repetitive swallowing. The mild attenuation or slowing preceding and following the seizure are other associated waveforms.

Clinical Significance
The ictal patterns of partial seizures usually are accompanied by a behavioral change indicating a true seizure, but sometimes no behavioral change is recognized to occur. The lack of recognized behavioral change does not mean that a seizure has not occurred. Complex partial seizures commonly produce behavioral change that may be overlooked by others because it is limited to impairment of memory and concentration. Deliberate cognitive testing during and after the episode may be the only way of determining if a complex partial seizure occurred. Even if testing is normal, a seizure may still have occurred, but it would be simple partial. Simple partial seizures are not evident if they are limited to a subjective experience. However, such seizures would be known by the patient to have occurred. If the patient is amnestic to the seizure, then the seizure, by definition, is complex partial.

Patterns that are identical to the ictal patterns of focal seizures also occur without any true behavioral or functional change. These "subclinical" or "electrographic" seizures are discussed in the ictal patterns of generalized seizures subsection. Beyond the occurrence of similar ictal patterns without true seizures, similar patterns also may produce seizures with disparate semiologies across different individuals (151), that is, the ictal pattern does not indicate the type of seizure manifestation with meaningful reliability. Furthermore, the ictal pattern often does not accurately indicate the true ictal onset zone or even its lateralization, as identified with invasive monitoring (152). Exceptions to this include focal beta frequency activity over a frontal lobe, which is a reliable indicator of the focus for frontal lobe epilepsy regardless of whether a lesion is present, and focal theta activity over a temporal lobe, which is a reliable indicator of the focus for temporal lobe epilepsy (153,154). For example, a specific pattern of phase reversals at the sphenoidal electrode that reach a frequency of 5 Hz or greater within 30 seconds correctly indicates a mesial temporal ictal onset in 82% of individuals who have it (154). Among localizations in general, patterns from temporal lobe epilepsy, and especially mesial temporal lobe epilepsy, are most likely to be focal, and those from parietal lobe epilepsy are the least likely to be focal (155,156).

Finally, seizures may occur without an ictal EEG change. Simple partial seizures, which by definition are not accompanied by impairment in memory, are the most likely to lack an EEG correlate. Only about 33% of simple partial motor seizures and about 15% of simple partial non-motor seizures have corresponding ictal patterns (157). Overall, ictal patterns are visible for between 20% and 30% of simple partial seizures that do not progress to complex partial seizures (158).

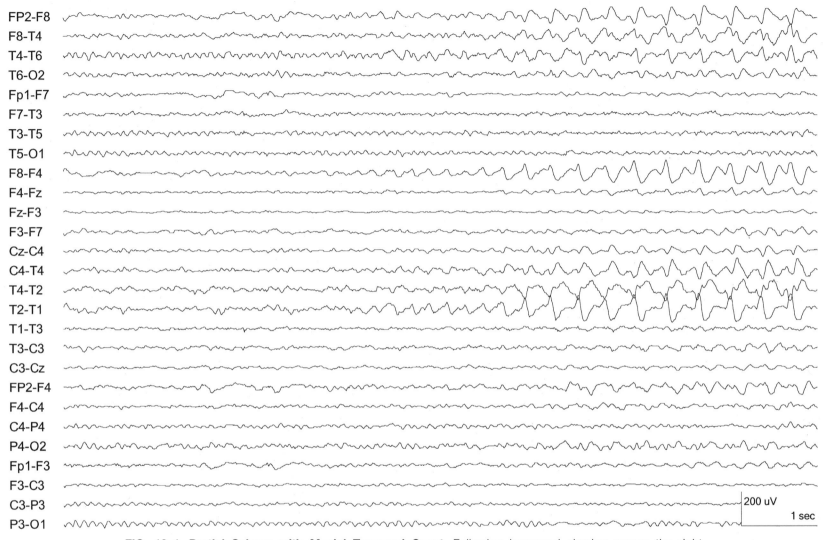

FIG. 13–1. Partial Seizure with Mesial Temporal Onset. Following increased slowing across the right temporal lobe, a 3-Hz phase reversing develops at the T2 and F8 electrodes. The rhythm evolves over the following 20 seconds (see continuation of figure) to reach a frequency of 6 Hz and encompass a larger right-sided field. The EEG corresponds to a complex partial seizure with occasional oral-buccal automatisms and intact verbal interaction. Right hippocampal sclerosis was identified following epilepsy surgery. Brief muscle artifact is present in the figure continuations. (LFF 1 Hz, HFF 70 Hz)

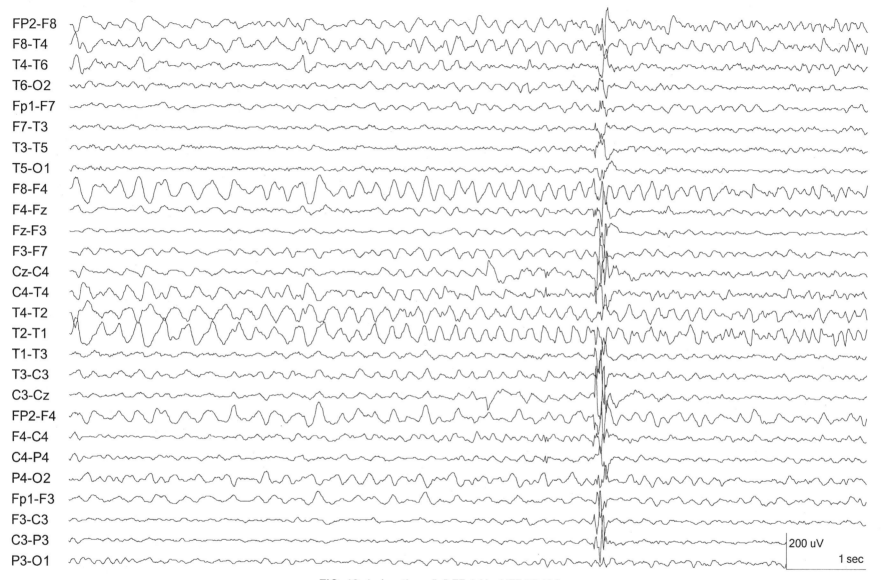

FIG. 13–1. *(continued)* (LFF 1 Hz, HFF 70 Hz)

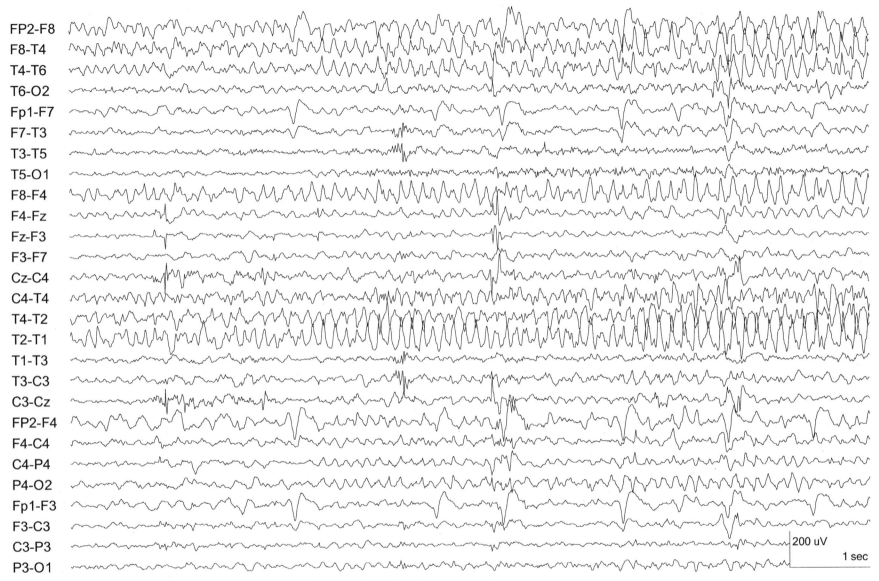

FIG. 13–1. *(continued)* (LFF 1 Hz, HFF 70 Hz)

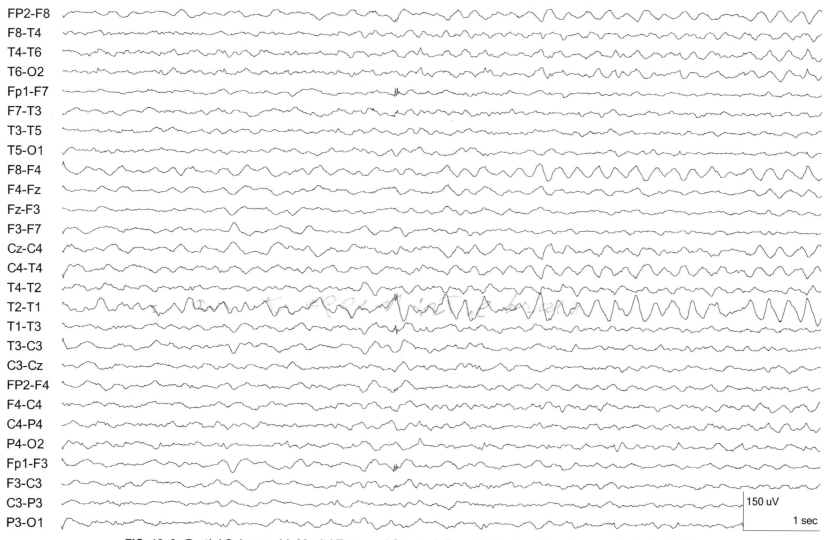

FIG. 13–2. Partial Seizure with Mesial Temporal Onset. Diffuse slowing transitions to more rhythmic slowing across the right temporal lobe with evolution in the following 10 seconds (see continuation of figure) to become more monomorphic and higher amplitude and to include a 4-Hz phase reversing rhythm at the T2 and F8 electrodes. The electroencephalogram (EEG) corresponded to a complex partial seizure with staring and unresponsiveness. Right hippocampal sclerosis was identified following resection for epilepsy surgery. (LFF 1 Hz, HFF 70 Hz)

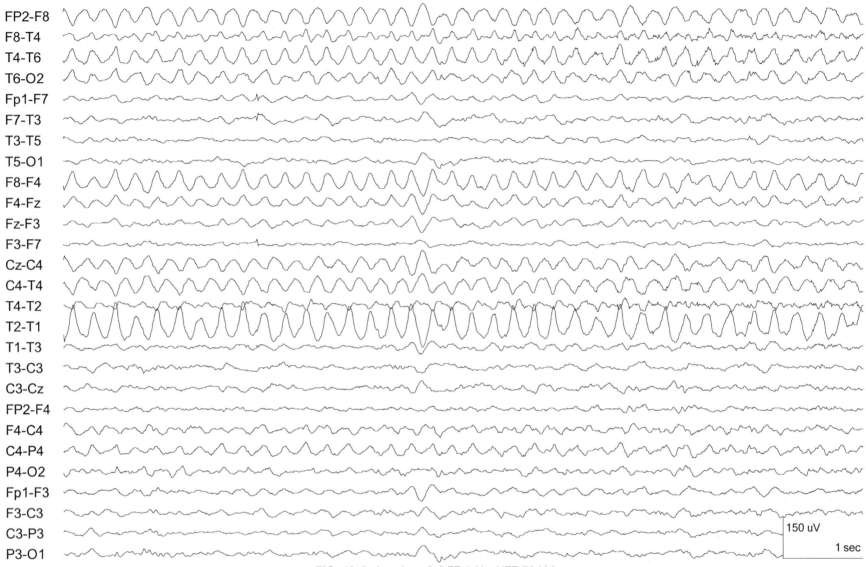

FIG. 13–2. *(continued)* (LFF 1 Hz, HFF 70 Hz)

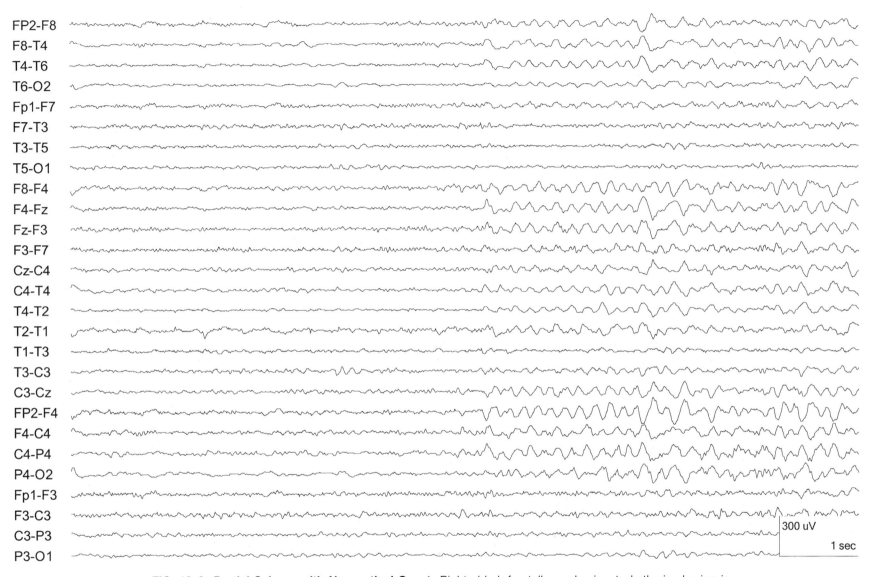

FIG. 13–3. Partial Seizure with Neocortical Onset. Right-sided, frontally predominant, rhythmic slowing is present at the onset and evolves (see p. 152) in morphology to become higher amplitude and include phase reversing spikes at the P4 electrode. The EEG corresponds to a complex partial seizure with versive gaze and head movements to the left prior to generalization. A right parietal astrocytoma was previously resected. (LFF 1 Hz, HFF 70 Hz)

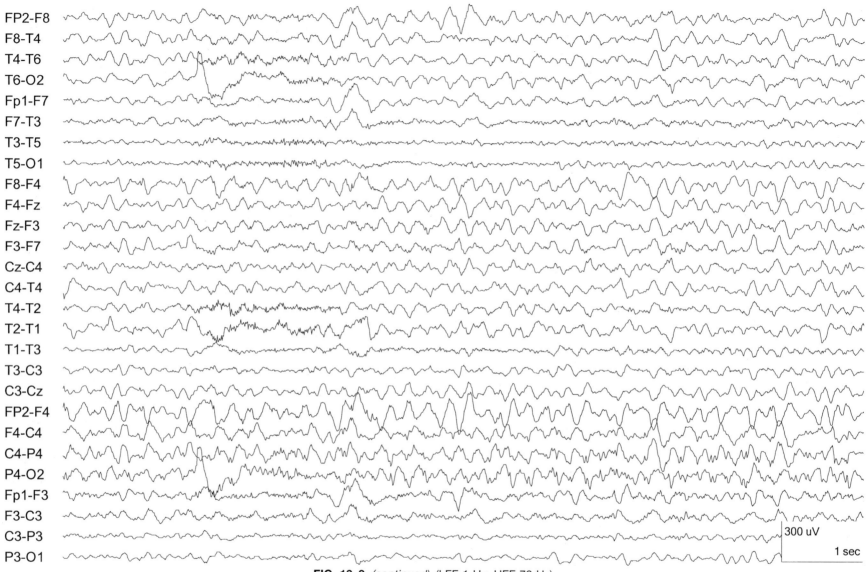

FIG. 13–3. *(continued)* (LFF 1 Hz, HFF 70 Hz)

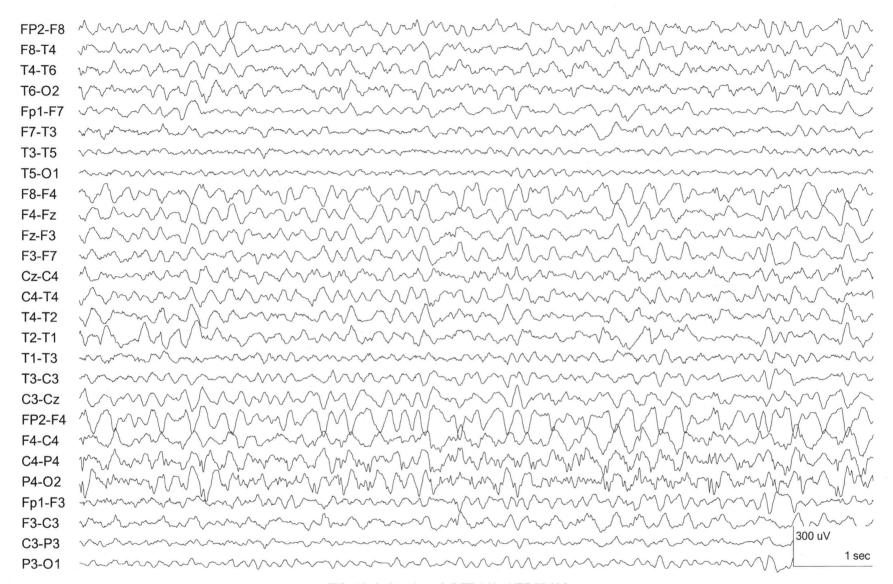

FIG. 13–3. *(continued)* (LFF 1 Hz, HFF 70 Hz)

ICTAL EPILEPTIFORM PATTERNS FOR GENERALIZED SEIZURES

Other Names
Subclinical seizure
Electrographic seizure
Epileptic recruiting rhythm

Types
Generalized spike and slow wave complex
Generalized paroxysmal fast activity
Slow spike and (slow) wave (complex)
Electrodecremental pattern
Epileptiform bursts

Description
The electrographic correlates to seizure onset for seizures that are generalized at their onset almost always have one of three types of generalized patterns: spike and slow wave complex, generalized paroxysmal fast activity (GPFA), or electrodecrement (Figs. 13–4, 13–5, and 13–6). From a low-amplitude and fast frequency onset, the pattern may demonstrate evolution with an increasing amplitude and a decreasing frequency that commonly remains in the beta frequency range. The ictal pattern also may progress to an epileptiform burst pattern, which commonly accompanies clonic activity. Rarely, an ictal pattern is solely generalized rhythmic slowing or a burst-suppression pattern (7).

The ictal generalized spike and slow wave complex (GSW) essentially is identical to the interictal spike and slow wave complex, except that it has a longer duration as manifested by a greater number of complex repetitions. The complex classically is triphasic with a negative spike followed by a negative slow wave but may be polyphasic because of a polyspike initiation. As an ictal correlate, the GSW occurs repeatedly without intervening background activity and has a duration usually at least 5 seconds (150). Shorter trains of GSW usually do not have a clinically evident behavioral change; thus, they do not meet the essential definition of a seizure. The repetition frequency varies with the type of epilepsy from less than 2.5 Hz at onset (slow spike and wave) for Lennox-Gastaut syndrome to 3 to 4 Hz at onset for childhood absence epilepsy. The wave is maximal over the midfrontal region and begins and ends more abruptly than the electrographic correlates of partial seizures. Essentially, it has little evolution other than the spike component's decreasing amplitude with successive repetitions (159). Occasionally with absence seizures, the spike component of the complex is not visible; thus, the ictal pattern assumes the appearance of paroxysmal, rhythmic delta frequency range activity (160). This waveform is described in more detail in Chapter 14.

The electrodecremental pattern's name is highly descriptive. This pattern is evident as a sudden and generalized attenuation. The tracing becomes nearly isoelectric across all channels. After a second or two, very fast low-voltage rhythmic activity usually develops (7,61). This activity gradually increases in amplitude and decreases in frequency over the subsequent few seconds and typically evolves into GPFA. GPFA also may begin without an electrodecremental onset. In such instances, it begins as a sudden manifestation of continuous rhythmic spikes at 20 to 40 Hz that may be accompanied by a minor attenuation. Thus, the electrodecremental pattern and GPFA have morphologic overlap with differences only in the degree of attenuation and the frequency of the fast activity. This similarity is in the onset and the evolution because GPFA typically evolves over 1 to 3 seconds to a lower frequency and a higher amplitude. Eventually it becomes repetitive spikes that are separate and not within one rhythm (7). As the individual spikes form, slow waves sometimes develop to form a pattern similar to the GSW mentioned previously. A more detailed description of GPFA is in Chapter 20.

Generalized seizures typically end in one of three ways: abruptly without any change to the ictal pattern, with continued evolution in wave morphology, or with disintegration of the ictal pattern. Typical GSW classically ends abruptly, just as it begins. The continued evolution is manifested by a gradual decrease in frequency and amplitude that often leads into postictal slowing, attenuation, or electrodecrement. The disintegration appears as a punctuation of the generalized epileptiform activity by suppressions or slowing with eventual replacement of the epileptiform activity by the intervening activity. Identifying the exact time of seizure resolution with evolution or disintegration is difficult and often inaccurate.

Distinguishing Features
Versus Artifact

Because generalized seizures often have generalized motor activity that creates high-frequency artifact, distinguishing between a seizure's electroencephalographic and EMG correlates commonly is necessary. GPFA differs from EMG artifact in its frequency and amplitude variability. GPFA is lower in frequency to the extent that individual spikes are visible. EMG artifact includes spikes of such high frequency that they blend together at the usual 10 seconds per page or display window. GPFA also is more consistent in its amplitude across a burst.

Even when an increase in amplitude is present across a burst, the increase is linear without significant decreases intermixed within it. Unlike GPFA, EMG artifact varies in amplitude and morphology as a function of the variation in the number of active motor units.

An exception to the expectation that EMG artifact is variable occurs with the EMG bursts that occur during the clonic phase of a generalized seizure. Because the movements during the clonic phase are brief and similar to one another, they produce an artifact with morphology that is consistently more similar to epileptiform polyspikes than typical EMG artifact. Simultaneous noncerebral EEG channels are helpful here. Differentiation also is possible through the evolution pattern of the bursts. As the clonic activity subsides the bursts subside in amplitude and develop a morphology that appears more like EMG artifact. Epileptiform bursts do not subside in this way. Their morphology evolves to become either more classically epileptiform with a clear spike or to become rhythmic slowing.

Postictal slowing, attenuation, or electrodecrement are features that sometimes are present and when present help differentiate an ictal pattern from artifact. However, both the presence and the absence of any of these features may not be entirely reliable as a distinguishing feature. Absence seizures are not followed by any change to the background activity, and motor activity that is nonepileptic but that resembles a generalized tonic-clonic seizure may lead to hyperventilation, which can produce slowing that continues after the episode ends.

Versus Burst-suppression Pattern

The bursts of a burst-suppression pattern resemble paroxysmal fast activity in their abrupt manifestation and high-frequency components. Furthermore, they are separated by suppressions that may resemble either ictal or postictal attenuations. Distinguishing these patterns is highly important in the clinical situation of a patient who is cognitively altered following a generalized cerebral insult. The importance rests in knowing whether to treat for status epilepticus. Making the distinction depends on the morphologic features of the bursts. Epileptic bursts are more monomorphic, stereotyped, and have greater rhythmicity, especially for the faster frequencies.

Versus Low-Voltage Electroencephalogram

Although the electrodecremental pattern is manifested by a low voltage, the decrease in voltage is brief and episodic and followed by stereotyped increases in amplitude with fast activity. The low-voltage EEG, as described in Chapter 17, is consistently low voltage. Indeed, an otherwise normal low-voltage EEG that has attenuations with electrodecremental pattern features may be including ictal events on the low-voltage background.

A more difficult differentiation is between the low voltage that occurs with normal behavioral arousal and the low voltage that accompanies a generalized attenuation or electrodecrement. This differentiation becomes irrelevant to determining if the pattern is epileptiform as the evolution to a clearly ictal correlate occurs. The differentiation is important to determine the exact moment at which a seizure begins; however, such a determination is rarely necessary and currently not possible with a conventional scalp EEG.

Versus Triphasic Waves

Generalized ictal patterns and triphasic waves (TW) share the features of component complexes with a triphasic morphology, occurrences in trains of several complexes, and overlapping repetition frequency ranges. Differentiating them often depends mostly on morphologic features. Ictal patterns are more often centered at the frontal midline and have a more sharply contoured initiating spike or sharp wave. However, the initiating discharge of atypical spike and slow wave complexes is the exception because it may be similar to that of TW. More helpful is the presence of evolution. TW do not evolve consistently. Occasional trains may have evolution, but the evolution is highly inconsistent in its features and its occurrence. Essentially, it is not stereotyped. Generalized ictal patterns include stereotyped evolution; however, the evolution may be minor for patterns like the 3 per second spike and slow wave complex of absence seizures. The typical evolution is a decrease in the spike amplitude, increase in the slow wave duration, and increase in polymorphic complexes.

Co-occurring Waves
Generalized motor seizures include a variety of artifacts, especially movement, EMG, and electrode artifacts. Mild attenuations, sometimes also called desynchronizations, often precede generalized motor seizures, and delta frequency slowing often follows.

Clinical Significance
Generalized ictal epileptiform patterns are always abnormal and are almost always accompanied by behavioral change (161). This change is the seizure, based on an exacting definition of seizures as abnormal behavior or experience

due to neuronal functional disturbance with excessive excitation and synchronization. Thus, ictal patterns without accompanying seizures are not truly ictal patterns and are termed subclinical seizures or electrographic seizures. Regardless of how much these terms are meant to be more precise, they are inherently flawed and oxymoronic because a seizure always has clinical features. Indeed, the language of an EEG lacks a universally accepted term to describe the patterns that most commonly accompany seizures.

The seizures that accompany generalized ictal epileptiform patterns may be generalized tonic-clonic, generalized tonic, generalized clonic-tonic-clonic, generalized atonic, myoclonic, absence, atypical absence, and epileptic spasms. Generalized ictal epileptiform patterns are not necessarily a sign of epilepsy. As signs of seizures, they reflect transient dysfunction and do not always indicate an intrinsic cerebral abnormality, that is, seizures provoked by cerebrally extrinsic conditions such as toxin exposures or metabolic abnormalities will be accompanied by the same patterns, and such seizures are, by definition, not indicative of epilepsy.

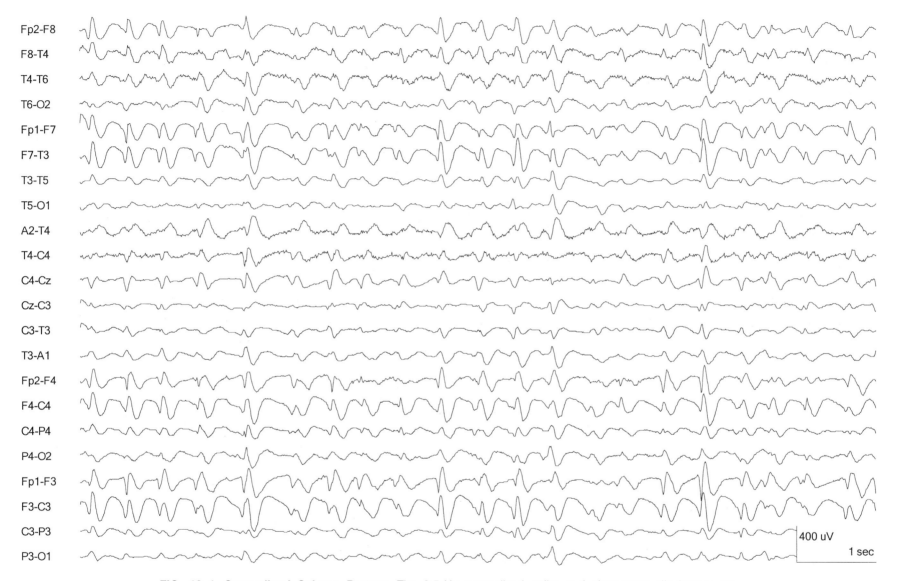

FIG. 13–4. Generalized Seizure Pattern. The 2.5-Hz generalized spike and slow wave discharges are continuous and do not evolve, which is a pattern that occurs during an atypical absence seizure. However, no behavioral change was noted during this segment. The EEG corresponds to symptomatic generalized epilepsy, a syndrome category in which this pattern also may occur between recognized seizures. (LFF 1 Hz, HFF 70 Hz)

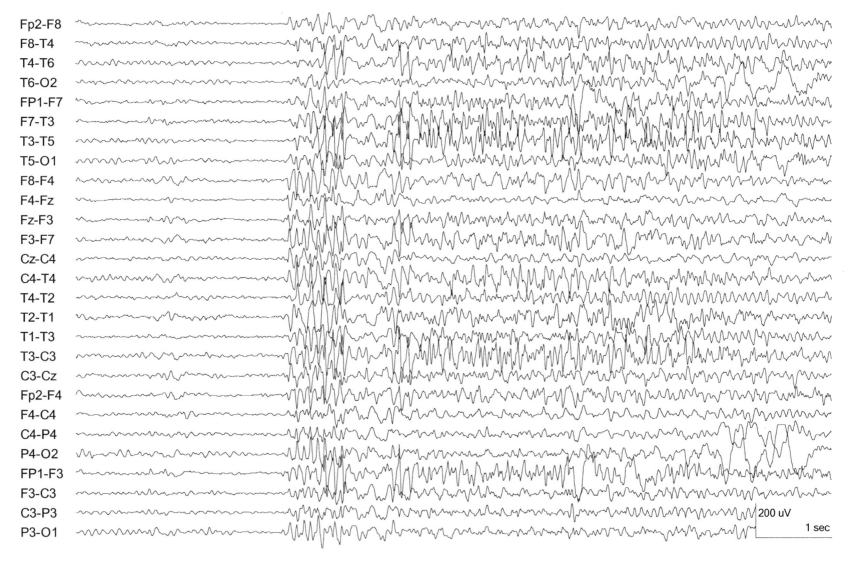

FIG. 13–5. Generalized Seizure. The ictal onset is abrupt with generalized, higher amplitude rhythmic 10-Hz activity and is followed (see figure continuation) by evolution into faster and more monomorphic activity. Muscle artifact eclipses the ictal rhythm by the end of the segment. The EEG corresponds to a generalized tonic clonic seizure due to juvenile myoclonic epilepsy. (LFF 1 Hz, HFF 70 Hz)

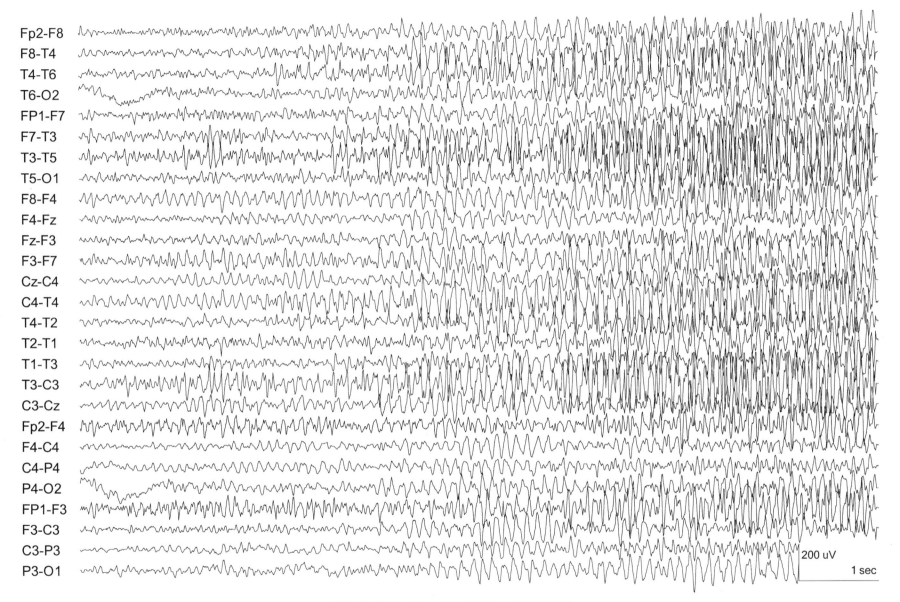

FIG. 13–5. *(continued)* (LFF 1 Hz, HFF 70 Hz)

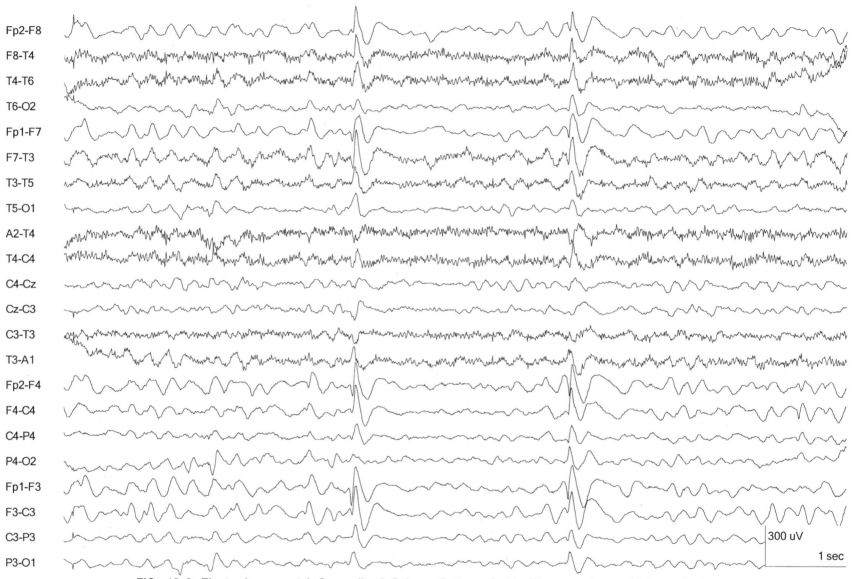

FIG. 13–6. Electrodecremental Generalized Seizure Pattern. Amid diffuse slowing, a high-amplitude, generalized sharp wave occurs and is followed by an immediate and significant decrease in background amplitude. No behavioral change was noted during this segment, and, unlike typical ictal electrodecrements, generalized paroxysmal fast activity does not evolve from the suppression. The EEG corresponds to symptomatic generalized epilepsy. The second high-amplitude sharp wave contrasts with the first by not being followed by an electrodecrement. (LFF 1 Hz, HFF 70 Hz)

CHAPTER 14

Interictal Epileptiform Discharges

FOCAL INTERICTAL EPILEPTIFORM DISCHARGES

Other Names
Localized interictal epileptiform pattern

Types
Spike
Sharp (wave)
Polyspike (complex)
Multiple spike complex
Spike and (slow) wave (complex)
Sharp and (slow) wave (complex)
Polyspike and (slow) wave (complex)
Rolandic discharges
Multifocal independent spike discharges (MISD)
Independent multifocal spike discharges (IMSD)

Description
Focal interictal epileptiform discharges (IEDs) appear as a variety of waveforms but almost always have four characteristic features. These are a field that extends beyond one electrode, a sharply contoured component, electronegativity on the cerebral surface, and disruption of the surrounding background activity (Figs. 14–1, 14–2, and 14–3). The sharply contoured component is either a spike or a sharp wave and may be incorporated in a complex with the sharply contoured element followed by a slow wave. Regardless of its form, the sharply contoured element of IEDs is usually asymmetric with a steeper rise to the peak than fall to the baseline (7). Less common than the complex of a single spike or sharp wave followed by a slow wave is a few successive spikes either in isolation or as a complex with a slow wave. This collection of a few spikes is termed a polyspike. A long polyspike run constitutes paroxysmal fast activity (PFA) and is discussed in Chapter 20. Unless it includes a polyspike, IEDs typically are triphasic. For isolated spikes or sharp waves, the three phases are a low-amplitude positive potential followed by the negative potential, which is visible as the sharply contoured wave, followed by another low-amplitude positive potential (61). The complex that includes a slow wave differs by having a fourth phase with much longer duration. The triphasic morphology is not a constant for IEDs because polyspikes have more than three phases and isolated spikes and sharp waves may be monophasic or diphasic. Regardless of which elements are included, focal IEDs disrupt the background by having a waveform that is dissimilar to the components of the surrounding activity. This difference usually is based in the IEDs frequency components, with the presence of faster activity, which produces the sharp contour, and an overall reduction in the number of superimposed frequencies. Fewer superimposed frequencies gives the IED a simpler morphology than the more complex admixture surrounding it. Although IEDs often also disrupt the background with a higher amplitude, this aspect is inconsistent enough that it is not a reliable characteristic.

Rolandic (also called centrotemporal) IEDs are a type of IED that is distinctive because of certain features and an association with a specific epilepsy syndrome, benign rolandic epilepsy (162). The most characteristic feature is an exception to one of the four general features of IEDs listed previously. This feature is polarity; rolandic IEDs may be surface positive (Figs. 14–4 and 14–5). The presence of a positive wave is due to a discharge orientation that is tangential to the cerebral surface. The electronegative potential of other IEDs arises from a perpendicularly oriented dipole within the crown of a gyrus, with the positive end pointing toward subcortical white matter and the negative end pointing toward the scalp. Because rolandic discharges are tangential, they classically manifest both ends of the dipole with a negative IED over the central to midtemporal region (C3/C4 to T3/T4) and a positive one that is midfrontal (F3/F4 to Fz) (163,164). Although this may be conceptualized as one dipole with both ends evident on the scalp, source analyses indicate two dipoles and functional magnetic resonance imaging (MRI) identifies more than one active region (165,166,167). Regardless, the dipole evident with scalp electroencephalogram (EEG) is oriented with the rolandic fissure. Rolandic discharges have several other common features including more often occurring with a triphasic morphology than other IEDs, occurring in short runs of 1.5 to 3 Hz, a greater increase in the number of occurrences with drowsiness than occurs with other IEDs, and a decrease in frequency with hyperventilation (7,168,169). They are unilateral in 70% of occurrences and bilaterally symmetric in the remainder. When unilateral, they typically alternate between hemispheres with an overall symmetry (150). The negative end of the dipole usually has a higher amplitude and typically is between 130 to 200 μV (170). Although often called rolandic spikes, rolandic IEDs have an average duration of 74 to 88 msec, so technically they are sharp waves (170,171).

Unlike rolandic IEDs, occipital IEDs do not have particularly distinguishing morphologic features but sometimes have an occurrence pattern related to visual stimulation. Especially in idiopathic focal occipital epilepsies, occipital IEDs occur most predominantly when visual fixation is not present. This is termed fixation-off sensitivity (FOS) and may be demonstrated with closure of the eyes, absence of ambient light, Frenzel lenses, and Ganzfeld stimulation (Fig. 14–6). More rarely, FOS may occur with symptomatic occipital epilepsy (172). Regardless of the etiology, the syndromes that produce focal FOS occipital spikes also sometimes produce generalized FOS IEDs. Like rolandic IEDs, occipital IEDs may be either unilateral or bilateral and often occur in repetition, which is rhythmic and usually has a frequency between 2.5 and 4 per second (173) (Fig. 14–7). Sleep has no consistent effect on occipital IEDs.

Positive waves with an IED morphology may occur at the vertex in two conditions other than benign rolandic epilepsy. These are cherry red spot myoclonus and the periventricular leukomalacia that occurs after a germinal matrix hemorrhage in neonates. Discharges that occur as repetitions in the range of 10 to 20 Hz are typical of cherry red spot myoclonus (174).

Distinguishing Features
Versus Fragment of Alpha Activity's Wicket Rhythm or Mu Rhythm

Fragments of the activity with a wicket or mu morphology resemble IEDs because of a sharply contoured component adjacent to a rounded component.

This appears similar to a diphasic spike and slow wave complex. Furthermore, wicket rhythm fragments occur over the temporal region, which is a common site for IEDs. Mu rhythm fragments occur centrally and may be mistaken for rolandic IEDs. Distinguishing these fragments of normal activity from IEDs relies on identifying the larger rhythms within the same portion of the EEG. Finding a rhythm of repeated waves with a morphology similar to the wave in question is strong evidence against the wave being an IED. Without the presence of a longer lasting and neighboring wicket rhythm or mu rhythm, a suspicious wave cannot be ascribed to be a fragment. Fragments rarely occur without the presence of the larger waveforms.

Versus Artifact

Several types of artifact appear similar to IEDs. The ones that are most similar are electrocardiographic (ECG), electromyographic (EMG), electrode pop, and lateral rectus spike with or without eye flutter.

ECG artifact may disrupt the EEG background activity similarly to an IED. Moreover, it is usually diphasic or triphasic with a phase that has a duration within the spike range. When it either occurs with a highly regular interval or can be compared to a channel specifically dedicated to an electrocardiogram, differentiating it from IEDs is straightforward. An episodic occurrence requires careful scrutiny of the morphology and location. ECG artifact almost always occurs in channels that include electrodes that are low on the head, especially ear electrodes. When a wave occurs in such a channel and has a perfectly conserved morphology and period, it is likely to be ECG artifact. IEDs show greater variation between occurrences than ECG artifact even when they recur as the same wave type, that is, they vary more in amplitude, duration, and contour than ECG artifact.

Only when EMG artifact occurs as individual muscle potentials is it similar to IEDs. This may occur as lateral rectus spikes or photomyogenic responses. Such potentials differ from IEDs by being more sharply contoured and having shorter durations. Unlike EMG artifact, spikes, which are the sharpest and briefest of IEDs, commonly are long enough in duration to separate the rising and falling phases. The rising and falling phases of EMG artifact usually appear to overlap when viewed with standard EEG parameters and, therefore, appears more like a vertical line. Like ECG artifact, EMG artifact is also highly conserved and tends to occur within certain regions. Lateral rectus spikes are lateral frontal and photomyogenic responses are broad frontal.

Electrode pop is due to the release of voltage that is stored across the gap between one electrode and the subjacent skin. Therefore, only one electrode is involved, which is very rare for IEDs. The morphology of electrode pop also is different from spikes by having a much steeper rise and much slower fall.

When the slow wave artifact of ocular flutter occurs in combination with the faster frequency artifact from eyelid movement, a compound wave results that appears to be a bifrontal spike and slow wave complex. Although the frontal poles may be the center of a spike and slow wave complex's field, this is an unusual location. When the bilateral spike and slow wave of a generalized IED has a phase reversal it usually is at F3 or F4. Focal spike and wave may occur at one frontal pole but does not have a bilateral symmetry. Spike morphology also may distinguish these waveforms. Because it is generated from muscle artifact, the spike of this simulated spike and wave complex is less stereotyped than the IED's spike. Lastly, true IEDs usually occur in states beyond light drowsiness, which is the state for ocular flutter. Even when the IEDs occur only with drowsiness, they continue to occur into stage II non–rapid eye movement (NREM) sleep.

Another compound wave results from the combination of the brief myogenic potential from the lateral rectus and the slow wave artifact from lateral gaze. This appears especially like an IED because the lateral rectus spike results from a single motor unit potential and is, therefore, relatively stereotyped across occurrences like the spike of an IED. It also occurs in the anterior temporal region, which is a region that often produces focal IEDs. Distinguishing lateral rectus spikes from IEDs depends on the lateral rectus spike's consistent low-amplitude, maximal field only at F7 and F8 and association with lateral gaze ocular artifact. IED spikes typically vary more in their amplitude and location, even if the variation is only minor and one electrode distance. A shifting asymmetry between F7 and F8 is not helpful because some individuals with temporal lobe epilepsy have bilateral independent temporal IEDs.

Versus Benign Epileptiform Transients of Sleep

Benign epileptiform transients of sleep (BETS) are more likely to be mistaken for focal IEDs than other transients because of their epileptiform morphology, field centered over the temporal lobes, and occurrence during sleep, a state with greater IED frequency. Distinguishing them from IEDs is much easier when they recur. Compared to BETS, IEDs tend to vary more in their morphology with inconsistent amplitudes and durations. IEDs also are more likely to have a prominent after-going slow waves, with an amplitude equal to or greater than the spike or sharp wave. Furthermore, focal IEDs tend to have narrower fields, which usually are limited to an electrode and its nearest neighbors and also may have co-localized but independently occurring focal slowing. The presence of such slowing indicates the region is abnormal and, therefore, is consistent with IEDs and not consistent with BETS. The occurrence of the same transient during wakefulness is also a distinguishing feature by eliminating the possibility of BETS. When a discharge consistent with a BETS occurs only once during a recording and no other suspicious finding is present, determining whether the transient is a BETS may not be possible. In such instances, the interpreter may rely on the basic tenet of EEG interpretation that undercalling abnormality is preferable to overcalling it. With this tenet, the interpreter may describe the transient within the report's body, state that the recording was normal, and state within the report's comment that the suspicious transient may have been BETS.

Versus Beta Frequency Activity and Breach Effect

The amplitude and frequencies of beta frequency range activity may spontaneously change during an EEG, and the coinciding of a sudden rise in amplitude and increase in frequency may appear as a spike. This occurs more commonly when a breach effect is present because of the breach region's greater amplitude and faster frequency components. Distinguishing IEDs from variations in the surrounding beta activity depends on identifying elements within the beta background that have morphologic similarities to the possible IED. If elements are similar and differ only in amplitude, then the wave needing identification is likely a variation in the background. The matter is complicated when a breach effect is present because IEDs may occur within a region of breach effect as a consequence of the trauma that led to the skull defect and because the trauma may have led to focal slowing within the region of the breach and the mixture of fast activity and slow waves may give the appearance of a spike and slow wave complexes.

Versus Lambda Waves

The characteristic triangular morphology and occurrence only with visual exploration distinguishes lambda waves from IEDs. IEDs more often are sharper than lambda waves and usually are not affected by eye opening or closure. FOS is the exception to this. In addition, IEDs usually become more frequent during sleep, a state during which lambda waves do not occur.

Versus Occipital Spikes of Blindness

Morphology provides the major means to differentiate occipital spikes of blindness (OSBs) from IEDs. However, significant overlap exists between these two patterns during mid childhood. The occipital location and increased frequency during sleep are not distinguishing because IEDs may have both of these features. The potential morphologic differences are most prominent in early childhood and adolescence with OSBs being sharper and lacking an after-going slow wave (61). When IEDs occur as spikes without a slow wave, they may be identified as IEDs if they resemble independently occurring sharp waves or spikes that are followed by slow waves. Thus, similarity with a more clearly identifiable IED may be helpful. Of course, the clinical history of blindness or a large scotoma from early life also is helpful. Moreover, when such waves occur in the context of later-life onset blindness, they are much more likely to be associated with seizures and, therefore, may not truly be OSBs (7).

Versus Paroxysmal Fast Activity

IEDs occur in several morphologies, including as polyspikes. Polyspikes are a train of spikes that usually are followed by a slow wave. Similar to PFA, they may be localized or generalized. When polyspikes occur without a slow wave, they are similar to PFA, and the distinction between these two patterns may be artificial or arbitrary because they have similar clinical significance. The only difference is duration. Classic polyspikes, as occur with slow waves, usually consist of only several spikes, so they rarely last longer than 0.5 seconds.

Versus Positive Occipital Sharp Transients of Sleep

The unvarying triangular morphology and consistent absence of an after-going slow wave distinguishes positive occipital sharp transients of sleep (POSTS) from IEDs. Even when they are sharp waves, IEDs usually are asymmetric and more sharply contoured than POSTS. Even though IEDs occur more frequently in sleep, they typically occur in wakefulness as well. Therefore, identification of a similar wave during wakefulness may help identify it as an IED and not a POSTS.

Versus Vertex Sharp Transients

Although they are rare, IEDs at the vertex occur. More common are parasagittal IEDs that occur within the region of off-center vertex sharp transients (VSTs). Regardless of their localization, IEDs typically have a sharper contour and lower amplitude than VSTs. They do not stand above the background activity as a characteristic feature but stand out through their sharpness against the slowing of drowsiness or sleep instead. When the IED is a rolandic spike, it has the additional differentiating feature of its characteristic morphology and polarity. Like the VST, classic rolandic spikes are triphasic; however, the first and third phases are less symmetric. Polarity also may distinguish rolandic spikes from VSTs. When a rolandic spike's tangential dipole is present, the positive end is central, which is the opposite polarity of the VST. Lastly, rolandic spikes that occur in repetitions do not appear as monophasic. They keep their triphasic morphology, and, furthermore, they often are separated by brief periods of background EEG activity.

Co-occurring Waves

When IEDs reflect a symptomatic focal epilepsy, co-localized focal slowing and attenuation may be present. When present, this is due to the dysfunction produced by the structural abnormality involved in the epileptogenic process. By definition, idiopathic localization-related epilepsies are not associated with underlying structural abnormality and do not have focal slowing.

IEDs occur in wakefulness and both forms of sleep but with a considerable difference in number and some difference in morphology. The stages of NREM sleep have the largest number of IEDs and increase in number with the later stages of NREM. Rapid eye movement (REM) sleep has the fewest number of IEDs, and wakefulness is between the two other states (175). In contrast, IEDs are most focal in REM sleep and least focal in NREM sleep.

Clinical Significance

IEDs are a sign of epilepsy, but like all diagnostic signs they are not infallible. However, the issue essentially is the quantitative reliability of IEDs as indicators of the risk for future seizures. Many large series have addressed this question, and the results are disparate. This partly may be due to different IED locations having different associations with epilepsy, with temporal IEDs having the highest and central IEDs in children having the lowest association. A meta-analysis of 19 studies that included 4,288 patients found sensitivity varied from 0.20 to 0.91 and the specificity varied from 0.13 to 0.99 (176). Differences in thresholds for abnormality among the readers accounted for 37% of the variance, and no other factor was found to explain the remainder. Overall, the meta-analysis found that the predictive value of an IED as a sign of epilepsy was greater when the EEG interpretation criteria were more restrictive. This recapitulates the conventional wisdom of erring toward underdiagnosing epilepsy when the clinical situation is not convincing.

Within healthy control populations, IEDs are present in 0% to 2.6% of individuals. Merging 12 studies of healthy adult that included a combined population of 59,496 subjects produces an overall positive rate of 0.2% (177,178). However, this positive rate includes both true and false positives because many of the studies did not follow the subjects forward to determine if seizures later developed. A retrospective study of 13,658 military recruits who had EEGs to evaluate for aircrew training reported spontaneous IEDs in the EEGs of 25 recruits (0.2%) and a photoparoxysmal response without spontaneous IEDs in another 44 (0.3%) (179). Of the 38 recruits with IEDs who were surveyed between 5 and 29 years later, only 1 definitely developed epilepsy. Another recruit died in a seizure-suspicious motor vehicle accident. Therefore, most IEDs in asymptomatic individuals are false positives and not indicative of epilepsy developing.

Hospital and EEG laboratory populations have higher rates of IEDs among individuals without epilepsy than healthy control populations, but this is due to conducting the survey with a group who has neurologic abnormalities sufficient to warrant obtaining an EEG even if the abnormality is not manifested by seizures (7). One such study of 521 patients over 10 years identified IEDs in the EEGs of 64 patients (12.3%) with 47 of these patients having acute or progressive cerebral disorders (180). A U.S. National Institutes of Health review of 6,497 patients without epilepsy identified 142 (2.2%) with IEDs (181). This group was followed clinically, and 20 (14.1%) subsequently developed epilepsy and those with progressive neurologic diseases were most at risk.

Within the epilepsy population, 90% have IEDs. However, the IEDs may be inconsistently present across multiple EEGs of single individuals. Overall, any one EEG of someone with epilepsy has about a 50% chance of demonstrating an IED (182). If two EEGs are performed, the chance of one of them showing an IED is about 75%. With three EEGs, it is 85%, and the likelihood asymptotes at about 90% with four EEGs. The likelihood of an IED varies across epilepsy syndromes and ages with the 50% rate representing focal epilepsy in young adults. EEGs of the elderly have the lowest sensitivity, and EEGs of children have a high sensitivity (183). However, the high sensitivity among children may be partly dependent on the age-related syndromes. This is typified by childhood absence epilepsy, which has IEDs on more than 75% of EEGs (182,184). Another primary generalized epilepsy, generalized tonic-clonic seizures on awakening, has a much lower rate of about 20%.

Despite the typical sensitivity of 50% for one EEG, IEDs are a powerful indicator of epilepsy in screened populations because of their much lower rate in healthy populations. As Goodin and Aminoff have shown, an IED on an EEG of a person whose history suggests epilepsy with 50% certainty would raise the certainty to 93% (182). However, the absence of IEDs would lower the certainty to 33%, which is less clinically helpful. This contrasts strongly with an unselected population, in which about 0.5% of members would have epilepsy. In this population, 94% of EEGs that have IEDs will be from individuals without epilepsy. Essentially, the positive predictive value of IEDs is greatly benefited by an increased prevalence of epilepsy in the tested population.

IED features have some bearing on the likelihood of seizures. Rolandic and occipital IEDs are usually clinically silent with only about half of children whose EEGs manifest either of these IEDs ever having a seizure (112,185,186). Because rolandic IEDs have autosomal dominant inheritance with a high penetrance, their presence may be considered as an incidental genetic finding (168). Contrasting with this is the pattern called MISD, alternatively called IMSD. This pattern is defined as the presence of spikes from both hemispheres and with three or more independent foci (Fig. 14–8). To be considered as arising from independent foci, spikes must have centers (phase reversals) two or more interelectrode distances apart. MISD is highly likely to be accompanied by epilepsy and is associated with frequent seizures that are not controlled with antiepileptic medications and often are generalized tonic-clonic seizures (9). It appears related to the generalized epileptiform abnormalities associated with severe bilateral cerebral dysfunction and may be a waveform that replaces the generalized childhood abnormalities (187,188). It commonly occurs in the context of mental retardation because it may be produced by metabolic or chromosomal abnormalities (189,190).

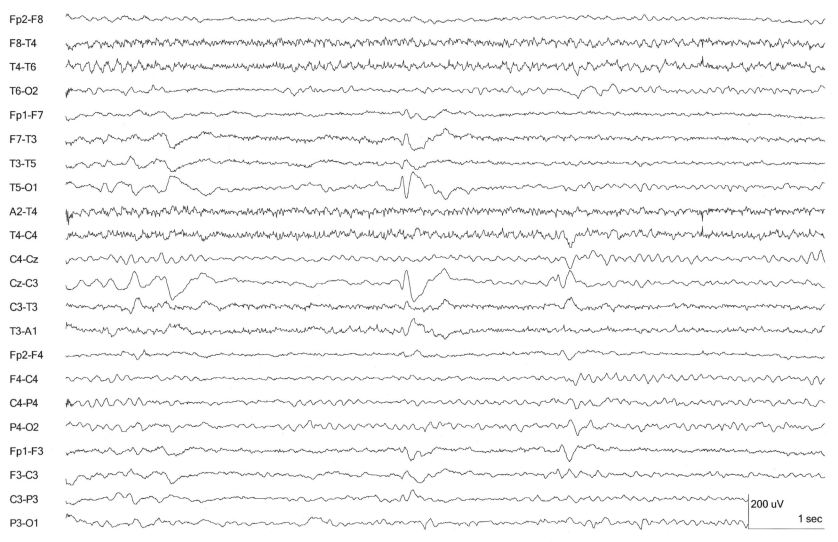

FIG. 14–1. Focal Interictal Epileptiform Discharge. A sharp and slow wave complex is present with a phase reversal at the T5 electrode and a field that includes the C3 and T3 electrodes. Left-sided slowing occurs at the beginning of the segment. Electrode artifact at the T4 electrode is 60 Hz and due to mismatched impedances. (LFF 1 Hz, HFF 70 Hz)

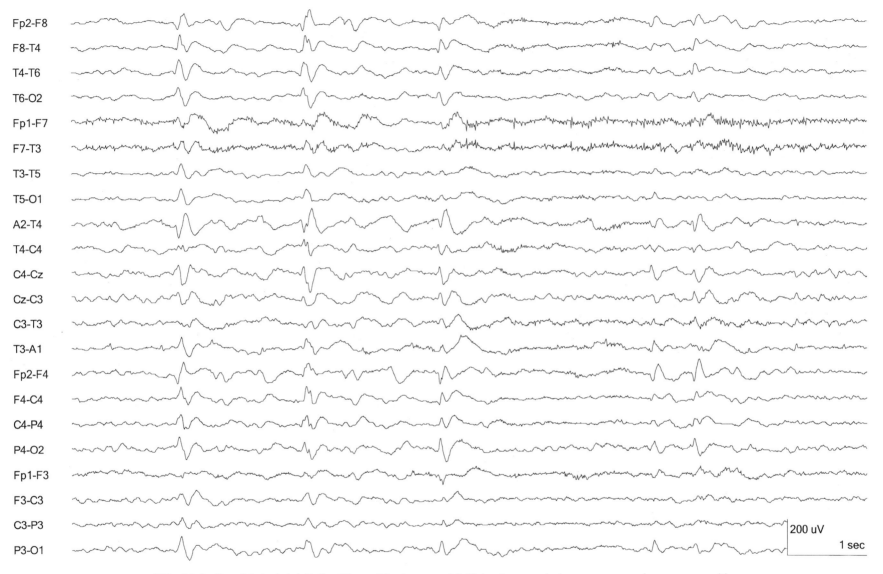

FIG. 14–2. Focal Interictal Epileptiform Discharges. Multiple sharp and slow wave complexes occur with minor variations in morphology. The phase reversals consistently are present at the F8 electrode and with fields that extend to include much of both hemispheres. The EEG corresponds to right lateral temporal lobe epilepsy, as supported by intracranial electrode recordings. Low-amplitude muscle artifact is present from the F7 electrode. (LFF 1 Hz, HFF 70 Hz)

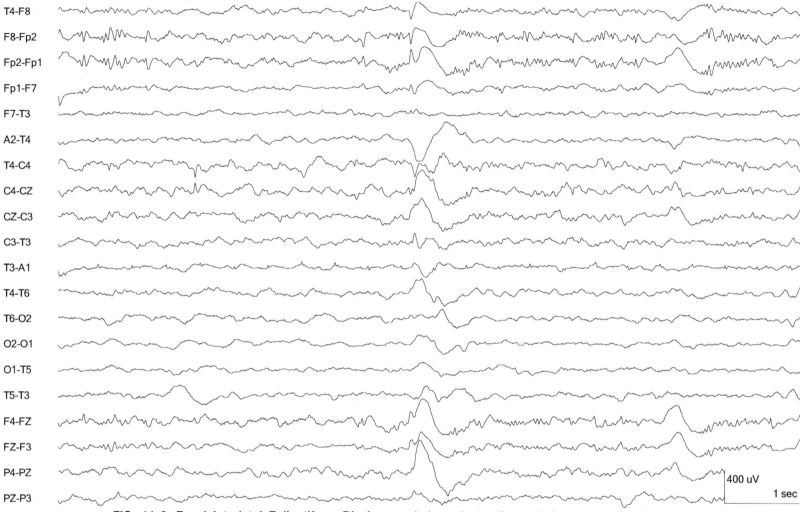

FIG. 14–3. Focal Interictal Epileptiform Discharges. Independent spike and slow wave complexes are present with phase reversals at the Fp2 and C4 electrodes. The C4 discharge's field is limited to one electrode while the Fp2 discharge's field includes the Fp1 and F4 electrodes. Asymmetric beta frequency activity co-localizes with the Fp2 discharges. (LFF 1 Hz, HFF 70 Hz)

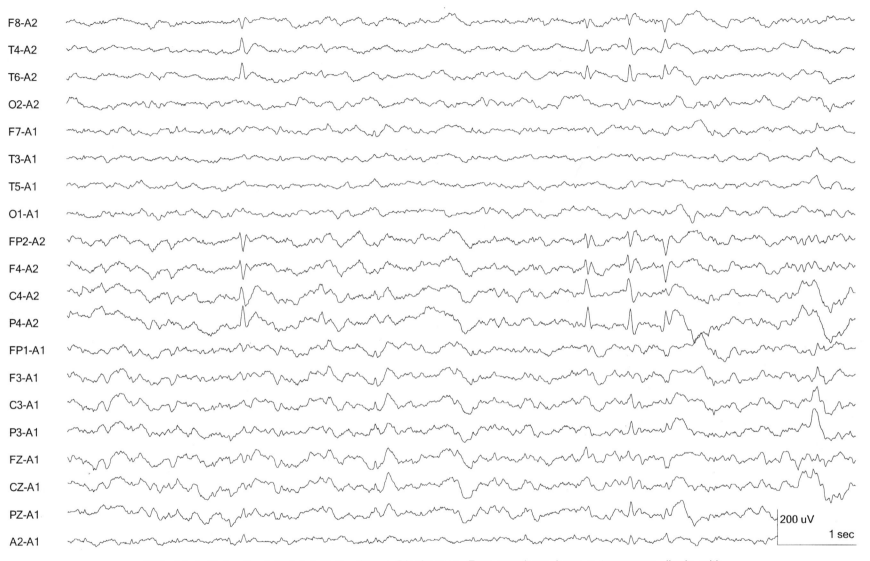

FIG. 14–4. Rolandic Interictal Epileptiform Discharges. Four transients have a transverse dipole with negativity over the right central and temporal regions and positivity over the right frontal region, as evident by a phase reversal in this referential montage. The occurrence of such transients in succession is typical of rolandic discharges. (LFF 1 Hz, HFF 70 Hz)

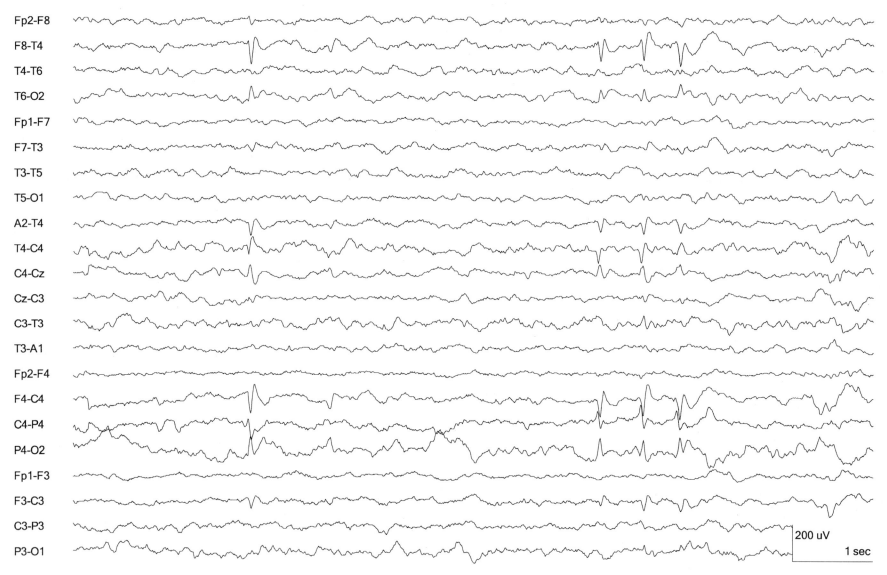

FIG. 14–5. Rolandic Interictal Epileptiform Discharges. The segment from Fig. 14–4 is presented in a bipolar montage for comparison. This montage obscures the transverse dipole but better depicts the classic rolandic discharge morphology. (LFF 1 Hz, HFF 70 Hz)

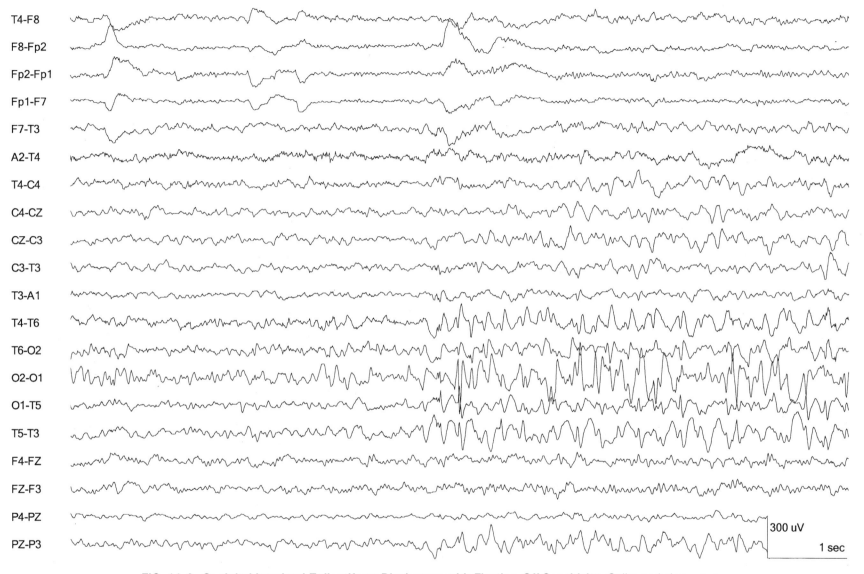

FIG. 14–6. Occipital Interictal Epileptiform Discharges with Fixation-Off Sensitivity. Spike and slow wave complexes with a phase reversals at the O1 and O2 electrodes occur in a train following eye closure, as is evident with eye blink artifact. (LFF 1 Hz, HFF 70 Hz)

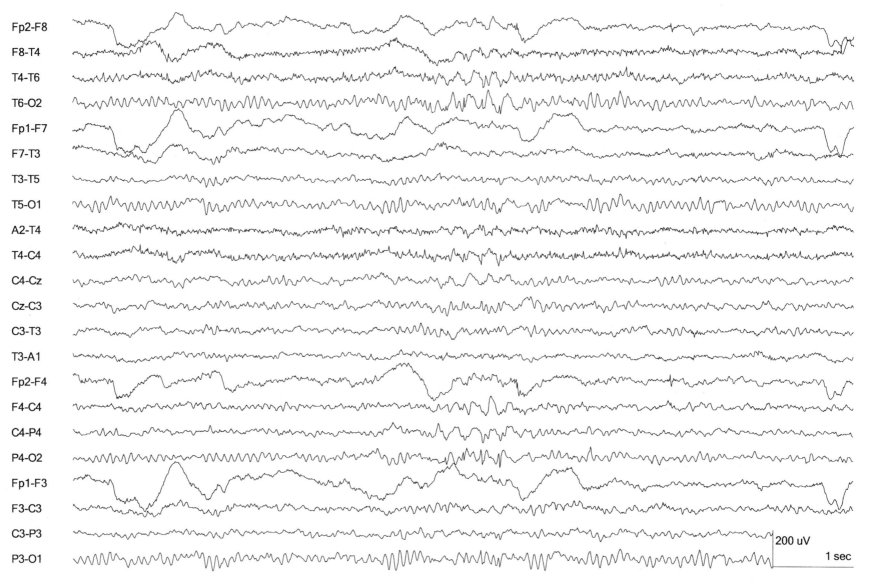

FIG. 14–7. Occipital Interictal Epileptiform Discharges. Three spike and slow wave complexes are centered at the O2 electrode and occur with a frequency of 4 Hz. The field extends anteriorly on the right and does not include the left occiput. (LFF 1 Hz, HFF 70 Hz)

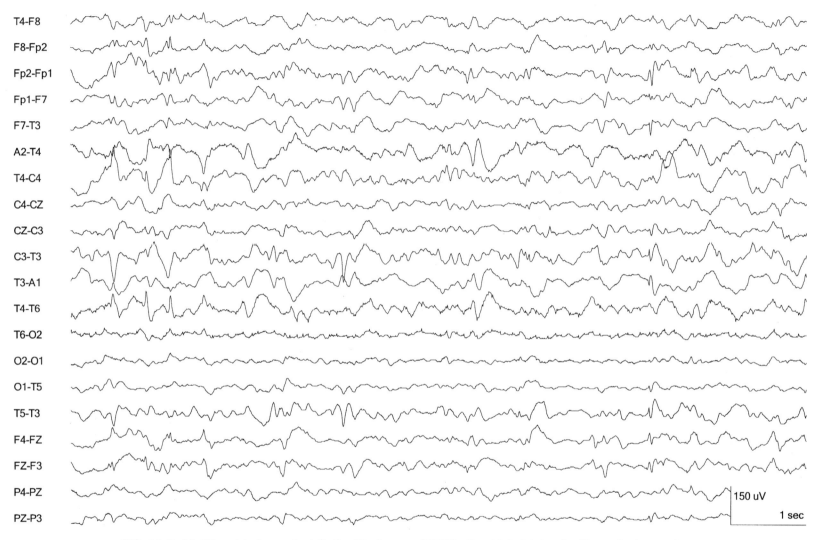

FIG. 14–8. Multifocal Independent Spike Discharges (MISD). Focal interictal epileptiform discharges have phase reversals at the Fp1, T3, and F8 electrodes. This segment meets criteria for MISD. (LFF 1 Hz, HFF 70 Hz)

GENERALIZED INTERICTAL EPILEPTIFORM DISCHARGES

Types

3 per second spike (and slow) wave (complex)
Atypical spike and slow wave
Slow spike and wave
Petit mal variant
Fast spike and wave
Polyspike and (slow) wave (complex)
Multiple spike complex
Spike and dome complex
Dart and dome complex
Hypsarrhythmia
Modified hypsarrhythmia
Secondary bilateral synchrony

Description

Generalized IEDs usually are not truly generalized across the entire scalp. Their field most commonly is maximal in the midfrontal region and extends to include the entire frontal region and some or most of the parietal region. The distribution across the temporal and occipital regions often is minimal (61) (Figs. 14–9, 14–10, 14–11, and 14–12). Phase reversals are present in about half of EEGs predominantly demonstrating generalized IEDs and occur most commonly at F3 and F4 and more rarely elsewhere in the rolandic and temporal regions (9), (191). Parietal phase reversals accompany a variant of the generalized IED in which the maximum field is posterior.

The morphology of generalized IEDs varies less than that of focal IEDs because it does not occur as individual spikes or sharp waves. Generalized IEDs typically occur as a complex including a sharply contoured wave (a spike or a sharp wave) and a slow wave but they may occur as bursts of successive spikes, which is termed generalized paroxysmal fast activity and is discussed in Chapter 20. When the sharply contoured wave is a spike or a polyspike, the morphology has been called spike and wave, spike and dome, and dart and dome. The spike and wave complex usually has a shorter duration than the form comprising a sharp wave followed by a slow wave and classically has a repetition frequency of 3 to 4 per second. The 3 per second repetition frequency functions as the overall demarcation between fast and slow forms. However, the repetition frequencies are not fixed over the time that a pattern is present, and patterns usually begin with complexes of shorter duration and slow in their repetition over their occurrence. A 3 per second spike and wave usually starts at 3.5 to 4 per second and ends about a second later at 2.5 to 3 per second (7).

A fast spike and slow wave complex begins at or above 4 per second and ends at about 3 per second (Fig. 14–13). A slow spike and slow wave (petit mal variant) complex usually begins between 1.5 and 2.5 per second and ends at about 1.5 per second (7,192) (Fig. 14–14). The slow spike and wave complex is termed an atypical spike and wave, and atypical spike and wave complexes may differ from the typical 3-Hz spike and in several features besides frequency. The atypical spike and wave classically may be asymmetric, asynchronous, and not frontally predominant; however, it also may be considered as present if the complex has a sharp wave instead of a true spike, begins or ends more gradually than the abrupt onset of typical form or has a phase reversal other than at the F3 or F4 electrode (1,7) (Fig. 14–15).

Typically, the spike of a spike and wave complex has an amplitude that is similar to or less than that of the slow wave. However, spikes that have amplitudes greater than the slow waves also occur. When the spike is low amplitude, it may appear as a notch in the slow wave's rising slope. Occasionally, the spike will not be visible for selected slow waves and the pattern appears to be rhythmic delta frequency range activity (193). In sleep, generalized IEDs are not as clearly formed with less regular slow waves, smaller fields, and slower repetition rates (9). However, they typically have a greater amplitude (194). The spike and wave complex may remain morphologically preserved across the life span but commonly becomes more atypical with aging (195).

Secondary bilateral synchrony (SBS) is an uncommon pattern of bilaterally synchronous spike and slow wave complexes that arise from a unilateral source (196). Thus, SBS is not an initially generalized pattern, but one that is due to discharge's spread over a large, bilateral field with the assumption of a repeating spike and wave pattern. The initiation and termination usually has an asymmetry consistent with their hemisphere of onset, but truly symmetric onsets also occur. The spike and slow wave complexes characteristically have a frontal predominance, a frequency typically less than 2.5 Hz, and a poorly formed morphology. Independent to the generalized IEDs, there commonly are focal IEDs with fields that indicate the SBS source, which most commonly is a frontal lobe (197). However, these focal IEDs must be distinguished from fragments of truly generalized IEDs, which may have phase reversals at F3 and F4 with a shifting asymmetry. Sometimes MISD is present. A review of an EEG database with 10,410 tracings recorded over 8 years identified 57 (0.5%) instances of SBS (197).

Hypsarrhythmia is a specific generalized interictal epileptiform pattern that typically occurs between the ages of 4 months and 2 years (7) (Fig. 14–16).

Rarely, it occurs as early as the neonatal period (198). Its compound name joins *hypselos,* Greek for "high," and arrhythmia, with reference to its characteristic disorganized background. Hypsarrhythmia usually has an amplitude between 200 and 400 µV but may be as high in amplitude as more than 1,000 µV. The disorganization is manifested by the absence of persistent rhythmic activity in any frequency range and the presence of asynchronous slow wave bursts amid a mixture of the frequency bands that are predominantly in the theta and delta ranges. The final characteristic feature of hypsarrhythmia is the presence of multifocal spikes or sharp waves. These IEDs and the background slowing may have a shifting asymmetry indicating an overall symmetry or may be consistently asymmetric. Consistent asymmetry supports the presence of focal pathology in the region of the greater slowing or frequent IEDs. Modified hypsarrhythmia is a term without as standard a definition as hypsarrhythmia but essentially suggests the absence of some typical features for hypsarrhythmia or a consistent asymmetry (7). When one feature is not present, it most commonly is the disorganization. In such instances, the background consists of rhythmic, generalized slow waves instead. Regardless of the type of hypsarrhythmia, the features that define this pattern are best seen during NREM sleep (199).

Distinguishing Features
Versus Phantom Spike and Wave

Some morphologic overlap exists between generalized IEDs and phantom spike and wave. However, the frequency and amplitude differences between these two patterns, especially compared to the record's background amplitude, are the best means to distinguish them from each other. Phantom spike and wave characteristically occurs at a rate of 6 per second and has a significantly lower amplitude. Less consistent but still possibly helpful features include phantom spike and wave's shorter duration and less generalized distribution (7).

Versus Secondary Bilateral Synchrony

Because of quick propagation or a focus that is invisible with scalp EEG, focal IEDs may appear bilaterally and thus resemble generalized IEDs. The relevance of distinguishing between SBS and generalized IEDs rests entirely on the importance of an accurate epilepsy syndrome diagnosis. Although the visible onset of individual occurrences for these two waveforms may be identical, SBS may be distinguished through asymmetries that are occasionally present but that have the same features with each occurrence (i.e., generalized IEDs have minimal, if any, overall asymmetry at the onset and SBS occasionally will have a unilateral lead-in that consistently is present on one side). The asymmetry in generalized IEDs is a shifting asymmetry with equal occurrences on each side. In addition, EEGs with SBS often demonstrate consistently asymmetric focal IEDs or background slowing, both of which is ipsilateral to the lead-in side. Finally, SBS usually has more variable morphology among the complexes, less rhythmicity, and a repetition frequency less than 2.5 per second (7). The presence of minor focal features in an EEG that otherwise appears to demonstrate generalized IEDS should not lead to certainty that SBS is present. Because EEGs with generalized IEDs are far more common than ones with SBS, a conservative approach should be used when considering SBS.

Co-occurring Waves
Generalized IEDs may occur in any behavioral state and have no consistently present co-occurring waves. However, generalized IEDs that occur in the context of symptomatic generalized epilepsies are associated with abnormally slow background activity or MISD (7). The generalized IEDs of primary generalized epilepsies occur amid normal background activity.

Clinical Significance
Generalized IEDs are hallmark signs of generalized epilepsy syndromes and may occur with both idiopathic generalized epilepsies (IGEs) and symptomatic generalized epilepsies (SGEs). Thus, they may reflect dysfunction that is solely manifested as seizures (idiopathic) and dysfunction that occurs due to diffuse cerebral pathology. Generalized IEDs that occur at 3 per second or faster typically indicate an IGE syndrome, such as childhood absence epilepsy, juvenile myoclonic epilepsy, and generalized tonic-clonic seizures on awakening. These IEDs occur in greatest number in the early morning (194). Childhood absence epilepsy's typical frequency is the 3 per second, and the fast spike and wave is more likely in juvenile myoclonic epilepsy. However, juvenile myoclonic epilepsy also may occur with the 3 per second pattern (7). Overall, IGE is a collection of epilepsies that usually first manifest in childhood and adolescence and usually respond to medical treatment with complete seizure control. Effective treatment often also decreases the number of IEDs (194).

The distinction between ictal and interictal generalized IEDs can be difficult because the waveform often is identical except in duration. Moreover, the likelihood of observing the cognitive impairment of an absence seizure increases with the duration of the wave, but some impairment may be present from the beginning of the first wave (200). Typically, a run of discharges lasting 3 seconds typically produces a loss of awareness (201). However, more subtle cognitive changes, such as memory or concentration impairment, also may accompany frequent generalized IEDs (202). Thus, wave duration is clinically significant.

Atypical spike and wave and hypsarrhythmia are indicative of SGE syndromes, which are conditions that present in childhood and are associated with seizures and developmental delay, with or without diffuse cerebral degeneration (7). The SGE syndromes typically include multiple seizure types and do not respond to medical treatment with complete seizure control. Lennox-Gastaut syndrome is the SGE associated with slow spike and wave, and infantile spasms/West syndrome is highly associated with hypsarrhythmia (199,203).

Although hypsarrhythmia is classified here as an interictal epileptiform pattern because of its association with an epilepsy syndrome, it may just as well be considered an abnormal background pattern because of its fixed presence in an EEG and its high association with developmental abnormality. Hypsarrhythmia typically occurs in the context of congenital brain malformations or metabolic abnormalities. The modified hypsarrhythmias are common and do not alter the prognosis (204).

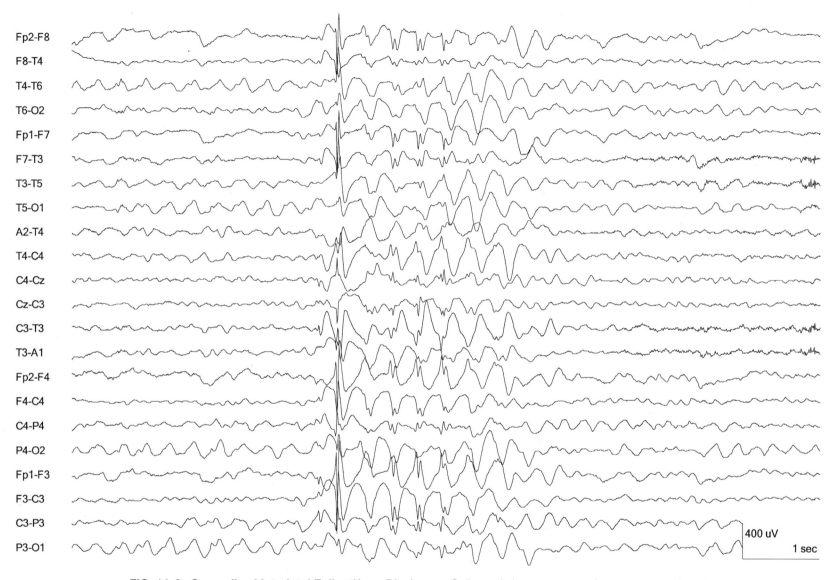

FIG. 14–9. Generalized Interictal Epileptiform Discharge. Spike and slow wave complexes are occurring at 3 Hz during hyperventilation, as is evident in the hypersynchronous background. The discharges follow a higher amplitude spike and have maximal amplitude and clearest morphology in the midline frontocentral region. (LFF 1 Hz, HFF 70 Hz)

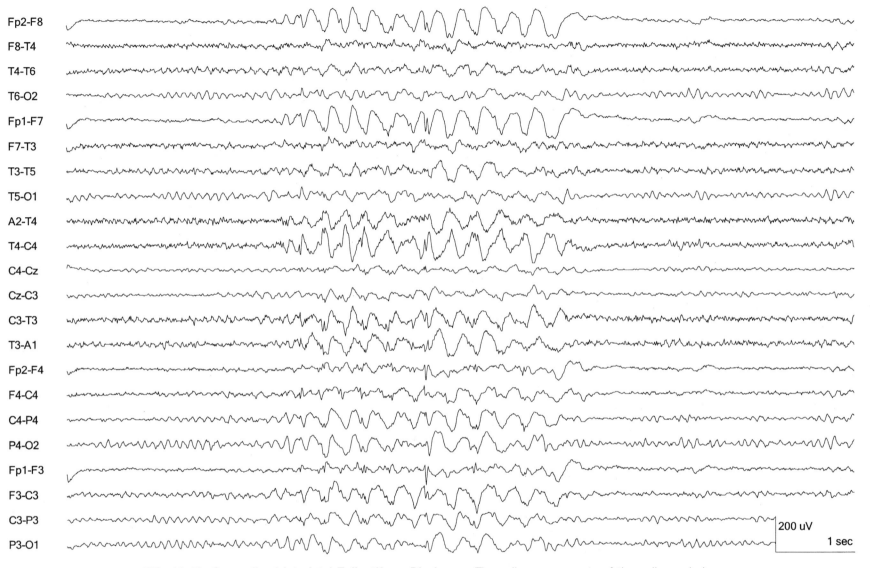

FIG. 14–10. Generalized Interictal Epileptiform Discharge. The spike components of the spike and slow wave complexes in this example of 3-Hz spike and wave complexes are not as clear as those in Fig. 14–9. However, the spikes still are visible and have a fixed temporal association with the slow waves. (LFF 1 Hz, HFF 70 Hz)

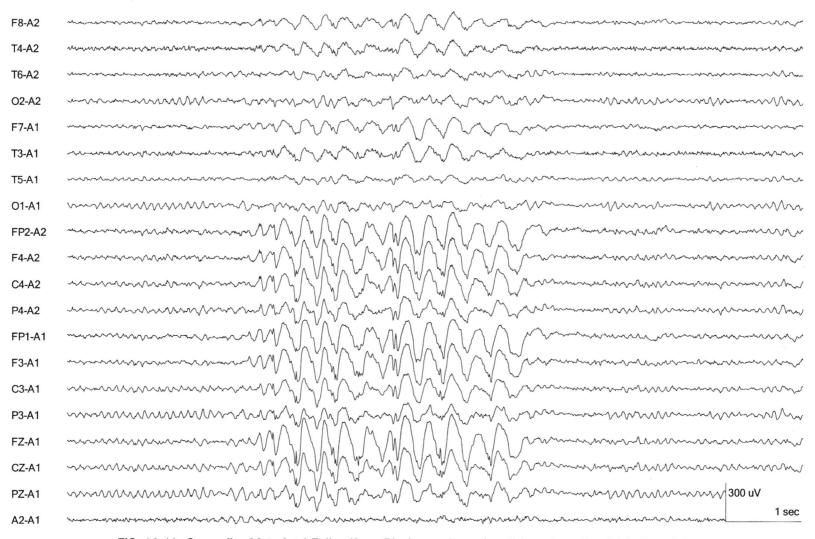

FIG. 14–11. Generalized Interictal Epileptiform Discharge. In a referential montage, the distribution of the generalized 3-Hz spike and wave complexes is more clearly present in the midline with an anterior predominance. This segment is the same as in Fig. 14–10 but in a different montage. (LFF 1 Hz, HFF 70 Hz)

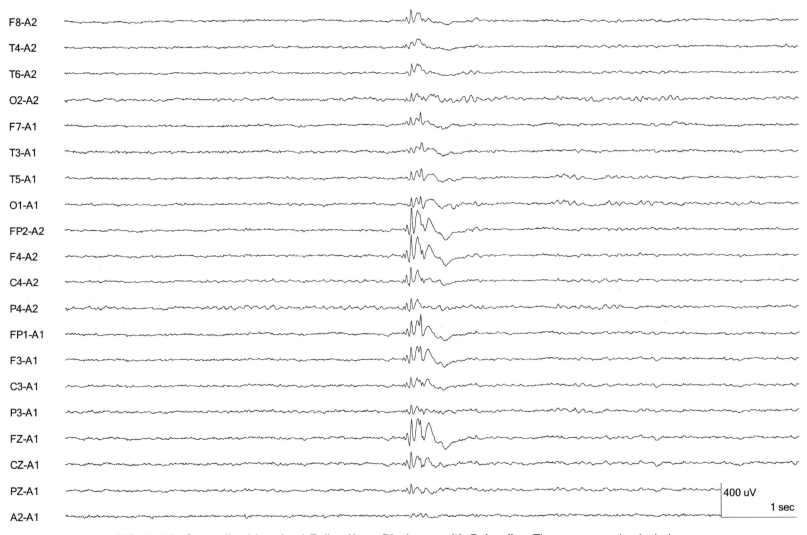

FIG. 14–12. Generalized Interictal Epileptiform Discharge with Polyspike. The wave complex includes a collection of several spikes of differing amplitude followed by a slow wave. The second complex includes one spike that rides on its preceding slow wave. (LFF 1 Hz, HFF 70 Hz)

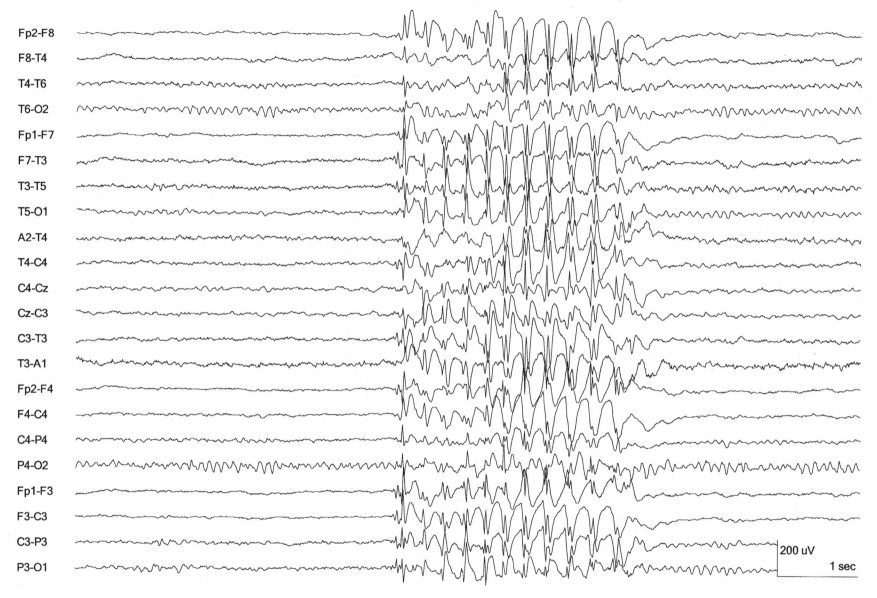

FIG. 14–13. Generalized Interictal Epileptiform Discharges. The wave complex has a frequency of 4 Hz and an onset with polyspikes. Compared to the 3-Hz spike and wave, the fast spike and slow wave complex more typically includes polyspikes. (LFF 1 Hz, HFF 70 Hz)

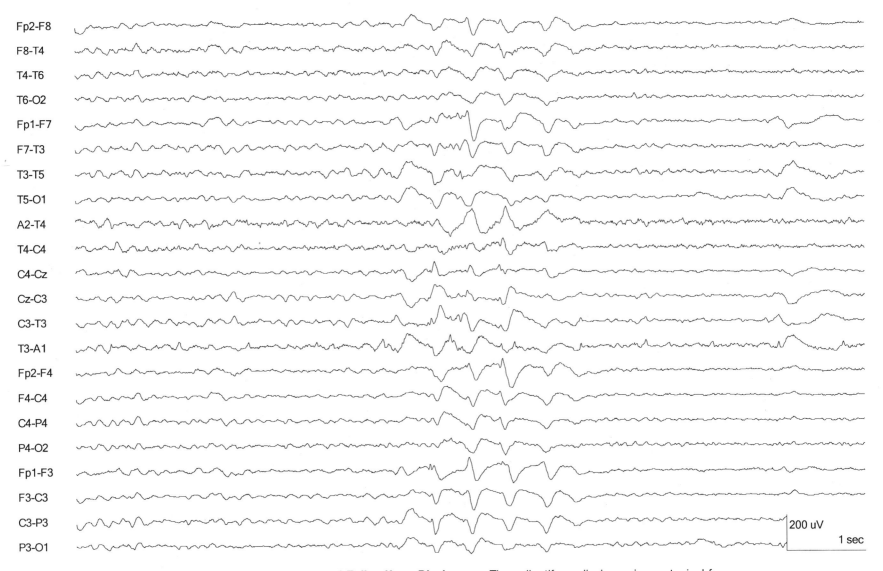

FIG. 14–14. Generalized Interictal Epileptiform Discharges. The epileptiform discharge is an atypical form of generalized spike and slow because of a frequency of 2 Hz, a poorly formed spike component, and consistent asymmetrically better formed morphology on the left side. Sharp waves with phase reversal at the T3 electrode have been noted in other segments, which raises the possibility of secondary bilateral synchrony. (LFF 1 Hz, HFF 70 Hz)

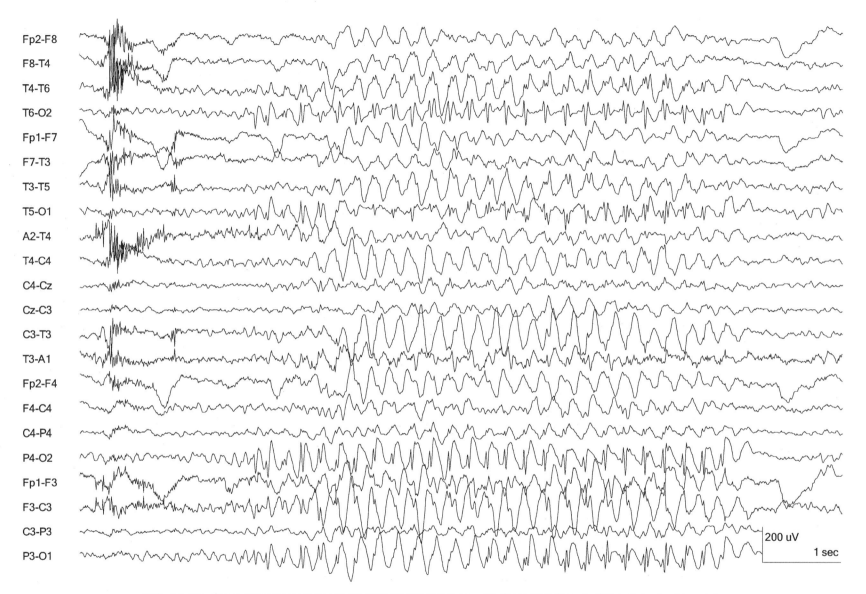

FIG. 14–15. Generalized Interictal Epileptiform Discharges with Occipital Onset. Other than the biooccipital onset, the pattern in this segment is similar to the typical, anterior 3-Hz spike and wave complex. The patient is a child with typical absence seizures. (LFF 1 Hz, HFF 70 Hz)

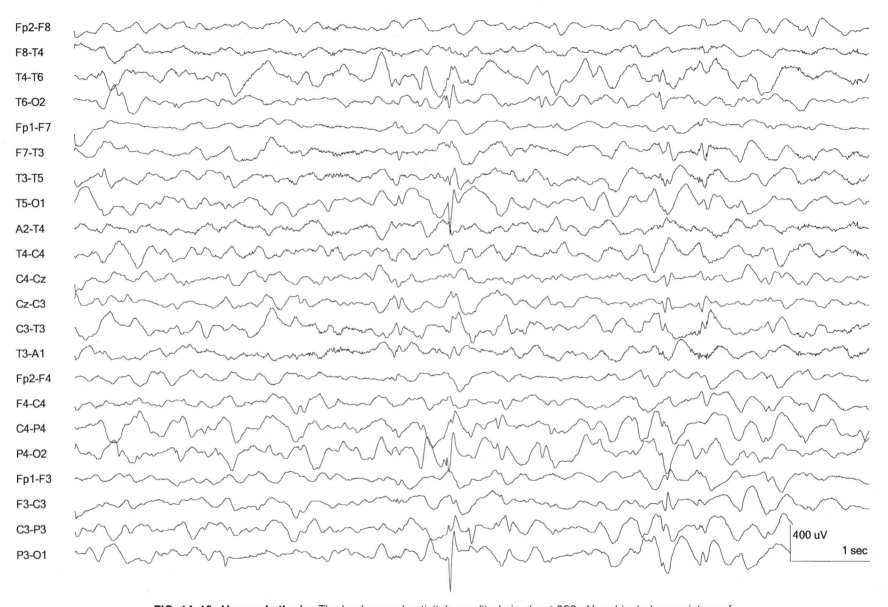

FIG. 14–16. Hypsarrhythmia. The background activity's amplitude is about 300 μV and includes a mixture of frequencies without consistent rhythms across scalp regions. Multiple spikes are present and have a bilateral posterior predominance. The most prominent spike has an amplitude of 700 μV in the P3-O1 channel. (LFF 1 Hz, HFF 70 Hz)

CHAPTER 15

K Complexes

K COMPLEXES

Other Names
K wave

Description
The K complex is a usually polyphasic transient at the vertex that occurs in stages II to IV of non–rapid eye movement (NREM) sleep (Figs. 15–1, 15–2, and 15–3). Sometimes, only two phases are visible. Most commonly, it immediately precedes a sleep spindle, and some definitions for it include the sleep spindle within its overall morphology (8). Other definitions stipulate that a sleep spindle must follow it. However, two standard definitions allow for it to occur in the absence of sleep spindles (1,205). Among its three or more phases, K complexes include a couplet of two waves of opposite polarity that are greater in amplitude than the surrounding background. The first wave of the pair is negative and usually has a shorter duration than the second. The duration for the K complex as a whole often is greater than 0.5 second and is required to be so when it used for sleep staging in polysomnograms. The distribution of the K complex is similar to that of the vertex sharp transient (VST) with its center at the vertex and possible extension of its field into the frontal, parietal, and temporal regions.

In infants, K complexes are greater in amplitude than at any other age with at least one phase commonly greater than 200 μV. However, the wave elements are not as sharply contoured as they become in childhood and remain through adulthood. Like sleep spindles, K complexes occur less often in late adulthood, even among neurologically healthy individuals (206).

Distinguishing Features
Versus Vertex Sharp Transient

The morphology of a K complex is more complicated than that of a VST, and this feature is the most differentiating. Although K complexes also have a negative phase reversal at the vertex, their morphology is polyphasic, longer in duration, less sharply contoured, and without as great an amplitude difference between the phases as VSTs have. Indeed, the polyphasic pattern of K complexes is more evident than the triphasic pattern of a VST because more than one of its phases has an amplitude greater than the background. Also like VSTs, K complexes occur individually; however, unlike VSTs, they do not occur in trains and often are immediately followed by a sleep spindle.

Co-occurring Waves
K complexes only occur in stages II to IV NREM sleep; thus, other features of these states always co-occur. These features are sleep spindles and background activity with principal frequencies that are in the theta or delta frequency ranges. Positive occipital sharp transients of sleep (POSTS) and VSTs, which first occur during stages I NREM sleep, also may be present.

Clinical Significance

Similar to VSTs, K complexes are normal phenomena that are provoked by various external stimuli (207,208). As such, they have been described as a response to stimulation that represents either a sign of arousal or of sleep maintenance (209–211). They appear to have a diffuse and varying cortical source despite their consistency in localization, and this fits with their interpretation as a long latency-evoked potential (212,213). Their most important difference from VSTs is their significance for sleep staging. Along with sleep spindles, K complexes are principal indicators of stage II NREM sleep. This differs from VSTs, which occur in stage I.

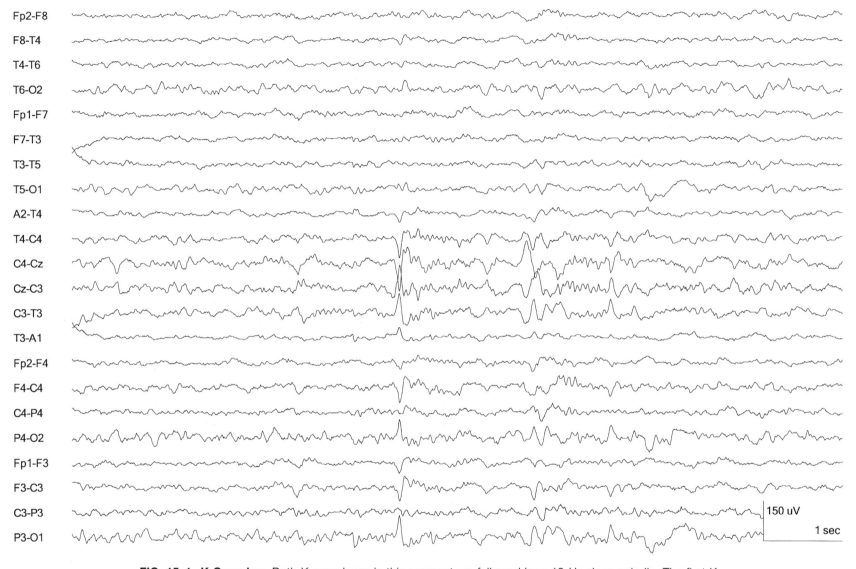

FIG. 15–1. K Complex. Both K complexes in this segment are followed by a 13-Hz sleep spindle. The first K complex is higher amplitude and has a more sharply contoured first phase. The second K complex is longer in duration and polyphasic. The second sleep spindle is followed by a low-amplitude vertex sharp transient. (LFF 1 Hz, HFF 70 Hz)

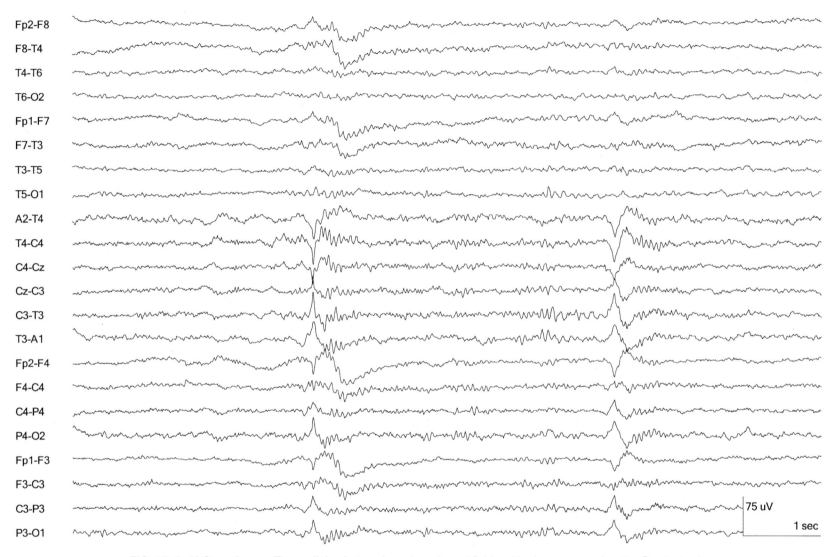

FIG. 15–2. K Complexes. These diphasic transients have broad fields with phase reversal at the Cz electrode and are followed by brief, 15-Hz sleep spindles. (LFF 1 Hz, HFF 70 Hz)

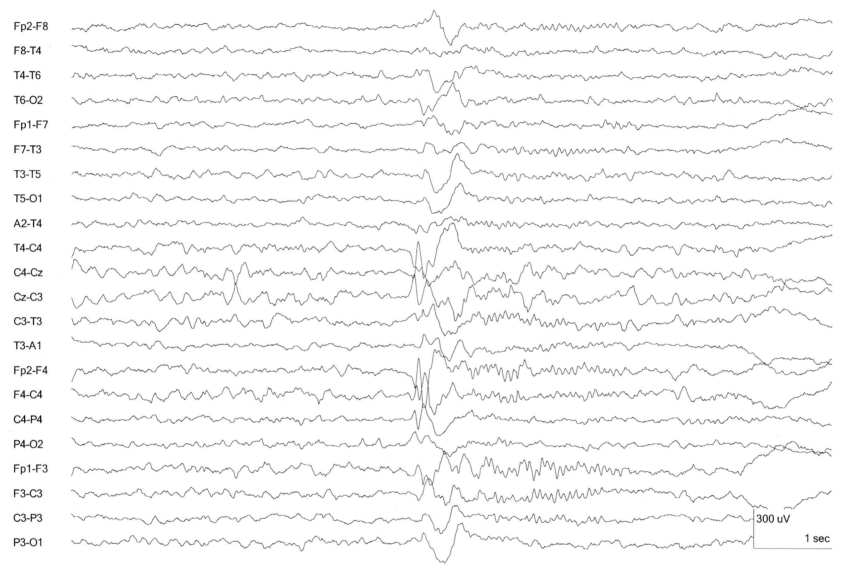

FIG. 15–3. K Complex. The polyphasic K complex has a duration of 600 msec and an amplitude of 450 µV in this bipolar montage. The spindle that follows is normal but unusually long with a duration of 1.5 seconds. A lower amplitude vertex sharp transient occurs earlier in the segment. (LFF 1 Hz, HFF 70 Hz)

CHAPTER 16

Lambda Waves

LAMBDA WAVES

Other Names
Sail wave

Description
Lambda waves are diphasic, or sometimes triphasic, occipital sharp waves that occur during visual exploration (Figs. 16–1 and 16–2). Therefore, they only occur during wakefulness and in a well-lit environment that includes visual details. Because of this need for visual details, they rarely occur under the conditions that most electroencephalograms (EEGs) are recorded, that is, lying supine and looking at a blank ceiling.

The prominent phase within the lambda wave gives the wave a triangular or saw-tooth morphology that resembles the Greek letter lambda (λ). Sometimes this phase is the only one that is evident, and the wave appears therefore monophasic. The prominent phase is positive and has an amplitude that typically is 20 μV and rarely greater than 50 μV. Its duration ranges from 100 to 200 msec, and the wave as a whole has a duration that typically is 200 msec and usually ranges from 150 to 300 msec. Lambda waves usually are bilaterally synchronous with a field that is centered at the occipital pole (O1 and O2 electrodes) and possibly extending to include the parietal (P3 and P4 electrodes) and posterior temporal regions (T5 and T6 electrodes). Because of the broad distribution, lambda waves are best recorded with channels that include posterior electrodes and have long interelectrode distances. Rarely, they occur unilaterally. When they are unilateral, there is a shifting asymmetry in occurrence that does not indicate an overall lateralization. Lambda waves usually occur as seemingly random and isolated transients but may recur at intervals of 200 to 500 msec.

Lambda waves do not occur before 1 year and are most common during the middle years of childhood. Between 1 and 3 years, lambda waves are larger and have longer durations, which may be up to 400 msec. Through childhood, they progressively become lower amplitude and shorter, with stabilization of their morphology in early adulthood. The prevalence of lambda waves between 3 and 12 years is about 80% (6). During the middle years of adulthood, the prevalence is about half of that during childhood.

Distinguishing Features
Versus Positive Occipital Sharp Transients of Sleep

The key distinguishing feature from positive occipital sharp transients of sleep (POSTS) is the state in which the wave occurs. Lambda waves occur only during wakefulness, and POSTS occur only during non–REM (NREM) sleep. Another difference is the likelihood of trains with repeating transients. POSTS commonly occur in trains, and lambda waves rarely do.

Versus Posterior Slow Waves Youth

Lambda waves and posterior slow waves of youth have the same localization, occur most commonly in the same childhood population, and are present only during wakefulness. The key distinction is the reproducibility of the posterior slow waves of youth with the eyes closed and their blocking when the eyes are opened. With sustained eye closure, lambda waves are not present. The morphologies of these two waves also are different. Lambda waves are briefer and more triangular than posterior slow waves of youth.

Versus Interictal Epileptiform Discharges

The characteristic triangular morphology and occurrence only with visual exploration distinguishes lambda waves from interictal epileptiform discharges (IEDs). IEDs more often are sharper than lambda waves and very rarely are affected by eye opening or closure. Furthermore, IEDs usually become more frequent during sleep, a state during which lambda waves do not occur.

Co-occurring Waves

Lambda waves are most likely to occur in the context of the saccades that occur with visual exploration; thus, they often are temporally linked to ocular artifacts due to blinking, lateral gaze, and lateral rectus spikes. Indeed, they may be time-locked to saccades, and when so, the delay averages 75 msec. In children, the association with blink artifact is especially strong. The occurrence lambda waves in attentive wakefulness creates an association to the presence of a posterior dominant rhythm (PDR). However, the PDR usually is inconsistently present when lambda waves occur because of the blocking related to eye opening. Individuals who have lambda waves are more likely to have a strong photic stimulation driving response.

Clinical Significance

Lambda waves are a normal phenomenon unless markedly and consistently asymmetric. The asymmetry may manifest as either an asymmetric bilateral field or through unilateral lambda waves that occur much more frequently on one side. Marked and consistent asymmetry indicates cerebral pathology on the side lacking lambda waves. Although the presence of lambda waves is associated with a strong photic stimulation driving response, these two phenomena have different cerebral generators. The basis of their association is clarified by the observation that pathologies that prolong the visual evoked potential latency also prolong the latency of the lambda wave (214). Based on this observation, lambda waves are believed to arise from changes in the afferent visual system during saccades. Regardless of their source, they are not statistically associated with a greater likelihood of IEDs (215).

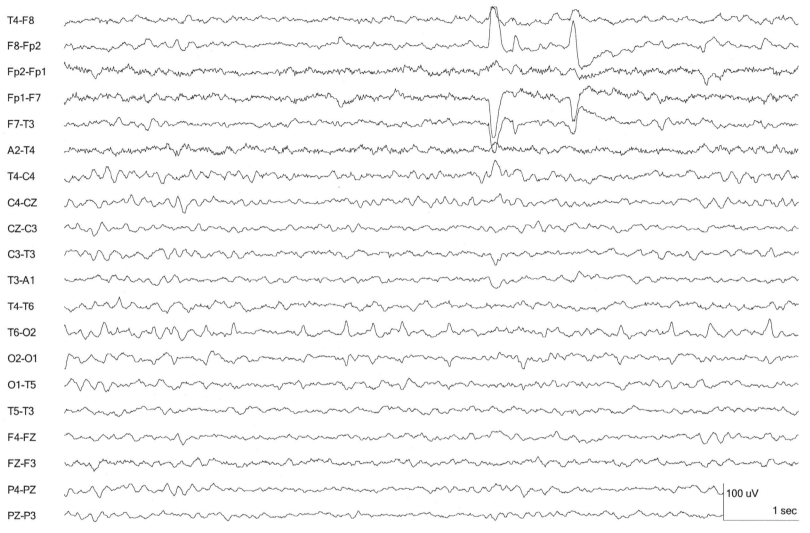

FIG. 16–1. Lambda Wave. Triangular waves with phase reversals indicating surface positivity occur at the O2 electrode. Eye blink artifact demonstrates the EEG reflects wakefulness despite the diffuse theta frequency activity. The EEG corresponds to visual scanning (LFF 1 Hz, HFF 70 Hz).

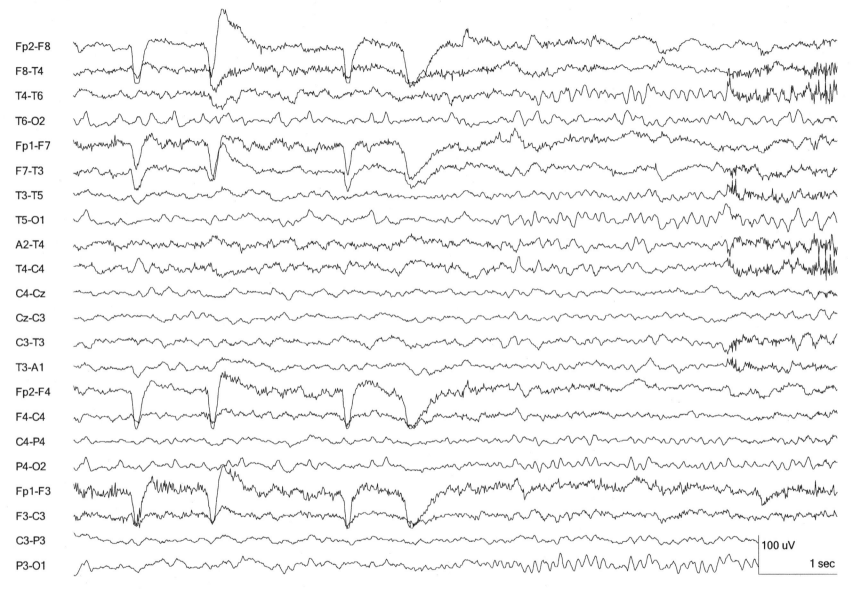

FIG. 16–2. Lambda Wave. Diphasic lambda waves occur across the occiput when the eyes are open and are absent after eye closure and return of the alpha rhythm (LFF 1 Hz, HFF 70 Hz).

CHAPTER 17

Low Voltage EEG and Electrocerebral Inactivity

LOW VOLTAGE EEG AND ELECTROCEREBRAL INACTIVITY

Other Names
Desynchronization
Suppression
Electrocerebral silence
Isoelectric EEG
Flat EEG

Description
A commonly used standard defines low-voltage activity as the persistent absence of any cerebrally generated waves greater than 20 μV (6). The value of 20 μV is arbitrary but effectively eliminates most spontaneous variations in amplitude that commonly occur in EEGs. Low-voltage activity usually extends beyond a focal region; and, it may be hemispheric, bilateral, or generalized (Fig. 17–1). Because an accurate measurement of amplitude is especially important when assessing for low voltage, channels with long interelectrode distances should be used. This decreases the likelihood of the appearance of low voltage due to broad, isoelectric fields by maximizing the likelihood that the channel's two electrodes are not both over the same activity. The amplitude of a broad, isoelectric field is more accurately determined by comparing the potential of an electrode within the field to one outside of it. Low-voltage EEGs sometimes contain high-frequency activity that is not apparent at usual sensitivities; thus, scrutiny of low-voltage periods at a high gain is warranted.

Depending on its cause, low voltage EEG may be a precursor to ECI (89). ECI is the extreme example of a low voltage EEG by lacking any visible cerebrally generated activity (Figs. 17–2 and 17–3). The absence of visible activity generally means the absence of potentials greater than 2 μV when reviewed at a sensitivity of 2 μV/mm. To be an accurate determination of any electrocerebral activity, an EEG performed to evaluate for ECI must be obtained under specific conditions (216,217). These are:

1. Eight or more scalp electrodes that includes midline coverage and one ear electrode
2. Electrode impedances between 0.1 and 10 kOhms
3. Interelectrode distances of ≥10 cm
4. Sensitivity of 2 μV/mm
5. Low-frequency filter 1 Hz or less
6. High-frequency filter 30 Hz or greater
7. Technologist testing of each electrode by physical manipulation
8. Somatosensory, auditory, and visual stimulation
9. Thirty or more minutes reviewed
10. Electrodes on extracerebral sites, including chest for electrocardiogram (ECG)
11. EEG recorded by qualified technologist

Distinguishing Features
Versus Artifact, Electrode

The artifactual loss of EEG signal from salt bridges or poor electrode contact is a focal phenomenon that often is not a consistent finding through an entire EEG. When the low amplitude is due to poor electrode contact, the finding occurs only in the channels that include the bad electrode. Therefore, the channels demonstrating low amplitude should be compared to determine if there is one electrode in common. Confirmation of the poor contact is possible by observing the EEG while physically manipulating the electrode. Salt bridges involve adjacent electrodes and manifest as a persistently low-amplitude signal that usually is limited to one channel. The problem arises from the undesired electrical connection between the electrodes and not with the electrodes individually. Therefore, other channels with each of the electrodes may be functional, and a plausible low-voltage field will not be present. Salt bridges also demonstrate very low frequency activity, which appears as undulations to the baseline at a frequency that is less than 1 Hz.

Versus Ictal Pattern

Unlike low-voltage activity that is not related to seizures, ictal patterns that manifest as decreases in EEG amplitude are brief occurrences that typically last fewer than several seconds. This is true regardless of the ictal pattern's field. Furthermore, such ictal patterns usually contain very fast frequencies and frequency evolution. Thus, reviewing the brief attenuation at a high sensitivity may provide additional confirmation of its epileptic basis.

Co-occurring Waves

Low voltage EEGs may occur in any context; thus, they have no specific accompanying waves. ECI commonly is accompanied by artifact. This is mostly due to the high sensitivity used during the review. In addition to a cardiac source, artifacts often include the electrical and mechanical devices that usually surround a patient with ECI.

Clinical Significance

Persistent and generalized low-voltage activity on an EEG may be a normal variant and has an increasing prevalence with advancing age. It is rare in childhood and reaches a prevalence of about 10% by middle adulthood (6,7).

Brief periods of generalized low voltage also may be a normal variant, caused by nervousness and anxiety, and may be a sign of a poor prognosis when recorded in the context of a coma (40,218,219). Establishing that low-voltage activity is present as a normal variant depends on eliminating each of the pathologic causes as possibilities.

Extracerebral pathology may produce low-voltage activity, and the distribution of the low voltage reflects the location of the pathology (220). Such pathologies include everything that impedes electrical fields and specifically may be scalp edema, subgaleal fluid collection, skull density changes that occur with conditions such as Paget's disease, and subdural hematomas (7,9). Focal and hemispheric low-voltage activity that is cerebrally generated is likely due to focal pathology that is limited to the cortex because subcortical white matter involvement produces slowing that is not low amplitude. Bilateral and generalized low-voltage activity is more likely to have an etiology that is degenerative or metabolic. Basal ganglia disease, and especially Huntington's disease, causes low voltage EEG (6). Between 30% and 60% of individuals with Huntington's disease have very low voltage EEG (221). Other associated diseases include Alzheimer's disease, Creutzfeldt-Jakob disease, and multiple sclerosis (7). Metabolic causes include hypothermia ($<25°C$), hyperthermia ($>42°C$), hypoglycemia (<18 mg/100 ml blood), hypothyroidism, abnormal parathyroid function, and chronic alcoholism (6,7,104,222). A sudden loss of generalized or bilateral voltage may occur with the onset of a seizure, hypoxia, or decerebration (7,223,224).

ECI is a confirmatory finding for brain death; however, it is more useful for excluding the diagnosis of brain death than for establishing it. Essentially, any evidence of electrocerebral activity excludes the diagnosis, but ECI may occur in circumstances other than brain death. The most common of such circumstances are sedative intoxication, profound hypothermia ($<17°C$), and the early period after a hypotensive or anoxic episode (225). The specified EEG criteria for ECI are intended to maximize the validity of the finding. However, a return of electrocerebral activity after ECI is possible, especially in children (226,227).

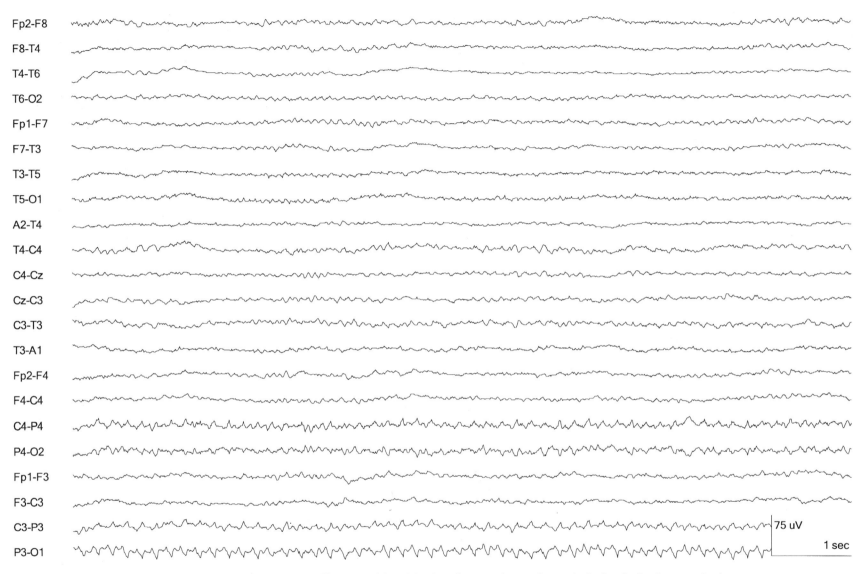

FIG. 17–1. Low Voltage. The diffuse 15-μV activity has frequencies and morphologies indicating cerebral origin. The 5-Hz notched activity that is predominantly present in the P3-O1 channel is artifact due to a hemodialysis machine's pump. The EEG corresponds to coma following hypotension (LFF 1 Hz, HFF 70 Hz).

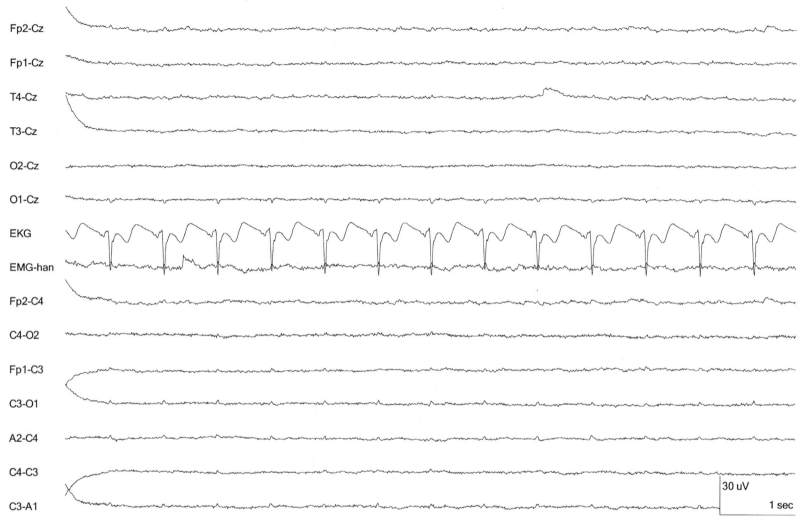

FIG. 17–2. Electrocerebral Inactivity. Recorded and depicted according to standard electrocerebral inactivity criteria, the highest amplitude activity are cardiac and electrode artifacts. The other activity is 2 μV or less. The EEG corresponds to clinically diagnosed brain death due to a large subdural hematoma (LFF 1 Hz, HFF 70 Hz).

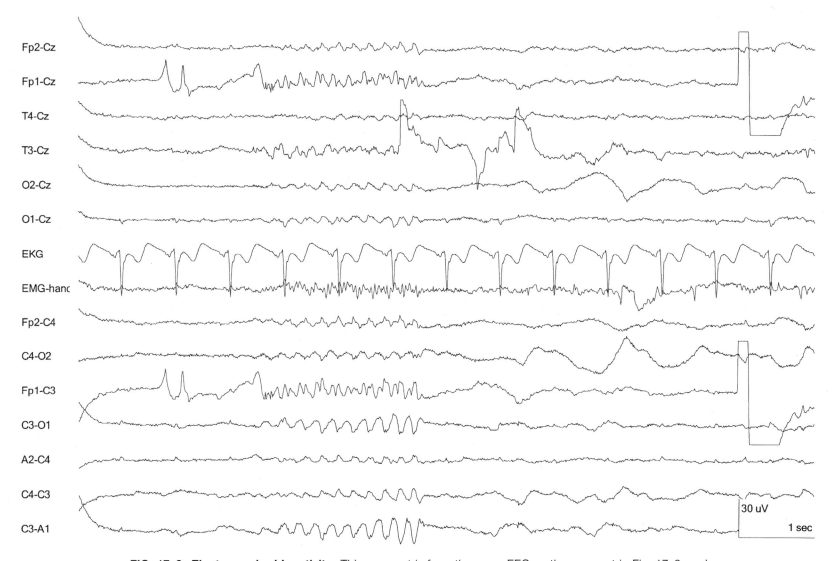

FIG. 17–3. Electrocerebral Inactivity. This segment is from the same EEG as the segment in Fig. 17–2, and includes 5-Hz and 1-Hz rhythmic artifacts that are preceded and accompanied by activity that is more clearly artifact because of its unusual morphology. The rhythmic artifact also is depicted in the EMG channel. Both artifacts and the high amplitude deflection in channels that include the Fp1 electrode are due to lead movement (LFF 1 Hz, HFF 70 Hz).

CHAPTER 18

Mittens

MITTENS

Other Names
None

Description
This pattern assumes the outline of a mitten through the partial superimposition of a sharp wave on the slope of a slow wave of the same polarity (Fig. 18–1). The overlap produces a notching in the pattern as a whole with the subsequent division of the pattern into a sharp wave thumb and slow wave hand compartment (8). The pattern occurs as individual waves that are centered in the frontal-central midline with extension into the parasagittal regions bilaterally. It has a duration that usually is about 400 to 500 msec and an amplitude that is high and equivalent to that of the surrounding delta frequency range activity. Anterior delta activity commonly is present because the pattern usually occurs during deep sleep. Mittens are best seen with referential montages.

Distinguishing Features
Versus K Complex

Similar to the K complex, mittens are individual complexes that occur at the midline during non–REM (NREM) sleep. They differ in morphology because the two major component elements of a mitten have the same polarity. The major elements of K complexes are two sharp waves of opposite polarity. The localization is somewhat differentiating because mittens typically are centered anterior to the vertex and K complexes are at the vertex.

Versus Interictal Epileptiform Discharge

The pairing of a sharp wave and a slow wave give mittens a description that resembles bilateral interictal epileptiform discharges (IEDs), but their morphology differs considerably from that of IEDs. The sharp wave element of a mitten has a longer duration and a less sharp contour then the initiating sharp wave of an IED. The inconsistency in the temporal relationship between the two component waves of a mitten also distinguishes it from an IED. The sharp or spike wave and the slow wave of IEDs have a relatively fixed temporal relationship with the initiating wave always occurring at the same distance from the slow wave's peak.

Co-occurring Waves
The electrographic features of stages III and IV NREM sleep accompany mittens. These include sleep spindles, K complexes, positive occipital sharp transients of sleep (POSTS), and generalized delta frequency range activity. The delta frequency background typically has sharply contoured features and bursts of anterior rhythmic activity (9).

Clinical Significance
Mittens now are considered normal variants, but they previously were believed to be markers of several diverse neurologic and psychiatric conditions including thalamic tumors, epilepsy, parkinsonism, and psychosis (228). The correlations to these clinical conditions were made in early electroencephalogram (EEG) research and focused on morphologic features of the mitten pattern, such as the duration of the thumb component (26). These correlations have not been replicated with more modern approaches.

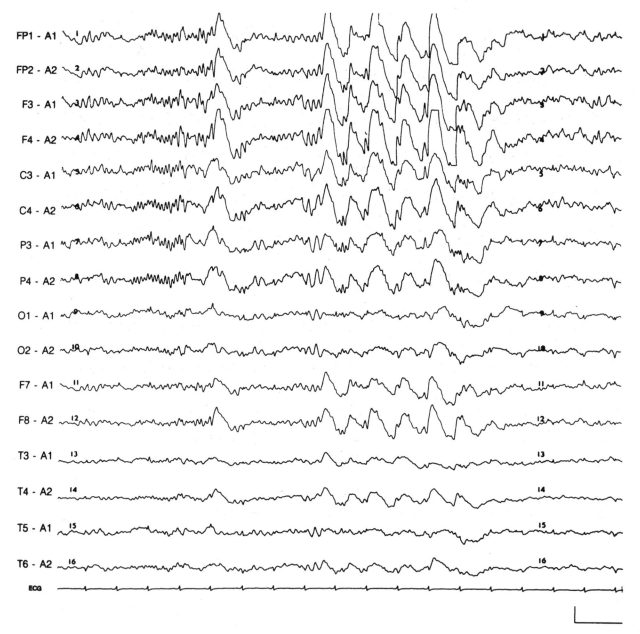

FIG. 18–1. Mittens. The superimposition of rhythmic slow waves and independent faster frequencies creates a "mitten" with a lower-amplitude shorter-duration wave producing the thumb compartment and the higher-amplitude slow wave producing the finger compartment (Calibration bars 1 sec and 70 μV). (From Blume WT, Kaibara M, Young GB. *Atlas of adult electroencephalography,* 2nd ed. New York: Lippincott Williams & Wilkins, 2002:1,140.)

CHAPTER 19

Occipital Spikes of Blindness

OCCIPITAL SPIKES OF BLINDNESS

Other Names
Needle spike

Description
Electroencephalograms (EEGs) of children who have blindness from birth or early infancy sometimes demonstrate unilateral or bilateral occipital spikes called occipital spikes of blindness (OSBs) (7) (Fig. 19–1). Less commonly and in conflict with the localization denoted by their name, OSBs occur within the parietal region (230). OSBs may be present as early as about 10 months but typically are low amplitude and very brief until about 2.5 years (231). By mid childhood their duration is increased and they may have an after-going slow wave. After-going slow waves usually are again absent by late childhood. In adolescence, the spikes become lower in amplitude and briefer in duration until they disappear by the end of adolescence (61,232). OSBs occur much more often during sleep, with 1-minute periods during which many may occur either individually or in bursts (233). Their amplitude usually is greater than the surrounding background activity's and usually is between 50 and 250 µV.

Distinguishing Features
Versus Focal Interictal Epileptiform Discharges

Morphology provides the major means to differentiate OSBs from interictal epileptiform discharges (IEDs). However, significant overlap exists between these two patterns in mid childhood. The occipital location and increased frequency during sleep are not distinguishing because IEDs may have both of these features. The potential morphologic differences are most prominent in early childhood and adolescence with OSBs being sharper and lacking after-going slow waves (61). When IEDs occur as spikes without a slow wave, observing similar transients that are longer in duration may help differentiate them through the process of identification by association, (i.e., waves of uncertain type that are similar to recognized waves are likely to be a variation of the recognized wave). Therefore, the occurrence of similar waves with an after-going slow wave or with a sharp wave's duration suggests that the wave needing identification is an IED. Of course, the clinical history of blindness from early life also is helpful. Moreover, when such waves occur in the context of later-life-onset blindness, they are much more likely to be associated with seizures and, therefore, may not truly be OSBs (7).

Co-occurring Waves
OSBs typically occur in EEGs that lack a normal alpha rhythm. In such EEGs, the alpha rhythm may be disorganized, impersistent, or absent (7,234).

Clinical Significance
The term blindness has been used with varying definitions in studies of OSBs and with inconsistencies among the studies regarding how severe the visual loss must be for OSBs to occur (233). Nevertheless, the trend is for complete visual loss having the greatest association with OSBs. Furthermore, OSBs occur most commonly when the visual impairment is due to a retinopathy that is present by early infancy. Overall, retrolental fibroplasia is most associated with OSBs, with an OSB prevalence of 75% between the ages of 3 and 14 years (231). Before 3 years, 35% have OSBs. The prevalence for other causes of bilateral blindness is less and is about 38% when all causes are included (230,234).

Because most children with OSBs have retinopathy and do not have epilepsy, OSBs are thought to be an innocuous result of noncerebrally generated blindness, possibly as a type of denervation hypersensitivity (61). However, an understanding of the significance of OSBs is complicated by the fact that they occur most commonly in the context of retrolental fibroplasia, which is associated with cerebral pathology. Furthermore, they occur more commonly if abnormal occipital slowing or multifocal IEDs are present or if the patient has mental retardation or epilepsy (234). Thus, they may be associated with noncerebral blindness and diffuse cerebral pathology and indirectly with seizures. Essentially, they may be an innocuous finding that occurs more readily in the context of occipital pathology than they do from purely ophthalmologic or ocular nerve abnormalities (235).

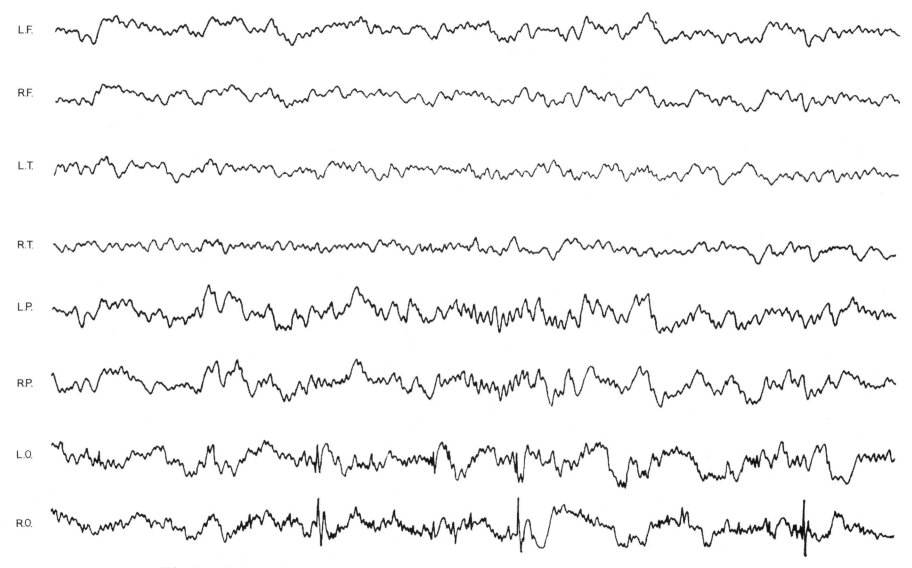

FIG. 19–1. Occipital Spikes of Blindness. Unilateral short-duration spikes are present at the occiput with occasional poorly formed after-going slow waves. The EEG corresponds to a 1-year-old with retrolental fibroplasia. (From Gibbs EL, Fois A, Gibbs FA. The electroencephalogram in retrolental fibroplasia. *N Engl J Med* 1955;253:1105, with permission.)

CHAPTER 20

Paroxysmal Fast Activity

PAROXYSMAL FAST ACTIVITY

Other Names
PFA
Rhythmic spikes
Fast paroxysmal rhythms
Beta band seizure pattern
Grand mal discharge (for generalized PFA)

Description
Paroxysmal Fast Activity (PFA) is a specific type of bursting beta frequency range activity that may be focal or generalized (236) (Figs. 20–1, 20–2, 20–3, and 20–4). Other than distribution, the two forms of PFA are similar in manifestation. PFA has a sudden onset and resolution and has a morphology that differs considerably from the surrounding background activity. A burst of PFA begins with the abrupt appearance of a fast, irregular rhythm that usually differs from the background by having a higher amplitude, often greater than 100 μV (237). Occasionally, the amplitude is decreased compared to the background and may be as low as 40 μV. Unless a seizure accompanies it, PFA remains fixed at the initial frequency or evolves with only a minor decrease in frequency. The decrease usually is a few cycles per second by the end of an occurrence. As is true for other electroencephalogram (EEG) patterns, seizures are accompanied by a greater amount of evolution. The amplitude and wave morphology typically does not change during an occurrence. The morphology is a repetition of monophasic waves with the sharp contour dictated by the high frequency. The frequency at the onset of a burst almost always is within the range of 10 to 25 Hz and usually is at least 15 Hz. The duration of PFA varies, especially for generalized PFA (GPFA). Localized PFA (LPFA) commonly lasts 0.25 to 2 seconds. GPFA usually lasts about 3 seconds but may last up to 18 seconds (82). Most GPFA runs that last longer than 5 seconds are accompanied by a seizure; thus, the EEG subsequently includes the very fast activity of seizure-related muscle artifact (83). Unlike LPFA, which may occur anywhere on the scalp, GPFA has a relatively consistent field with a maximum in the frontal or frontal-central regions bilaterally. Although it often is generalized or at least includes the majority of both hemispheres, GPFA may be limited in distribution to the bilateral frontal or frontal-central region.

Sleep is the state in which PFA is most likely to occur, but it is not unusual in wakefulness. Compared to sleep, GPFA that occurs in wakefulness is longer in duration on average and more likely to have accompanying ictal behavior. Hyperventilation and photic stimulation are not activating for PFA (159). PFA most commonly occurs in the age range of older children to young adults.

Distinguishing Features
Versus Muscle Artifact

Muscle artifact and PFA both develop abruptly and include high-amplitude, very fast activity. They differ in their frequency components. Muscle artifact contains a greater number of frequencies and, therefore, appears more disorganized. This basis in a superimposition of fast frequencies also makes muscle artifact appear slightly different with each occurrence. PFA has a more organized morphology that is stereotyped among occurrences.

Versus Beta Activity

Normal beta activity differs from PFA by typically beginning and ending gradually, even if only over a second. The abrupt change in amplitude and frequency components makes PFA more identifiable as a distinct pattern amid ongoing background activity.

Versus Polyspike Interictal Epileptiform Discharges

Interictal epileptiform discharges (IEDs) occur in several morphologies, including as polyspikes. Polyspikes are a train of spikes that usually are followed by a slow wave. Similar to PFA, they may be localized or generalized. When polyspikes occur without a slow wave, they are similar to PFA, and the distinction between these two patterns may be artificial or arbitrary because they have similar clinical significance. The only difference is duration. Classic polyspikes, as occur with slow waves, usually consist of only several spikes; thus, they rarely last longer than 0.5 seconds.

Versus Fourteen and Six Positive Bursts

When fourteen and six positive bursts (14&6) occur in their faster frequency form (~14 Hz), they are similar to LPFA because they also develop abruptly and typically last less than 1 second. They differ by having a very broad field and an arciform morphology that points in the positive direction. LPFA usually has a field that covers a region and rarely extends across a region. The significant evolution from about 14 Hz to about 6 Hz that a 14&6 occasionally demonstrates is another key differentiating feature. However, the 14&6 does not typically slow during an occurrence.

Versus Spindles

Spindles usually contain slightly slower frequencies than PFA, but there is overlap between the two patterns. Nevertheless, the faster frequency of PFA (>15 Hz) is the feature that is most useful for differentiation. Morphology and state are other differentiating features. Spindle morphology includes a variable amplitude during an occurrence with maximal amplitude at the midpoint. Spindles also are limited to one state, non–REM (NREM) sleep. Although more common in sleep, PFA may occur in wakefulness. PFA also sometimes includes frequency evolution with a minor slowing in frequency during a burst.

Co-occurring Waves

Both generalized and localized PFA occur most commonly in EEGs that have at least mildly abnormal, generalized slowing. More commonly, the background has moderate slowing. EEGs with PFA almost always also have other types of epileptiform abnormality, specifically spikes, sharps, or complexes of either a spike or a sharp with a slow wave. These other epileptiform abnormalities may immediately follow PFA. The other IEDs often demonstrate multiple localizations and meet the criteria for multifocal independent spike discharges (MISD).

Clinical Significance

PFA is an epileptic pattern that, depending on its duration, is either an interictal or ictal abnormality (238). It is not included in the interictal or ictal chapters (Chapters 13 to 14) only because of its morphologic and clinical differences from other epileptiform abnormalities. PFA occurs most commonly in the context of seizures that are generalized at their onset and manifesting a symptomatic generalized epilepsy (SGE), and Lennox-Gastaut syndrome in particular (238,239). Epilepsies that are not symptomatic generalized rarely demonstrate PFA, but it has been reported to occur rarely with posttraumatic epilepsy (61). PFA's greater prevalence with SGE results in its association with abnormally low IQ and other neurologic deficits, evident structural abnormality, and poorly controlled seizures of multiple types (27,240). However, it may occur in individuals with normal intelligence. Among the seizure types, PFA occurs with generalized motor seizures, which may be tonic, clonic, or tonic-clonic (7).

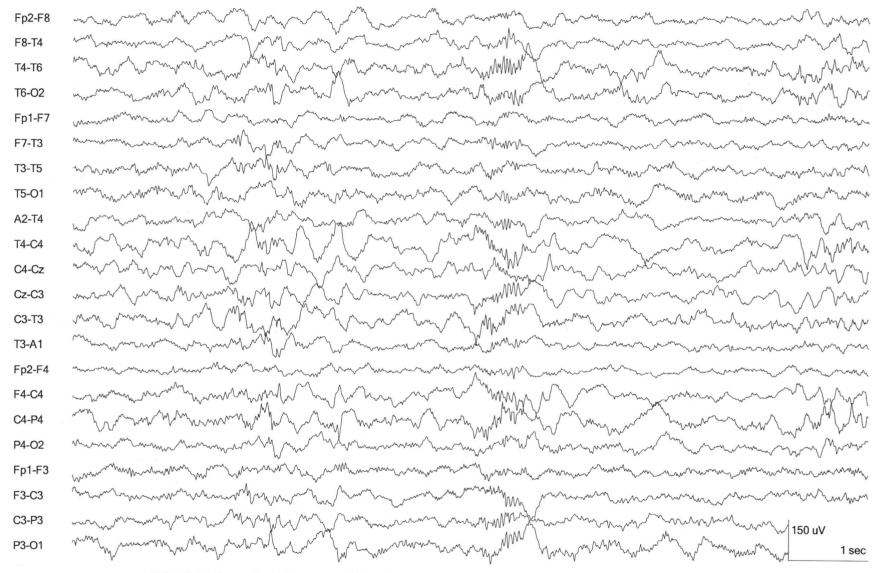

FIG. 20–1. Generalized Paroxysmal Fast Activity. The burst of fast frequency activity is asymmetric with right-sided predominance. The background activity also is asymmetric because of attenuation across the left side. The EEG corresponds to an 11-month-old with infantile spasms (LFF 1 Hz, HFF 70 Hz).

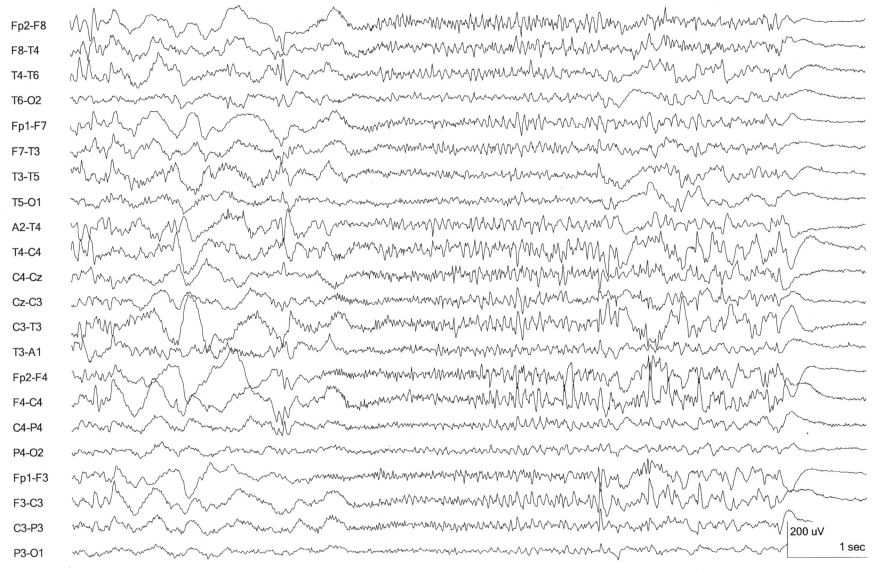

FIG. 20–2. Generalized Paroxysmal Fast Activity. The pattern begins with its lowest amplitude and highest frequency and subsequently evolves with increasing amplitude and decreasing frequency. Its resolution is followed by generalized attenuation. This EEG was interictal and corresponds to a symptomatic generalized epilepsy (LFF 1 Hz, HFF 70 Hz).

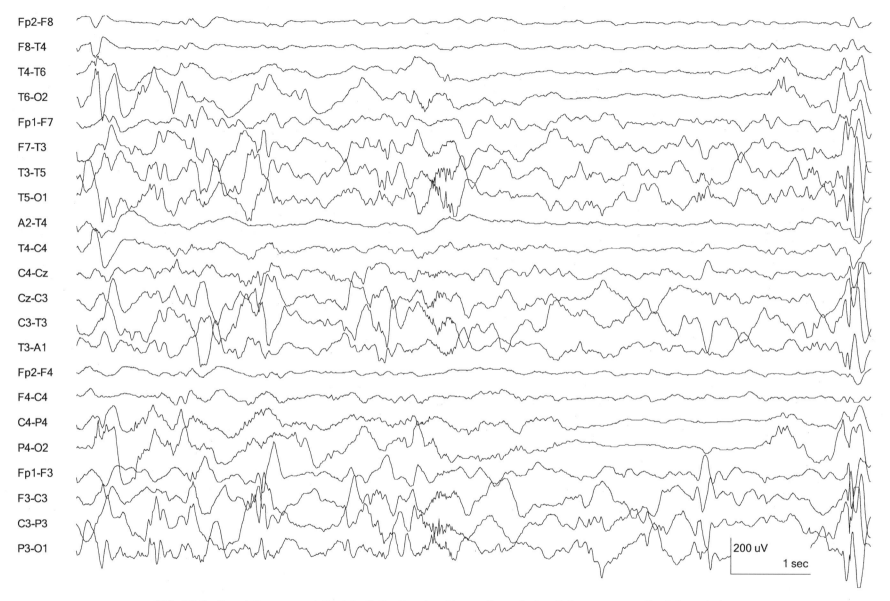

FIG. 20–3. Focal Paroxysmal Fast Activity. Bursts of low-voltage, fast activity occur over the left posterior quadrant and co-localize with high-amplitude, polymorphic slowing and focal spike and sharp waves. The EEG corresponds to right hemimegalencephaly (LFF 1 Hz, HFF 70 Hz).

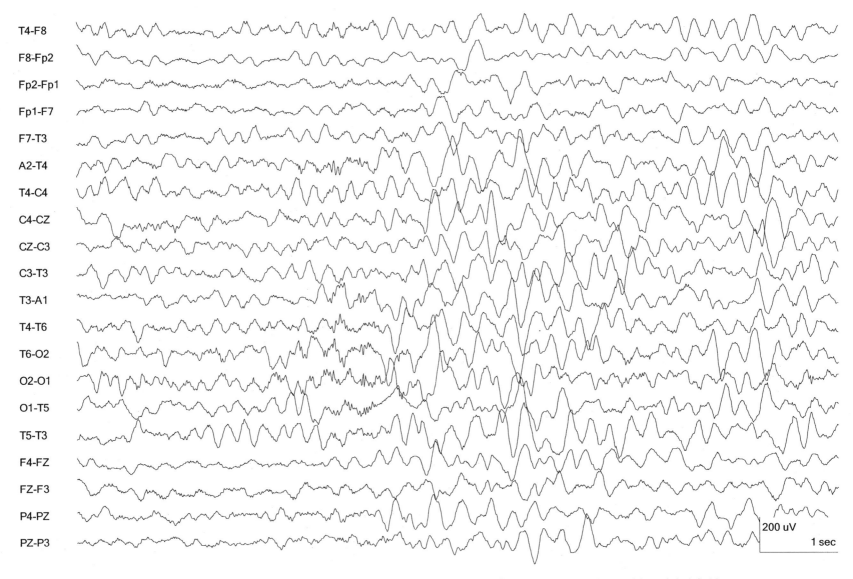

FIG. 20–4. Focal Paroxysmal Fast Activity. Low-amplitude, high-frequency activity has a bi-occipital field and durations of less than a second. The hypersynchronization that follows the burst is of unclear significance and may be an arousal response. The EEG corresponds to a toddler with normal imaging and an idiopathic epilepsy (LFF 1 Hz, HFF 70 Hz).

CHAPTER 21

Periodic Epileptiform Discharges

PERIODIC LATERALIZED EPILEPTIFORM DISCHARGES

Other Names
PLEDs
Recurrent sharp waves
Periodic sharp wave complexes

Description
Similar to interictal epileptiform discharges (IEDs) and triphasic waves (TW), periodic epileptiform discharges (PEDs) classically are triphasic with a sharply contoured wave followed by a slow wave. However, their significance is distinct despite their similar waveform. PEDs are an uncommon electroencephalogram (EEG) pattern with an overall incidence between 0.4% and 1% in EEG laboratory series (241). They usually have a singular focus which is a form called periodic lateralized epileptiform discharges (PLEDs) (Figs. 21–1 and 21–2). This focus may be anywhere on the scalp and contrary to the name may be at the midline (Fig. 21–3). The term periodic epileptiform discharges at the midline has been proposed to avoid the oxymoron, but it is not commonly used (242). Although a triphasic morphology is most characteristic, PLEDs may have one to several phases (243). Their total duration usually is between 100 and 300 msec, and their amplitude usually is greater than the background and in the range of 100 to 300 µV (61,221,244). However, morphology is not the essential feature of PLEDs; a conserved recurrence pattern is. As the term *periodic* in the name indicates, PLEDs recur but do so with varying degrees of regularity. They may be highly regular with an interval that is almost constant, and, alternatively, they may recur without a set interval. Regardless of which type, the recurrence pattern almost always is conserved throughout an EEG. With regard to PLEDs, the term *pseudoperiodic* has been used with two definitions. Traditionally, it refers to greater variation in wave morphology among recurrences, but it currently is more commonly used to indicate greater variation in interdischarge interval (245). Recurrence frequencies for PLEDs commonly fall in the range of one transient every 0.5 to 4 seconds. Usually, they recur at least every 2 seconds (7). Low-amplitude slow activity usually separates PLEDs.

Distinguishing Features
Versus Electrocardiogram Artifact

A diphasic or triphasic morphology and a periodic occurrence are features that PLEDs and electrocardiogram (ECG) artifact share. Differentiating these waves is straightforward when comparison to an ECG channel is possible. When an ECG channel is not present, the regularity of the intervals between the transients is the key distinguishing feature. PLEDs usually are not nearly as regular in their interval as ECG artifact. This is especially true because the conditions for obtaining an EEG do not produce significant changes in heart rate. Other distinguishing features are distribution and frequency. Although ECG artifact may be unilateral, it often is bilateral and PLEDs are not bilaterally synchronous. Bilateral periodic epileptiform discharges (BiPEDs) are bilaterally synchronous, but they have large, bifrontal fields. ECG artifact usually is maximal in the two temporal regions. Frequency is a less reliable means for differentiation. Most ECG artifact will be at 1 Hz or faster because a heart rate slower than 60 beats per minute is atypical. In contrast, PLEDs usually occur with intervals greater than 1 second. However, the interval between PLEDs varies, especially across different etiologies.

Versus External Device Artifact

When an external device causes intermittent artifact, it often has a regular interval and may be similar to PEDs in its periodicity. However, this type of artifact rarely has the diphasic or triphasic morphology of PEDs and usually has a distribution that is highly unusual for PEDs. External device artifact often does not have a distribution consistent with cerebrally generated waves. Instead, it may be generalized or confined to specific electrodes.

Versus Interictal Epileptiform Discharges

Because PLEDs may have morphologic features of IEDs, differentiation depends on the presence of periodic recurrence. IEDs also may recur but most commonly do so sporadically. Recurring discharges that are separated by intervals that range from less than 1 second to greater than several minutes are likely to be IEDs. Although PLEDs may be absent for portions of an EEG, they typically recur at least every few seconds when they are present.

Co-occurring Waves

The clinical states that produce PLEDs usually also cause background slowing with either disorganization or synchrony. Either type of slowing is abnormal and contrasts with normal background activity. Because of close temporal associations with myoclonus, muscle and movement artifact may be time-locked with PLEDs (221).

Clinical Significance

PLEDs are a sign that usually indicates a focal pathology that is acute or subacute, almost always affecting cerebral cortex, and more likely to occur in the context of co-existing metabolic abnormality (61,246–248). Exceptional cases of PLEDs due to caudate or thalamic pathology or purely metabolic abnormality have been reported (249–251). Overall, the significance of PLEDs is the same in children as in adults when considered in the context of their underlying cause (252,253).

PLEDs usually last days to weeks and rarely may last years (7,61,254). Their occurrence is accompanied by co-localized focal deficit in about 80% of instances (232). Cortical stroke is responsible for almost half of the incidence of PLEDs, and tumors and infections are each responsible for almost another 20% (118,255). Among strokes, embolism and watershed distributions are more likely to produce PLEDs than thrombosis and single vessel territo-

ries. Strokes with a watershed distribution are more likely to produce PLEDs at the midline. Other causes include cerebral infections (especially viral), prion diseases, extraaxial hematomas, and epilepsy (254–257). Less commonly, they are caused by Alzheimer's disease; mitochondrial disease; multiple sclerosis; and intoxication with medications including baclofen, lithium, levodopa, and ifosfamide (258–261). Trauma without subsequent hemorrhage is a rare cause for PLEDs (96). Regardless of the cause, PLEDs indicate a clinically significant risk for seizures and may sometimes evolve into ictal rhythms (7). Whether or not the PLEDs evolve into an ictal rhythm, seizures occur in up to about 80% of patients with PLEDs, with focal motor seizures as the most common seizure type to occur (232,244,255,262). The seizures are not usually generalized and may be subtle, especially because 20% of those with PLEDs are comatose and almost all of the remaining 80% have impaired consciousness.

Among infectious diseases, herpes simplex encephalitis (HSE) is the most likely to produce PLEDs; most HSE cases demonstrate PLEDs at some point along their course (263). This is almost always within a week of the onset of symptoms, with disappearance of the PLEDs often within 2 weeks after the onset (264). PLEDs due to HSE almost always are centered over one or both temporal lobes. When they are bilateral, they usually are synchronous or time-locked. Their recurrence interval commonly is 1.5 to 2.5 seconds, and they are almost always within the interdischarge interval range of 1 to 5 seconds (61,264). Furthermore, the interdischarge interval of PLEDs due to viral encephalitides varies significantly less than for other PLED etiologies, but considerable overlap limits the specificity and usefulness of this feature (265). Influenza B and LaCrosse virus are other causes for encephalitis that produce temporal PLEDs (266,267).

Among prion diseases, Creutzfeldt-Jakob disease (CJD) more commonly has PLEDs, and PLEDs are a useful sign to help distinguish CJD from other dementias or progressive encephalopathies (268). Between 67% and 100% of CJD cases demonstrate PLEDs for a self-limited period of time during the disease course (258,269). The PLEDs of CJD are somewhat distinctive because of short interdischarge intervals. In CJD, PLEDs typically recur every 0.5 to 2 seconds, and a rate greater than 1 per second is faster than what typically occurs from other etiologies. The PLEDs of CJD usually are hemispheric with a focal predominance when they first manifest, which may be several months after the clinical onset (258). They tend to be present only during wakefulness and may or may not be accompanied by myoclonus (61). Over months, the PLEDs evolve into BiPEDs with a lower amplitude and greater interdischarge interval. They then are absent as the EEG progresses to more diffuse suppression or polymorphic low delta frequency activity.

Controversy surrounds the issue of whether PLEDs truly are an ictal pattern and merit treatment as seizures. The matter extends beyond the association of PLEDs with simple partial motor seizures and into the common clinical situation of the presence of PLEDs and cognitive impairment with the question of whether nonconvulsive status epilepticus is present (270). Functional imaging studies with positron emission tomography (PET) and single-photon emission computed tomography (SPECT) demonstrate hypermetabolism and hyperperfusion of regions generating PLEDs, and resolution of the imaging abnormalities accompanies clinical improvement with antiepileptic medications (271–274). However, these reports may reflect individual cases more than the norm. Prospectively ob-tained serial EEGs of patients with clinically overt SE may identify PLEDs associated with ictal rhythms and as the only epileptiform abnormality, therefore, as the ictal pattern (275) (Fig. 21–4). One reasonable synthesis of this information could hold that PLEDs are a sign of increased likelihood for seizures and their presence should lead to a more careful ascertainment if seizures are present but that they do not warrant treatment with antiepileptic medications when clinical seizures are not present. An important clinical fact is that patients with PLEDs as an ictal pattern do not uniformly have a poor prognosis. However, the presence of PEDs in the context of status epilepticus indicates a poor prognosis regardless of the etiology for the seizures (276).

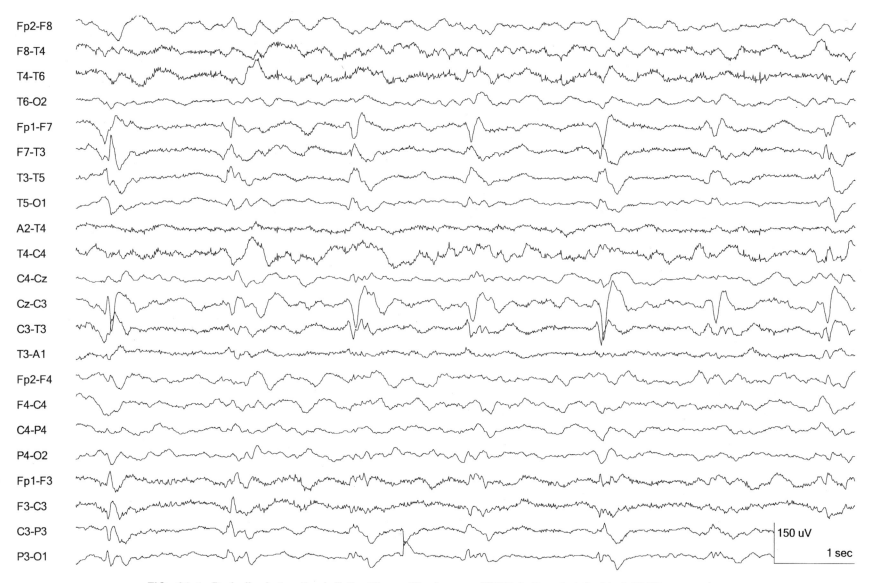

FIG. 21–1. Periodic Lateralized Epileptiform Discharges (PLEDs). Broad, left-sided PLEDs occurring with an interval of about every 1½ seconds in the context of bilateral background slowing. The EEG was obtained after a generalized seizure with brief postictal right-sided paralysis (LFF 1 Hz, HFF 70 Hz).

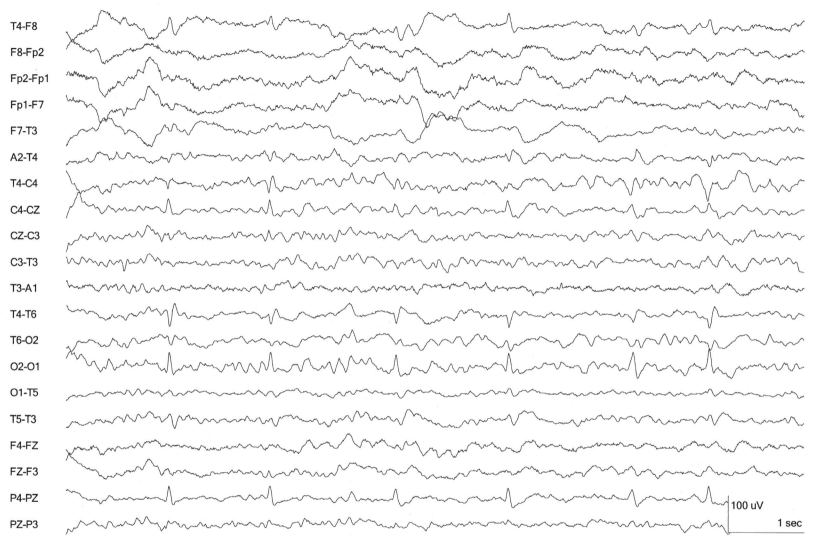

FIG. 21–2. Periodic Lateralized Epileptiform Discharges (PLEDs). The right posterior PLEDs do not emerge from the background as clearly as the PLEDs in Fig. 21–1, and they more closely resemble electrocardiographic (ECG) artifact. However, the field and variability in the morphology and interval are unlike ECG artifact. Slow roving eye movement artifact is present frontally (LFF 1 Hz, HFF 70 Hz).

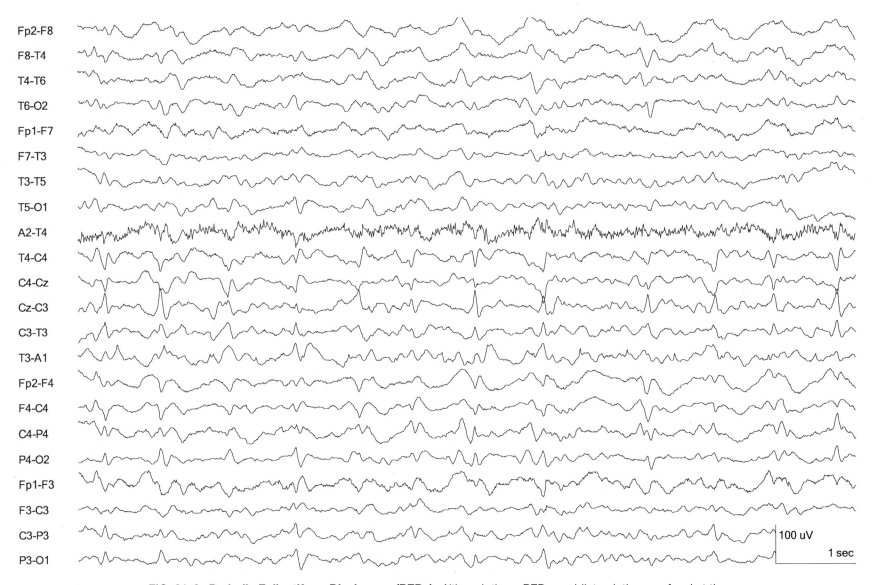

FIG. 21–3. Periodic Epileptiform Discharges (PEDs). Although these PEDs are bilateral, they are focal at the vertex and not truly bilateral periodic epileptiform discharges (BiPEDs). Their 800-msec interval is consistent with the underlying diagnosis of Creutzfeldt-Jakob disease. The patient presented with a clumsy gait and had a magnetic resonance imaging (MRI) scan that demonstrated abnormal signal in parietal parasagittal cortex and bilateral putamens (LFF 1 Hz, HFF 70 Hz).

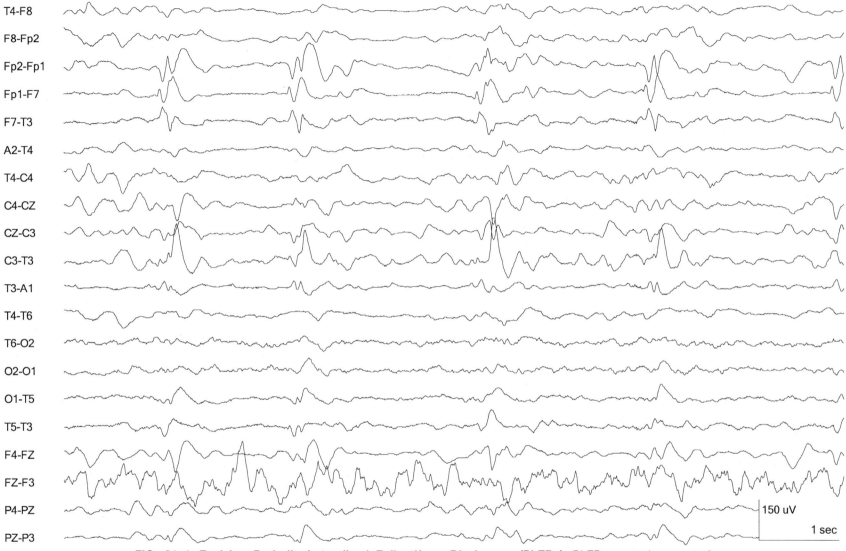

FIG. 21–4. Evolving Periodic Lateralized Epileptiform Discharges (PLEDs). PLEDs occurring every 2 seconds over the left central region evolve into a co-localized 10-Hz rhythm. Although the 10-Hz rhythm continued to evolve similar to an ictal rhythm, no behavioral correlate was noted. The background is diffusely slow. The patient was comatose with multiple medical problems and multifocal cerebrovascular disease. Poor contact of the F3 electrode is producing artifact (LFF 1 Hz, HFF 70 Hz). *Continued*

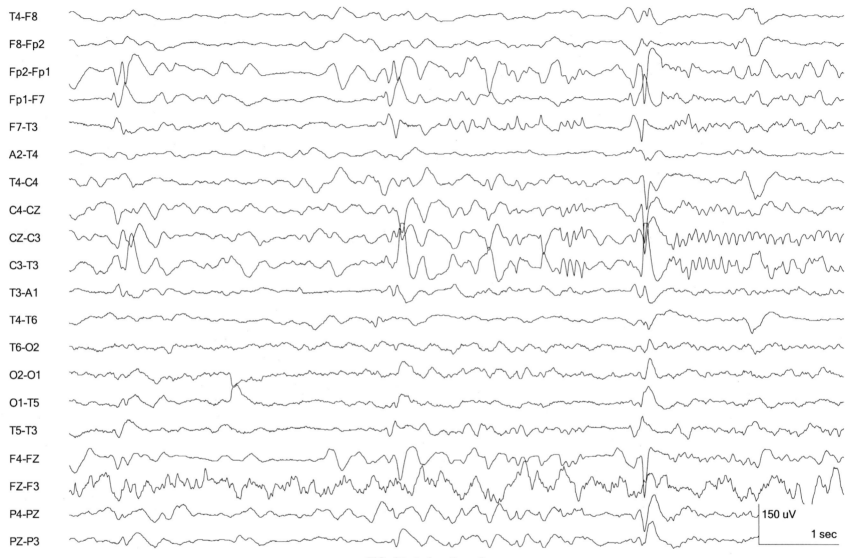

FIG. 21–4. (continued)

BILATERAL INDEPENDENT PERIODIC LATERALIZED EPILEPTIFORM DISCHARGES

Other Names
BIPLEDs
Cerebral bigeminy

Description
Implicit to their definition, PLEDs have a singular focus. However, an EEG may demonstrate PLEDs arising from more than one region. When this occurs, both hemispheres commonly are involved and the pattern is called BIPLEDs (7) (Fig. 21–5). Commonly, there are two foci, but multifocal BIPLEDs also occur (277,278). To be considered independent, each of the PLED patterns within the one EEG must be asynchronous and have a different localization. Independent PLEDs usually also differ in morphology and recurrence rate (9). The descriptive features for the waves of BIPLEDs are the same as for PLEDs.

Distinguishing Features
See PLEDs.

Co-occurring Waves
See PLEDs.

Clinical Significance
The causes of BIPLEDs are the same as for PLEDs but are skewed toward the more multifocal or diffuse etiologies (7,232,279,280). Together, cerebral infections and anoxia are the etiologies in most cases (281). This association is manifested in a lower rate of focal deficit and a greater rate of coma and death than is observed with PLEDs. Among those with BIPLEDs, focal deficit occurs in about 10% and coma in about 70%. BIPLEDs have mortality rates of about 60%, which is about twice the overall rate for PLEDs (280,281). Seizures are less common with BIPLEDs, with an incidence of about 30% (232). BIPLEDs due to HSE often develop sequentially, with the initial side of infection first manifesting PLEDs and first having them resolve (264).

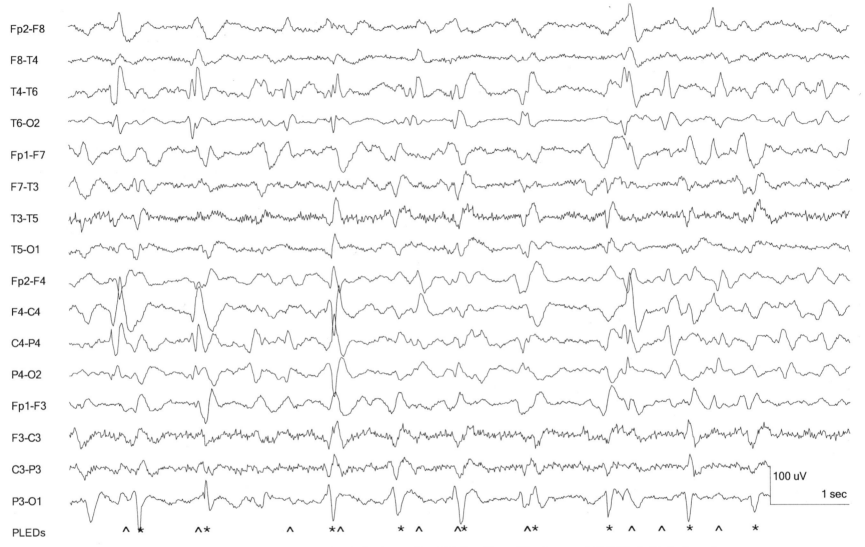

FIG. 21–5. Bilateral Independent Periodic Lateralized Epileptiform Discharges (BIPLEDs). Periodic epileptiform discharges are present with foci over the right posterior temporal and left posterior parasagittal regions. In addition to location, the two patterns are differentiated by morphology and asynchronous occurrence. The occurrences of the right-sided periodic lateralized epileptiform discharges (PLEDs) are indicated by the carets (^), and those of the left-sided PLEDs by the asterisks (*). The EEG corresponds to coma related to multifocal cerebrovascular disease and multiple metabolic abnormalities (LFF 1 Hz, HFF 70 Hz).

BILATERAL PERIODIC EPILEPTIFORM DISCHARGES

Other Names
BiPEDs
Generalized periodic epileptiform discharges

Description
When periodic epileptiform discharges occur symmetrically and synchronously across both hemispheres, they are termed BiPEDs (Figs. 21–6 and 21–7). These are distinguished from BIPLEDs, which have bilateral, asynchronous, and lateralized PEDs. Although several features differ, BiPEDs may be considered a generalized form of PLEDs and BIPLEDs may be considered as a multifocal form. Although they are generalized, BiPEDs tend to be maximal in the midfrontal region (61). Compared to PLEDs, BiPEDs usually contain less sharply contoured elements prior to the slow wave, and their etiologies vary in amplitude, duration, and interdischarge interval to a larger extent than PLEDs. Much of the variation is attributable to subacute sclerosing panencephalitis (SSPE), which is associated with BiPEDs of very high amplitude, longer duration, and long interdischarge interval (Fig. 21–8). The BiPEDs of SSPE have an average amplitude of 500 μV and commonly range from 100 to 1,000 μV (61). However, they may be as high as 1,500 μV. Their duration ranges from 0.5 to 3 seconds, and they commonly recur every 3 to 20 seconds (7,128). Early in the course of SSPE, BiPEDs may recur as infrequently as every 5 minutes (282). The occurrence of BiPEDs with such long interdischarge intervals is so characteristic of SSPE that it is pathognomonic (283). Another characteristic feature of BiPEDs in SSPE is asynchrony with about 15% of instances having marked asymmetry to the PED (284). BiPEDs due to diffuse etiologies other than SSPE, such as cerebral anoxia, usually have recurrence rates and amplitudes similar to PLEDs.

Distinguishing Features
Versus Burst-Suppression Pattern

Similar to burst-suppression pattern (BSP), BiPEDs constitute an abruptly recurring pattern that includes spikes or sharps and higher amplitude than the background. Furthermore, many clinical situations that produce BSP instead may be accompanied by BiPEDs. Differentiating these two patterns rests mostly on morphology. Unlike the bursts of BSP, BiPEDs typically have a more conserved morphology that also includes a recurring relationship between sharply contoured transients (spikes or sharp waves) and slow waves. Moreover, the relationship among the wave elements is epileptiform with the slow wave following a sharp wave or one or more spikes. Occasionally, bursts are morphologically conserved, but they comprise multiple sharply contoured waves and slow waves without the epileptiform pattern (90).

Versus Triphasic Waves

Although BiPEDs are typically generalized, they usually have a frontal predominance that is similar to the frontal field of TW. The wave morphology and the recurrence pattern are the two principal differentiating features. As epileptiform discharges, BiPEDs are triphasic in morphology; however, their waveform is more similar to epileptic discharges than is the waveform of TW. As such, BiPEDs have a more sharply contoured initiating spike or sharp wave and an overall shorter duration. They also differ from TW by recurring with brief intervals of background activity separating the individual waves. Thus, BiPEDs recur as individual discharges, which differs from the trains of repetitions found with TW. Furthermore, the intervals between the individual waves that comprise BiPEDs tend to be similar in duration. This gives BiPEDs their periodicity. The intervals between trains of TW are inconsistent. TW's usual occurrence with an anterior-to-posterior (AP) lag is another differentiating feature. This is manifested by a slightly earlier occurrence of each wave in the more anterior channels.

Co-occurring Waves
The background activity accompanying BiPEDs usually is disorganized, generalized theta or delta frequency range activity (7,61). When anoxia is the cause for the BiPEDs, the background may be continuously or episodically suppressed or demonstrate electrocerebral inactivity (ECI). Although BiPEDs often are best formed in the waking state, the EEG may not show clear evidence of wakefulness without direct comparison to behavioral sleep. When compared, wakefulness may demonstrate a greater component of frequencies in the alpha range.

Especially with SSPE, the epileptiform discharges are almost always accompanied by myoclonus. However, the muscle or movement artifact of the myoclonus may be displaced from the epileptiform discharge by 200 to 800 msec, and the displacement may be either to before or after the discharge.

Clinical Significance
Similar to other abnormal and generalized EEG patterns, BiPEDs are produced by diffuse pathologic conditions. However, BiPEDs tend to occur with the

diffuse pathologies that are more likely to produce structural change to the brain (285). This contrasts with TW or frontal intermittent rhythmic delta activity (FIRDA), which classically are more likely to accompany potentially reversible metabolic abnormalities. Cerebral anoxia, HSE, CJD, SSPE, and rarely Alzheimer's disease all produce BiPEDs but do so at different points along their natural histories. Cerebral anoxia is associated with BiPEDs soon after the injury and when it has been sufficiently severe to produce coma. Although it is a nonprogressive encephalopathy, cerebral anoxia's EEG may progress from BiPEDs to diffuse theta or delta frequency activity, BSP, or ECI. Like PLEDs, BiPEDs usually are a temporary pattern that accompanies acute and subacute states. The direction of the progression is more prognostic for recovery than the presence of BiPEDs alone because BiPEDs do not indicate as poor a prognosis as BSP or ECI (286). HSE and CJD progress to BiPEDs from PLEDs, so BiPEDs reflect a more severe state and relatively later point in the disease course. In the late stages of CJD, BiPEDs are replaced by BSP or attenuated activity. BiPEDs occur late in the course of Alzheimer's disease. The EEG during much of the course of Alzheimer's disease demonstrates generalized slowing that progressively worsens. For SSPE, BiPEDs are a nearly specific sign of the second stage of the disease and accompany the time when clinical diagnosis becomes more clear (61). The initial stage of SSPE is accompanied by diffuse slowing and less severe neurologic impairment. By the third stage, the BiPEDs are absent, the background comprises diffuse attenuation or a BSP, and neurologic impairment is severe.

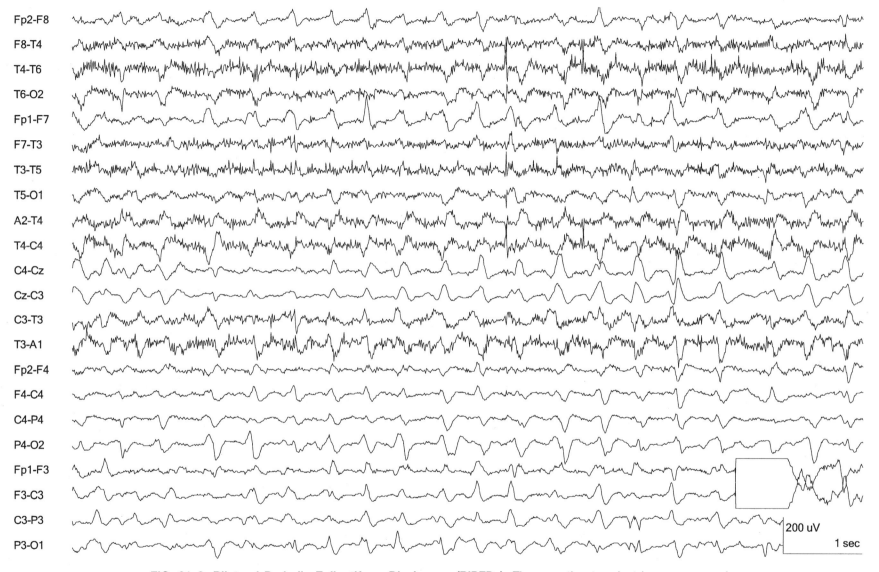

FIG. 21–6. Bilateral Periodic Epileptiform Discharges (BiPEDs). The repeating transient has a preserved morphology and interdischarge interval and is bilaterally synchronous without focus. Unlike an ictal pattern, the BiPEDs are not evolving. The EEG corresponds to a coma due to multiple medical problems that resolved with treatment (LFF 1 Hz, HFF 70 Hz).

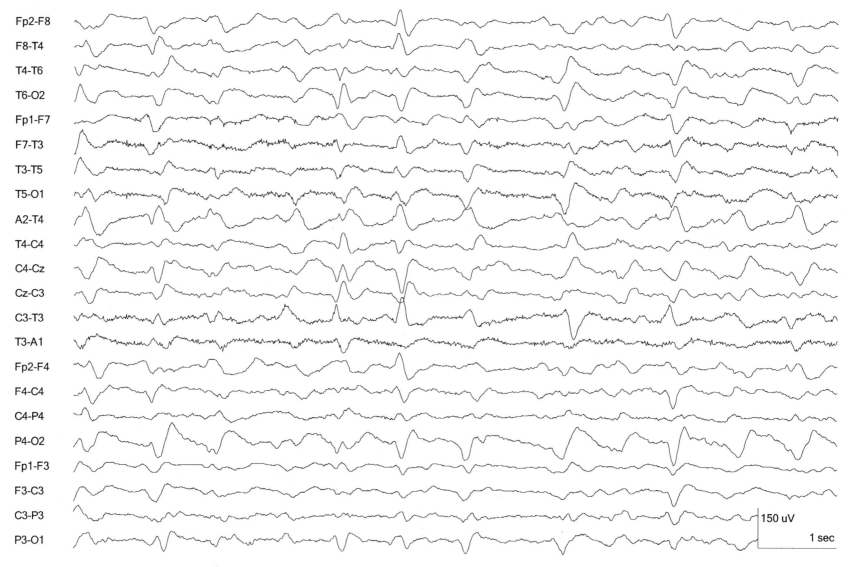

FIG. 21–7. Bilateral Periodic Epileptiform Discharges (BiPEDs). The transients have an interval that varies slightly and a bilateral field that is inconsistently symmetric, but the preserved morphology, recurrence pattern, and overall distribution are typical of BiPEDs. The EEG corresponds to encephalopathy due to cardiac insufficiency (LFF 1 Hz, HFF 70 Hz).

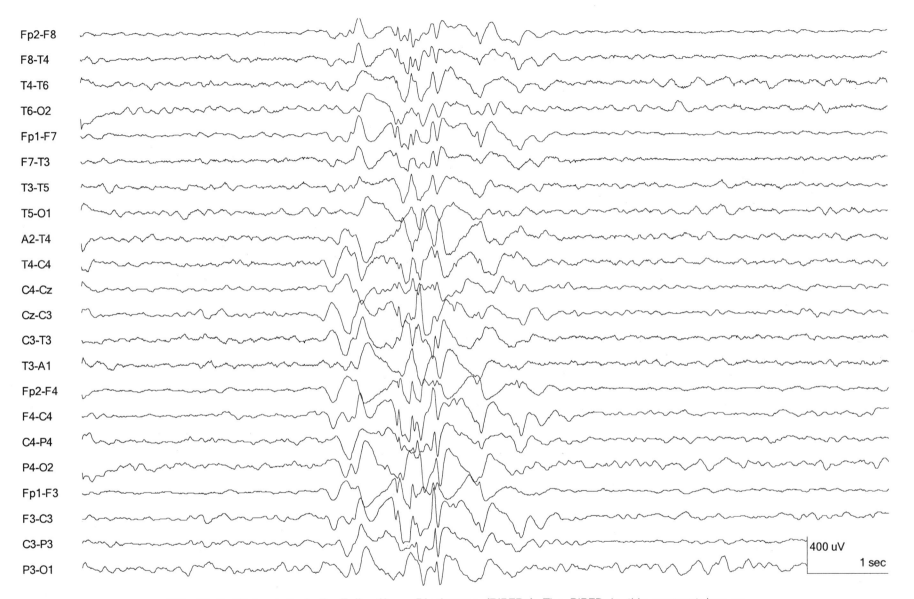

FIG. 21–8. Bilateral Periodic Epileptiform Discharges (BiPEDs). The BiPED in this segment has an approximate amplitude of 550 μV and recurs with similar morphology every 10 to 20 seconds. The EEG corresponds to subacute sclerosing panencephalitis and is the same patient as in Figs. 10–3 and 10–4 but was obtained 3 weeks earlier than Fig. 10–3 (LFF 1 Hz, HFF 70 Hz).

CHAPTER 22

Phantom Spike and Wave

PHANTOM SPIKE AND WAVE

Other Names
6 per second spike and (slow) wave
Miniature spike and wave
Wave and phantom spike
Larval spike and wave

Description
The phantom spike and wave (PhSW) takes its name from the low-amplitude, often not clearly discernible, spike within a repeating spike and slow wave complex (Fig. 22–1). To clarify the meaning of the name, the alternative "wave and phantom spike" also has put forward. When the spike element is visible and the frequency is 6 per second, the PhSW is easily distinguished from any other wave. However, the absence of a discernible spike is the most likely cause for misidentification. Without the spike, the wave appears to be a paroxysmal 6-Hz rhythm.

Morphologically, the pattern is similar to the 3 per second spike and wave complex that may accompany primary generalized epilepsies and it has been called a miniature version of the 3 per second pattern. The crucial differences simply are the faster frequency, which usually is 5 to 6 per second, and the low amplitude of the spike and the wave. However, these differences are not inviolable and some overlap exists with generalized interictal epileptiform discharges (IEDs). That is about 25% of PhSW patterns have repetition rates of 4 per second, which is a common rate for generalized IEDs, and generalized IEDs may have low-amplitude spikes that may appear as notches within the slow wave. The spike of PhSW is more consistently small and has an amplitude that usually is less than 40 µV and a duration that usually is shorter than 30 msec. About 25% of spikes are less than 25 µV, which is why the spike sometimes is not visible. The slow wave of PhSW typically is less than 50 µV; thus it differs more significantly from the higher amplitude slow waves of generalized IEDs than does the spike.

The typical manifestation of PhSW is as a bisynchronous burst that lasts up to 2 seconds, but this manifestation segregates into two types. The two types are distinguished according to four features: amplitude of wave, location of wave, gender of patient, and state of patient. One form is called waking, high amplitude spike, anterior, male (WHAM), and the other is called female, occipital, low amplitude spike, and drowsy (FOLD). High-amplitude spikes are defined as greater than 45 µV. Although PhSW usually is either frontally or occipitally predominant, about 20% of occurrences are generalized.

PhSW is an uncommon pattern that occurs slightly more often in women. Overall, it occurs during 0.5 to 1% of electroencephalograms (EEGs). The age range during which it is most likely to occur is adolescence and young adulthood, with an occurrence rate in this group of 2.5%. The pattern may occur in wakefulness and sleep, but it is most likely to occur in drowsiness.

Distinguishing Features
Versus Fourteen and Six Positive Bursts

When fourteen and six positive bursts (14&6) occurs bisynchronously at 6 Hz, it is similar to the PhSW's posterior variant (137). Both patterns occur in children during drowsiness and have durations typically less than 2 seconds. The distribution of the field is the key distinguishing feature; PhSW is maximal along the midline and 14&6 is lateralized. Other differentiating features are the PhSW's diphasic morphology and low-amplitude spike. The 14&6 pattern is monophasic.

Versus Hympnopompic and Hypnagogic Hypersynchrony

Hypersynchronizations into the theta frequency range during state changes between wakefulness to drowsiness share a theta range, sinusoidal, bifrontal pattern with the PhSW, but the two patterns may be differentiated through their amplitude and distribution. Hypersynchrony usually has an amplitude greater than the preceding background and a distribution that is generalized. Hypersynchrony also often recurs during the same recording, and it usually does so without occurring at the same frequency. Therefore, finding several similar waves during the state transitions that differ in frequency may indicate hypersynchronization as the underlying entity. Furthermore, hypersynchrony that is well formed enough to mimic PhSW usually occurs in early childhood, an age at which PhSW is uncommon.

Versus Interictal Epileptiform Discharges

Frequency and morphologic overlap exists between generalized IEDs and PhSW. The amplitude difference between these two patterns, especially compared to the record's background amplitude, is the best means to distinguish them from each other. Less consistent, but still possibly helpful features, include PhSW's shorter duration and less generalized distribution (7).

Co-occurring Waves

Electrographic features of drowsiness may accompany PhSW. These may include slowing or absence of a posterior dominant rhythm, slow roving ocular movements, theta frequency activity in the central or temporal regions, and beta in the central region. However, PhSW may occur in any state; thus, the signs of drowsiness are not necessarily present. About 22% of EEGs with PhSW also demonstrate 14&6, and about 20% have epileptiform abnormality, either 3 per second spike and wave or focal spikes. The WHAM form is the type that more commonly has co-occurring epileptiform abnormality.

Clinical Significance

The prevalence of epilepsy is increased among individuals with PhSW with about 50% of such individuals having epilepsy, but these estimates arise from clinical EEG lab series and not from random populations (287). Thus, they are based on a population with a higher prevalence of epilepsy than the population as a whole. Between the two forms of PhSW, WHAM has a greater prevalence of epilepsy with a rate of about 80%. The rate for the FOLD form is about 30%. Part of the increased rate for the WHAM form may be due to overlap with the frontal fast spike and wave complex (usually 4 to 5 Hz) that may accompany primary generalized epilepsies. About half of the epilepsies that accompany PhSW are manifested by generalized tonic-clonic seizures. However, WHAM PhSW may briefly impair cognition alone. Reaction time is increased at the times of WHAM PhSW discharges.

The administration and withdrawal of sedatives and diphenhydramine also may produce PhSW (61,288).

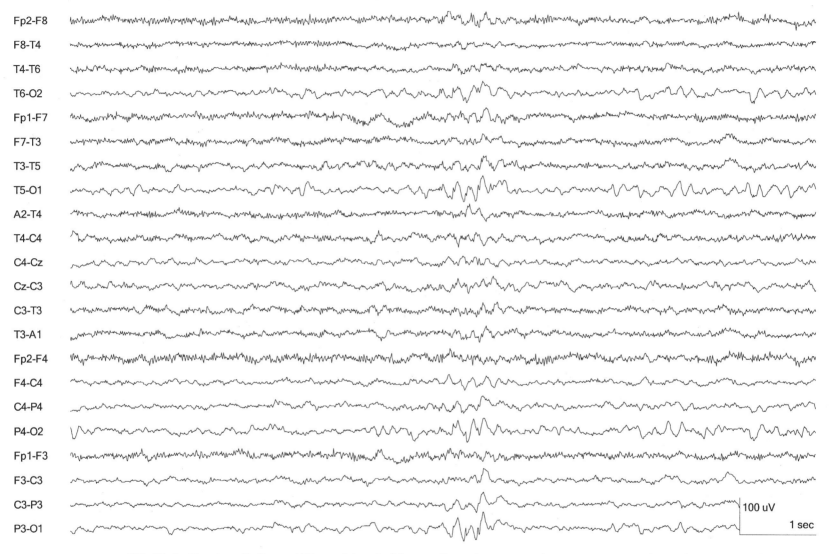

FIG. 22–1. Phantom Spike and Wave. A burst of three spike and wave complexes occur across the occiput over a period of almost a half second. The location of the discharges, the female gender of the patient, and the drowsy state, which is reflected in the background, are consistent with the female, occipital, low-amplitude spike, and drowsy (FOLD) form of phantom spike and wave. The waves average 45 µV and, therefore, are borderline for low amplitude (LFF 1 Hz, HFF 70 Hz).

CHAPTER 23

Photic Stimulation Responses

PHOTIC DRIVING RESPONSE

Other Names
Occipital driving response

Description
Visual stimulation with a flashing strobe commonly produces sharply contoured, positive, monophasic transients that follow each stimulation by 80 to 150 msec. This is called a photic driving response (7) (Figs. 23–1 and 23–2). The transients usually have the same frequency as the stimulation but also may be a harmonic or a subharmonic of it (Fig. 23–3). Photic driving responses are best elicited with the eyes closed or with stimulation using red light (143). The stimulation frequency that is most likely to produce a response varies with age and usually is close to the frequency of the individual's alpha rhythm but not necessarily the same frequency (10). Moreover, the photic driving response's amplitude is maximal with stimulation frequencies close to the alpha rhythm's frequency and decreases with greater differences between the stimulation frequency and alpha rhythm. Supporting this association with the alpha rhythm, the photic driving response may be seen in individuals as young as 3 months, which is about the age when an alpha rhythm first develops. However, the alpha rhythm in infants and young children is not within the alpha frequency range. It is in the theta range, and the frequencies that elicit the photic driving response also are in the theta frequency range until early childhood when the alpha rhythm reaches the alpha frequency band (13). In general, photic driving responses may occur at frequencies as broad as from 5 to 30 Hz, and stimulation frequencies less than 3 Hz rarely produce a response (7).

The field of the photic driving response is mainly bilateral occipital but may extend to include the posterior temporal regions. Extension to more anterior regions is uncommon but occurs. The driving response's amplitude is low until about 6 years and is similar to that of the alpha rhythm from youth to middle adulthood. In later adulthood, the amplitude decreases. Also similar to the alpha rhythm, photic driving responses may be asymmetric with greater amplitude on the right (9).

Distinguishing Features
Versus Lambda Waves

Morphologically, photic driving responses are similar to lambda waves and appear more similar if they occur inconsistently, such that they do not have a fixed interval. Identifying transients as a photic driving response depends on notation on the electroencephalogram (EEG) record that indicates the photic stimulation frequency and the moments that the strobe discharges.

Versus Photomyogenic Response

Although the photomyogenic response usually has an anterior field, occasionally it includes head movements that produce posterior artifact from contact between the head and the surface below it. Because the posterior artifact is due to movement and not individual motor unit potentials, they may be blunt enough to resemble the photic driving response. Furthermore, they will be time-locked with stimulation like the photic driving response. Differentiation depends on morphology and field. Neither the morphology nor the field of the driving response waveforms vary during one stimulation or among multiple stimulation frequencies, whereas the photomyogenic response movement artifact's waveform and location depends on the more variable movement of the head.

Versus Photoparoxysmal Response

When the photic driving response is a harmonic of the stimulation frequency, the elicited transients have the duration of spikes. However, the absence of after-going slow waves is a straightforward differentiating feature from epileptiform discharges. Identifying if a harmonic relationship exists by comparing the transient's frequency to the stimulation frequency also may differentiate these waves because photoparoxysmal responses usually do not occur with frequencies related to the stimulation frequency. Furthermore, extension of the response beyond the stimulation is helpful because this does not occur with photic driving responses.

Co-occurring Waves

When photic stimulation is performed during wakefulness with eyes closed, an alpha rhythm is present within the region of the driving response. Frontal artifact that is synchronized with the stimulation also may be present, as is produced by either an electromyographic response or a photoelectric effect.

Clinical Significance

A bilateral photic driving response at a frequency close to the patient's alpha rhythm is a normal phenomenon but is not necessary for an EEG to be considered normal. The absence of a photic driving response is a common normal variant that is more common in the elderly (7). Medications may affect whether a photic driving response is present; adrenergic blocking drugs augment the response and adrenergic stimulants diminish it (289,290). A photic driving response at a frequency less than 3 Hz may be abnormal with significance similar to focal slowing, and a response at a frequency greater than 20 Hz may be associated specifically with migraine (291). Asymmetry to the photic driving response is not necessarily abnormal and should be compared to the symmetry of other EEG features, such as the alpha rhythm. If the driving response's asymmetry is consistent with the normal asymmetries in other features, then it most likely also is normal. In the absence of another asymmetry, asymmetric photic stimulation responses may be a sign of abnormality. However, they also may be due to gaze deviation away from the strobe or atypical calcarine cortex anatomy with a subsequent abnormal dipole orientation. Moreover, abnormal asymmetry does not indicate which side is abnormal. Decreased amplitude may result from destructive lesions, and increased amplitude may result from irritative ones. An abnormal unilateral loss of a photic driving response is more easily interpreted and indicates pathology ipsilateral to the side without the response.

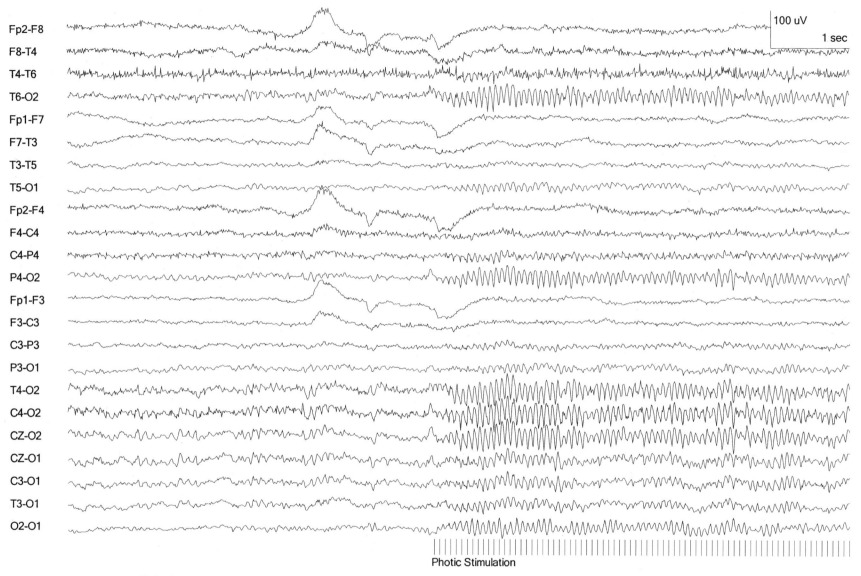

100 uV

1 sec

Fp2-F8
F8-T4
T4-T6
T6-O2
Fp1-F7
F7-T3
T3-T5
T5-O1
Fp2-F4
F4-C4
C4-P4
P4-O2
Fp1-F3
F3-C3
C3-P3
P3-O1
T4-O2
C4-O2
CZ-O2
CZ-O1
C3-O1
T3-O1
O2-O1

Photic Stimulation

FIG. 23–1. Photic Driving Response. Photic stimulation at 14 Hz begins where noted and produces 14-Hz bioccipital driving with a minor amplitude asymmetry. Blink artifact precedes the stimulation (LFF 1 Hz, HFF 70 Hz).

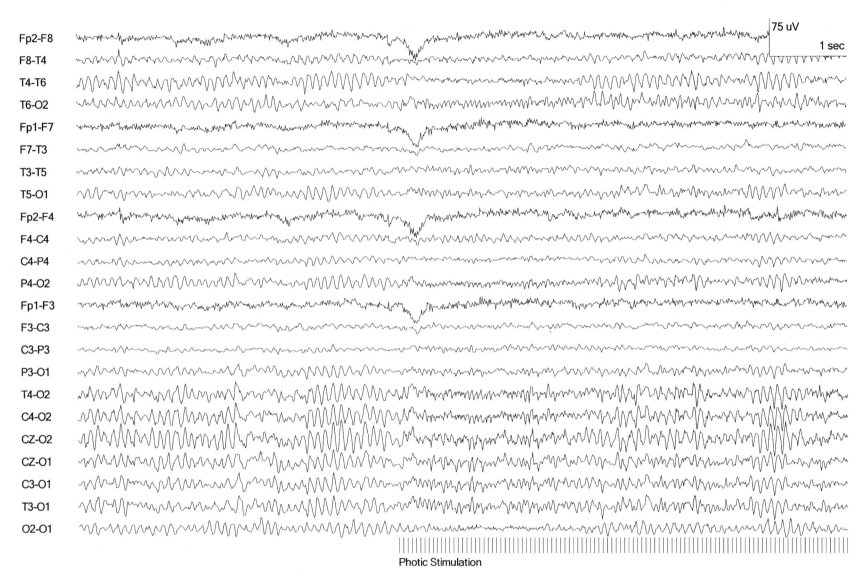

FIG. 23–2. Photic Driving Response. Photic stimulation at 18 Hz begins where noted with an 18-Hz driving response and slows to a subharmonic of 9 Hz after 2 seconds. The driving response replaces the alpha rhythm that precedes it. The blink artifact at the start of stimulation indicates a startle response because the eyes remain closed during stimulation (LFF 1 Hz, HFF 70 Hz).

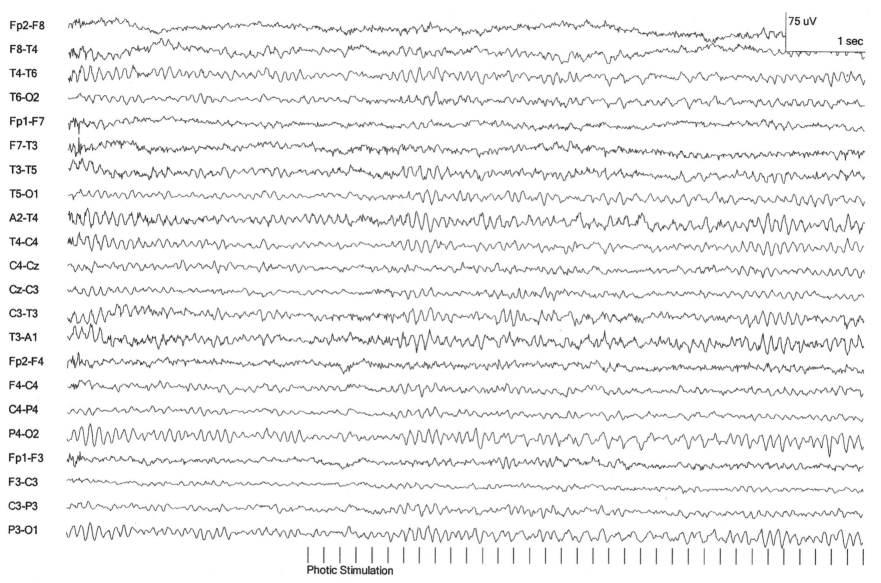

FIG. 23–3. Photic Driving Response. A poorly formed 5-Hz driving response becomes evident shortly after photic stimulation at 10 Hz begins. The response is less clear in this montage, because it does not include channels with an occipital reference and double distance electrodes (LFF 1 Hz, HFF 70 Hz).

PHOTOPAROXYSMAL RESPONSE

Other Names
Photoconvulsive
Photoepileptiform

Description
The photic stimulation procedure that produces a photic driving response also may elicit epileptiform discharges (Figs. 23–4 and 23–5). Such an occurrence is termed a photoparoxysmal response. Photoparoxysmal responses most commonly occur with stimulation frequencies higher than the alpha rhythm's frequency and are more easily elicited when stimulation is performed with the eyes opened and delivered to binocular central vision. Like the photic driving response, red light is most effective (292). In general, 15 Hz is the frequency most likely to elicit a photoparoxysmal response with the eyes opened and 20 Hz if the eyes are closed (143).

The epileptiform discharges do not recur at the same frequency as the stimulation and may vary in their frequency during a burst. They almost always have a spike and slow wave or polyspike and slow wave morphology and a bilateral, synchronous field (143). However, the field is not always occipital. Instead, it may be generalized or maximal over bilateral frontal or central regions. Generalized photoparoxysmal responses are more likely to occur with children. Regardless of the field, photoparoxysmal responses may outlast the stimulation by several seconds, and the occurrence of this has no clinical significance (7,293). With repeat stimulation, the threshold for eliciting a photoparoxysmal response decreases and the trains of discharges become longer and are more likely to have accompanying clinical signs, such as myoclonus, impairment of consciousness, or a generalized seizure (9).

Distinguishing Features
Versus Photomyogenic Artifact

Because photoparoxysmal responses may have a maximal field frontally, their field may overlap with that of photomyogenic artifact. Furthermore, photomyogenic artifact has a spike-like morphology due to its basis as individual motor unit potentials. Differentiating the two patterns depends on morphologic differences and the degree of association between the transients and the flashing stimulation. Photomyogenic artifact is very sharply contoured and lacks aftergoing slow waves. Furthermore, it almost always occurs across a broad range of stimulation frequencies, commonly at almost every stimulation frequency used, and does not persist beyond the period of stimulation. This contrasts with photoparoxysmal responses that typically occur at one or two stimulation frequencies and may continue beyond the stimulation interval. Complicating the process of distinguishing these waveforms is the possibility of the two occurring simultaneously. Generalized seizures that follow photoparoxysmal responses also may follow brief bursts of myoclonus with myoclonus' associated photomyogenic artifact.

Versus Photic Driving Response

When the photic driving response is a harmonic of the stimulation frequency, the elicited transients have the duration of spikes. However, the absence of after-going slow waves is a straightforward differentiating feature from epileptiform discharges. Identifying if a harmonic relationship exists also may differentiate these waves because photoparoxysmal responses usually do not occur with frequencies related to the stimulation frequency. Furthermore, extension of the response beyond the stimulation is helpful because this does not occur with photic driving responses.

Co-occurring Waves
Because photoparoxysmal responses are associated with generalized epilepsy syndromes, generalized interictal epileptiform discharges (IEDs) may occur independently to the responses. These most commonly have a frequency of 4 to 5 Hz (150). Photoparoxysmal responses are accompanied by muscle and movement artifact if myoclonus occurs.

Clinical Significance
Although photoparoxysmal responses may occur in individuals without spontaneous seizures (13,294), they usually represent an interictal epileptiform abnormality (294). However, their specificity as an epileptiform abnormality is less than IEDs because they are more common in the general population than other IEDs. They have been found in about 2% of healthy adult volunteers and are more common in children (178). As a sign of epilepsy, photoparoxysmal responses are somewhat nonspecific and are present in the EEGs of 1% to 10% of patients with epilepsy (295–297). The highest rate appears to be in the age range from mid childhood through adolescence. Among epilepsy syndromes, they are most common in the idiopathic and symptomatic generalized syndromes (7,298). Juvenile myoclonic epilepsy has the highest prevalence of

photoparoxysmal responses with approximately 17% of patients demonstrating one (299). However, localization-related epilepsies in which the abnormality is occipital also may produce a photoparoxysmal response. Unilateral photoparoxysmal responses are more indicative of an occipital lobe epilepsy than a idiopathic generalized syndrome (143). Symptomatic generalized epilepsies also may manifest photoparoxysmal responses, with such responses common in Unverricht-Lundborg disease (106). Furthermore, high-amplitude photoparoxysmal responses to stimulation at less than 3 Hz often indicate neuronal ceroid lipofuscinosis. Lastly, photosensitive reflex epilepsies are associated with photoparoxysmal responses.

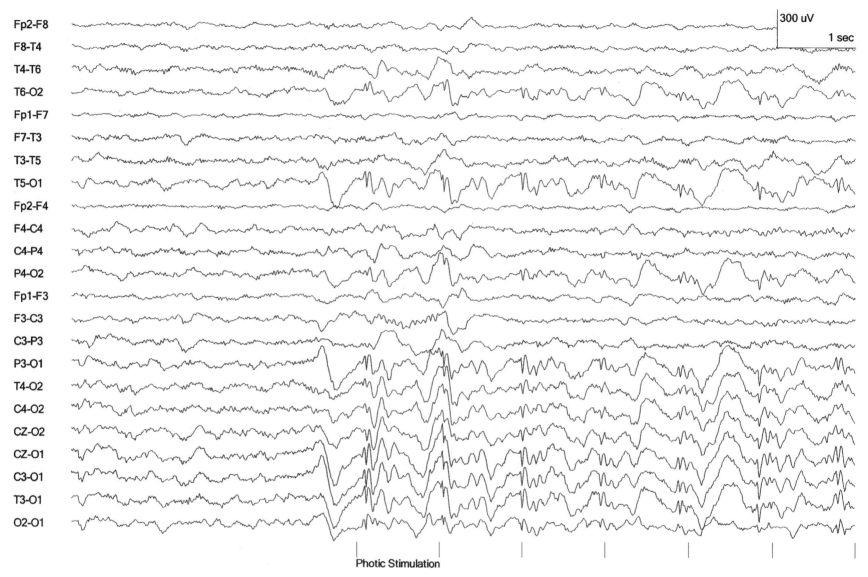

FIG. 23–4. Photoparoxysmal Response. Shortly after 1-Hz photic stimulation begins, individual spike and slow wave complexes develop at the same frequency. The background activity is diffusely slow due to sleep in this infant with normal development and the occurrence of one seizure (LFF 1 Hz, HFF 70 Hz).

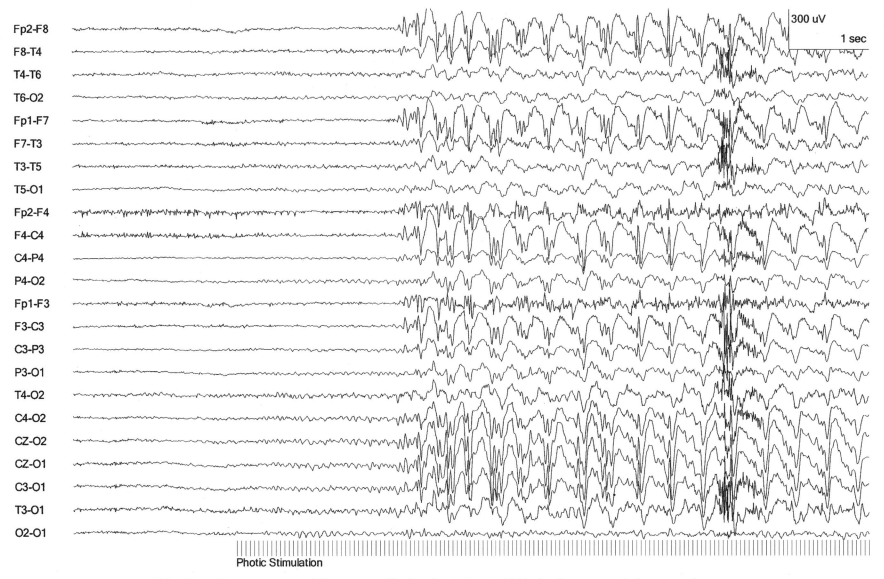

FIG. 23–5. Photoparoxysmal Response. Photic stimulation at 18 Hz begins were noted and produces a bifrontal spike and wave complex that initially has a frequency of 5 Hz and quickly slows to 3 Hz. Light-headedness was reported during the photoparoxysmal response, but no signs of a seizure were present (LFF 1 Hz, HFF 70 Hz).

Positive Occipital Sharp Transients of Sleep

POSITIVE OCCIPITAL SHARP TRANSIENTS OF SLEEP

Other Names
POSTS
Lambdoid waves
Occipital sharp waves of sleep
Rho waves

Description
Positive occipital sharp transients of sleep (POSTS) are what they are named. These transients first occur in late stage I non–REM (NREM) sleep (deep drowsiness) and may persist into slow wave sleep. They are most frequent during the first 30 minutes after sleep onset, and the occurrence of POSTS in REM sleep is rare. Their waveform is characteristic with a positive polarity sharp wave with phase reversal almost always at either the O1 or O2 electrode (Figs. 24–1 and 24–2). They may be either monophasic or diphasic and have a triangular shape with symmetric rising and falling phases. When they are diphasic, the positive peak is prominent and followed by a negative potential of lower amplitude. Their field usually extends across the bilateral occiput and generally is asymmetric. An amplitude asymmetry of 60% is common. Amplitudes usually are between 20 and 75 μV (8), and durations usually are between 80 and 200 msec. They may occur as individual transients and usually recur without periodicity and with a separation of more than 1 second. Just as often, they occur in a train that rarely lasts more than 2 seconds and has up to four to six POSTS per second.

POSTS rarely occur before 3 years and are typically poorly formed in young children. They are most common from adolescence through middle adulthood and become uncommon after 70 years (300). Overall, they are a common finding; the electroencephalograms (EEGs) of about 50% to 80% of healthy adults demonstrate POSTS (301,302).

Distinguishing Features
Versus Cone Waves

POSTS are similar to cone waves in their triangular morphology, occipital distribution, and occurrence in NREM sleep. However, they differ by having a shorter duration, which is typically less than 200 msec, and not demonstrating positivity at the center of their field, which POSTS demonstrate with phase reversals. Cone waves occur only from infancy to mid-childhood, which is a younger age range than POSTS. Unlike cone waves, POSTS also may be diphasic.

Versus Lambda Waves

Morphologically, POSTS are very similar in morphology and distribution to lambda waves. Their key distinguishing feature is the state in which they occur. Lambda waves are produced with active visual exploration, and POSTS only occur in sleep. Another difference is the likelihood of trains with repeating transients. POSTS commonly occur in trains, and lambda waves rarely do.

Versus Interictal Epileptiform Discharges

The unvarying triangular morphology and consistent absence of an after-going slow wave distinguishes POSTS from interictal epileptiform discharges (IEDs). Even when they are sharp waves, IEDs usually are asymmetric and more sharply contoured than POSTS. Although IEDs occur more frequently in the sleep, they typically occur in wakefulness as well. Therefore, identification of a similar wave during wakefulness may help identify it as an IED and not a POSTS.

Co-occurring Waves

POSTS first occur in late stage I NREM and may persist through deeper stages of NREM sleep. Therefore, the surrounding record depicts sleep with a background of diffuse theta to delta frequency range activity, vertex sharp transients, K complexes, and the absence of an alpha rhythm.

Clinical Significance

POSTS are a normal and common finding in individuals with intact central vision (302). They are absent in individuals with visual acuity less than 20/200 but are present in those with constricted visual fields and normal acuity. Their basis may be related to a functional "playback" of visual experiences for processing during sleep (26). This is based on their similarity to lambda waves and the absence of POSTS in individuals with severely impaired central visual acuity (302). However, POSTS differ from lambda waves by lacking an association to oculomotor activity; thus, the similar appearance may be misleading with regard to their functional significance. If they are indeed an indicator of visual playback, the playback is not associated with NREM dreaming because POSTS do not occur more frequently during this experience.

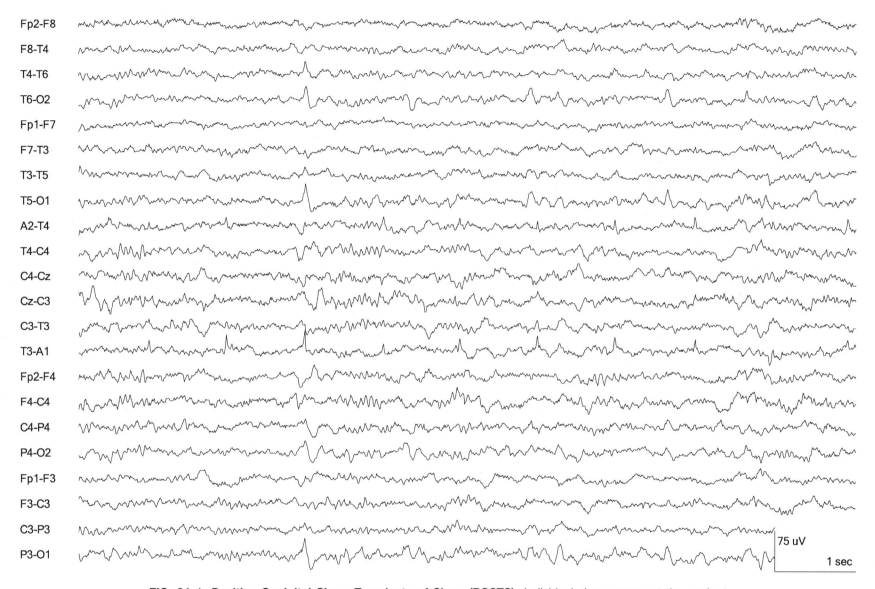

FIG. 24–1. Positive Occipital Sharp Transients of Sleep (POSTS). Individual sharp waves at the occiput have the typical morphology of POSTS, but their end-of-chain location hampers localization and determination of polarity (LFF 1 Hz, HFF 70 Hz).

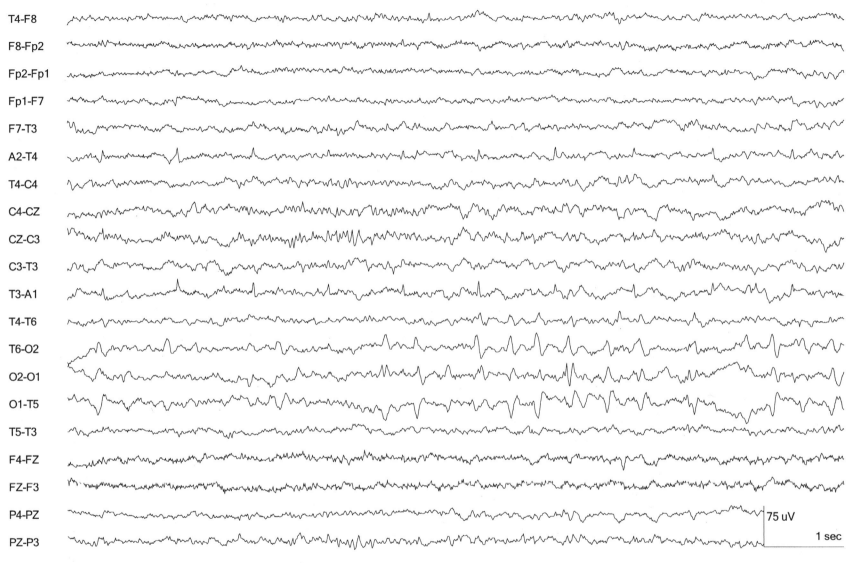

FIG. 24–2. Positive Occipital Sharp Transients of Sleep (POSTS). In a montage that includes a posterior circumferential (hatband) chain, POSTS are more clearly surface positive with foci that shift between the O1 and O2 electrodes. The POSTS in this segment occur in succession but are not in a typical train because of intervening background activity (LFF 1 Hz, HFF 70 Hz).

CHAPTER 25

Posterior Slow Waves of Youth

POSTERIOR SLOW WAVES OF YOUTH

Other Names
Delta de la jeunesse
Youth waves
Polyphasic waves

Description
Posterior slow waves of youth (PSWY) are slow waves that only occur amid the alpha rhythm (AR) (Figs. 25–1 and 25–2). They may either disrupt the AR or be superimposed on it. Similar to the AR, PSWY have a posterior field that is maximum at the occipital poles and present only with the eyes closed in a relaxed wakeful state. They are most clearly depicted with bipolar montages and in channels that include both central and occipital electrodes (14). Their morphology is variable, with durations that usually are between 0.35 and 0.5 seconds and without a consistent polarity (13). Most commonly, they appear as sporadic, interspersed slow waves and may occur in clusters of individual transients that are separated from each other by one to several seconds (7). Less often, they occur in trains, which usually are composed of two or three waves with a frequency of 2 to 3 Hz. Like individual PSWY, the individual waves within a train may vary in duration and morphology, and, because of this, the trains may appear as one polyphasic transient (13,303). Individual PSWY also may appear to be a polyphasic transient if they follow faster background activity. PSWY usually are symmetric and bisynchronous across the occiput but may occur with minor lateralization to one hemisphere. However, they should be symmetric overall with a similar number occurring with right and left lateralizations. An asymmetry greater than 50% is abnormal (14).

As the name indicates, PSWY have a peak prevalence in the young. They occur most commonly between 6 and 12 years and are rare before 2 and after 21 years. Occurrences between 2 and 6 years and between 12 and 21 years are not rare. About 15% of electroencephalograms (EEGs) obtained between 16 and 20 years demonstrate PSWY (14). PSWY are more common in females.

Distinguishing Features
Versus Slow Alpha Rhythm Variant

Similar to the slow alpha variant, PSWY occur only within the AR. However, it may be differentiated by its frequency and morphology. The slow alpha variant is a subharmonic of the AR, with a frequency that is half of the AR's. Therefore, the slow alpha variant is a regular rhythm with a frequency that is at least 4 Hz when the AR is normal. More commonly, the frequency is closer to 5 Hz. Even when PSWY occur in trains, the repetition is not regular due to the varying morphology and the frequency rarely is in the theta range.

Versus Abnormal Delta and Theta Slowing

Abnormal occipital slowing and PSWY are similar in frequency and in the occurrence as individual waves and as repetitions. However, PSWY differs by being present only when the AR also is present. Although abnormal slowing often is best represented in wakefulness because of the greater contrast between itself and the faster frequencies of wakefulness, abnormal occipital slowing is present when the eyes are open and the AR is absent.

Versus Interictal Epileptiform Discharge

Individual waves and brief trains of PSWY occasionally appear as an individual, polyphasic epileptiform transient because of the fusion with faster activity or the morphologic variability of the waves constituting the train. The presence of a polyphasic transient with epileptiform appearance only amid the AR does not provide an irrefutably differentiating feature because the interictal epileptiform discharges (IEDs) of some forms of epilepsy occur only with the eyes closed. The absence of focal slowing of the background also does not always differentiate the two patterns because the focal IEDs of idiopathic epilepsies are not associated with co-localized slowing. Recurrence of the pattern with the same morphology is one means to determine if the wave is an IED. IEDs most often have stereotyped features, and PSWY resembling polyphasic transients are composed of a random succession of waves. The morphology of the apparent slow wave in the polyphasic transient provides another differentiating feature. Because polyphasic transients that are truly PSWY have superimposed alpha activity, faster frequencies ride on the slow wave. The slow wave of an epileptiform complex do not demonstrate a mixture of frequencies.

Versus Intermittent Rhythmic Delta Activity

PSWY resemble occipital intermittent rhythmic delta activity (OIRDA) in distribution, wave duration, and occurrence in childhood. Similar to the waves constituting IRDA, PSWY typically have durations of 0.35 to 0.5 seconds. However, PSWY occur individually and with varying morphology, so they do not have the essential regular, rhythmic features of OIRDA. Furthermore, PSWY interrupt the AR; thus, they are not accompanied by the diffuse slowing that typically is OIRDA's background activity.

Co-occurring Waves
The AR is the key and only consistently accompanying wave.

Clinical Significance
PSWY are a normal variant and have no clinical significance when present or absent.

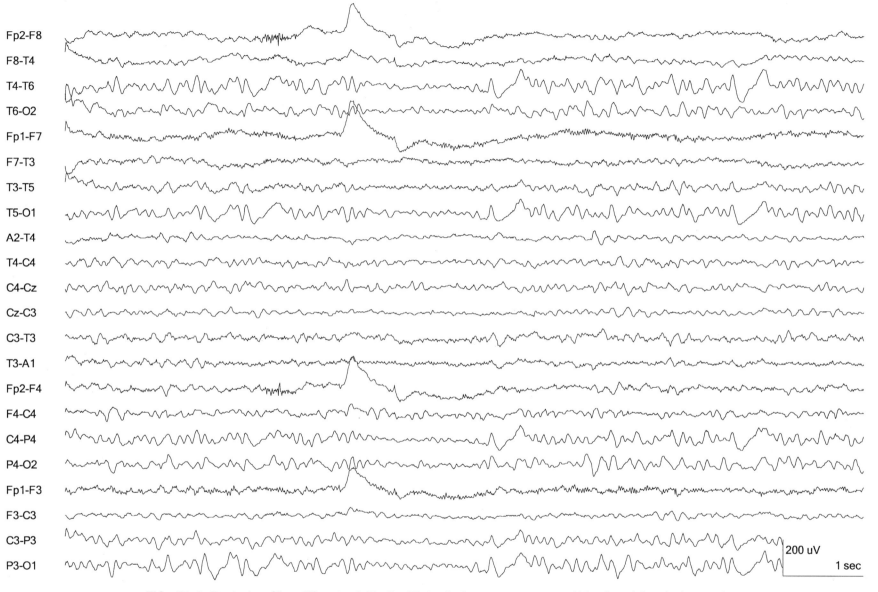

FIG. 25–1. Posterior Slow Waves of Youth. Bilateral slow waves occur within the alpha rhythm and are absent in the middle of the segment when the alpha rhythm is briefly blocked by eye opening (LFF 1 Hz, HFF 70 Hz).

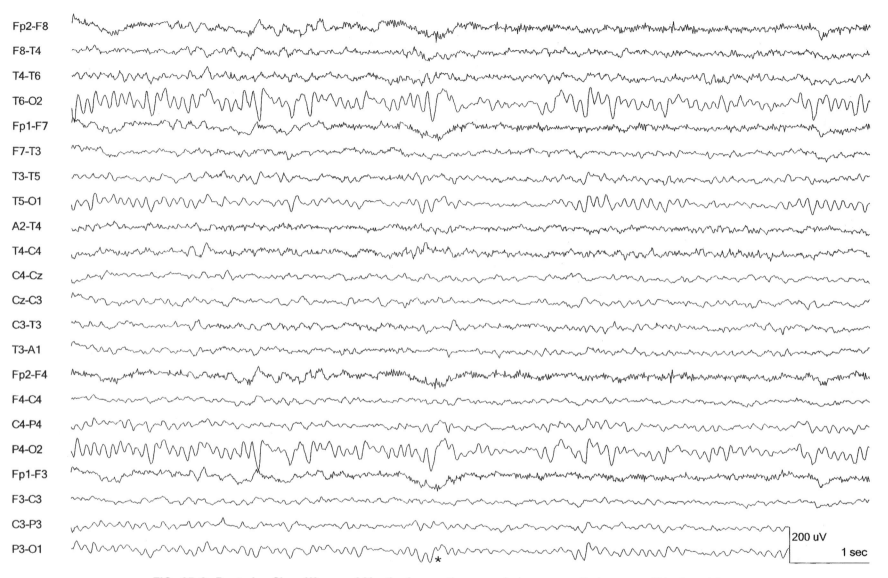

FIG. 25–2. Posterior Slow Waves of Youth. Among the several slow waves that occur within the alpha rhythm, the slow wave that occurs about halfway through the segment (at asterisk) has the best morphology and depicts the resemblance between an interictal epileptiform transient and a posterior slow wave of youth fused with a component from the faster background activity (LFF 1 Hz, HFF 70 Hz).

CHAPTER 26

Saw-Tooth Waves of REM Sleep

SAW-TOOTH WAVES OF REM

Other Names
Saw-toothed waves
Dents de Scie

Description
The rapid eye movement (REM) stage of sleep is defined by low-voltage mixed-frequency electroencephalogram (EEG) background activity, characteristic REMs, and low-amplitude electromyographic activity (205). It also commonly includes brief bursts of regular 3- to 7-Hz activity over the midline, which are called saw-tooth waves (7) (Fig. 26–1)(Fig. 26–2). Typically, the frequency is in the higher end of this range. The waves have an amplitude less than 50 μV and a duration of about 5 seconds. Although they originally were described as frontal or central, a more recent investigation found them to be consistently maximal at the vertex with a potential distribution that decreases equally in both the anterior and posterior directions (304). Essentially, their field is similar to that of vertex sharp transients and K complexes. Saw-tooth waves have a morphology that is triangular with superimposed faster frequencies that sometimes give the appearance of an increasingly steep rise and fall around the apex (9). However, this morphology is best appreciated with an epoch time (page duration) of 30 seconds, which is the standard duration used for polysomnograms and three times that of the usual EEG.

Distinguishing Features
Versus Cigánek Rhythm

The Cigánek rhythm shares a central localization with saw-tooth waves and has a typical frequency that overlaps with the upper end of saw-tooth waves' frequency range, but it may be distinguished based on morphology and the behavioral state in which the waves occur. The waves constituting a Cigánek rhythm usually are sinusoidal and are arciform when they include a sharp component. Furthermore, the Cigánek rhythm occurs in drowsiness; thus, they may be distinguished by the accompanying waves that indicate this state, including an intermittent alpha rhythm, central beta frequency activity, slow eye movements, and occasional blinks. Moreover, the Cigánek rhythm does not occur in REM sleep; thus, unlike REM sleep, they also may be accompanied by muscle artifact.

Versus Intermittent Rhythmic Delta Activity

When it occurs at the slower end of its possible frequencies, saw-tooth waves are in the delta range and also are similar to frontal intermittent rhythmic delta activity (FIRDA) with a midfrontal maximal field. However, their field differs from FIRDA in morphology and distribution. FIRDA lacks the sharp contour of saw-tooth waves, is less symmetric in the anterior to posterior direction, and extends more laterally in the frontal regions. Furthermore, FIRDA occurs irrespective of behavioral state; thus, it may be accompanied by electrographic evidence of wakefulness or, at least, muscle activity. Muscle activity artifact is minimal in REM sleep.

Versus Ocular Artifact

Because they occur during REM sleep, saw-tooth waves must be distinguished from the ocular artifact of REM sleep. Differentiation is based on their field and rhythmic morphology. Saw-tooth waves have a field that usually extends beyond the frontal region; thus, it is more posterior than eye movement artifact. They also have a sharply contoured rhythmic pattern, which REMs do not have. When electrodes are placed slightly lateral to each eye with one electrode above one eye and the other below the other eye, lateral and vertical eye movements produce a phase reversal on a bipolar montage. This also distinguishes the two because saw-tooth waves do not have this phase reversal.

Co-occurring Waves

Saw-tooth waves accompany or precede the REMs; thus, they are temporally associated with ocular artifact (26). The ocular artifact of REM is most clearly identifiable with electrodes that are placed to produce a phase reversal, as described already. The background activity at the time of saw-tooth waves is that of REM, with the absence of an alpha rhythm and the presence of diffuse alpha to theta frequency range activity.

Clinical Significance

Saw-tooth waves of REM are normal phenomenon and have no clinical significance in either the presence or absence. They are present in about 60% of normal REM sleep EEGs (305).

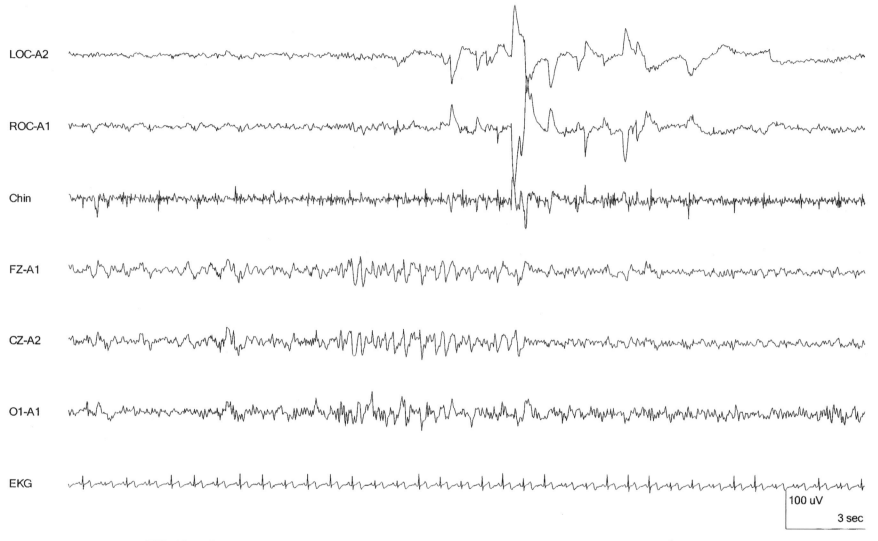

FIG. 26–1. Saw-tooth Waves of REM Sleep. A rhythm of sharply contoured, central, slow waves occurs in the context of saccadic lateral eye movements and decreased chin EMG activity. All three findings are characteristic of REM sleep. The montage includes the relevant channels from a polysomnogram and is presented as the standard 30-second epoch (LFF 1 Hz, HFF 70 Hz).

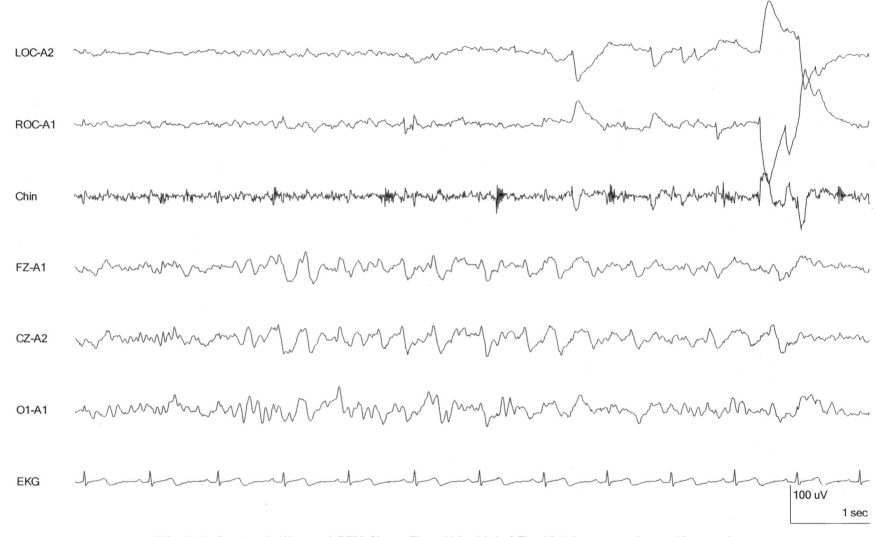

FIG. 26–2. Saw-tooth Waves of REM Sleep. The middle third of Fig. 26–1 is presented as a 10-second epoch. In this routine adult EEG time scale, the saw-tooth waves lose their characteristic morphology, but the phasic chin movements, which are a feature of REM sleep, are more apparent (LFF 1 Hz, HFF 70 Hz).

CHAPTER 27

Spindles

SPINDLES

Other Names
Sleep spindles
Sigma waves
Sigma activity

Description
Spindles are a type of rhythmic burst that occur at the vertex in stages II to IV of non–REM (NREM) sleep (Figs. 27–1 and 27–2). Their amplitude characteristically varies during the burst with the lowest amplitudes at the spindle's beginning and end and the maximal amplitude at about the midpoint. This shape lends the pattern's name *spindle* because it appears similar to a spindle of wound thread or string. Spindles begin and end abruptly and contain a single, unchanging frequency that typically is between 12 to 14 Hz but may be between 11 and 15 Hz. When they occur later than early childhood, they are localized to the vertex with a frequency of 13 to 14 Hz during light sleep and are displaced frontally with a slower frequency during deep sleep (9,26) (Fig. 27–3). Overall, they should remain symmetric along the parasagittal midline; thus, consistent lateralization indicates abnormality on the side lacking spindles.

Spindles change considerably as a function of age from their first occurrences at about 2 months until about 2 years. During infancy, spindles have an arciform morphology, are present unilaterally or asynchronously in the frontal regions with an overall symmetry among occurrences, have durations of up to 10 seconds, and recur as often as every 10 seconds (Figs. 27–4 and 27–5). More commonly, they last 2 to 4 seconds and recur less often. After the first year, they transition into a sinusoidal, bisynchronous, central, and shorter rhythm. After age 2 years, asynchronous spindles indicate abnormality.

Regardless of age, spindles typically are lower in amplitude than the surrounding background slow activity. Nevertheless, they usually are the predominant wave in their region when they occur because they are not superimposed on background slow waves or other activity. Although they are not superimposed, sometimes they appear fused to an immediately preceding K complex, and occurrences following K complexes are common for spindles. Their amplitude is maximal in adolescence and decreases through adulthood (13,26,306,307). They typically occur least often in late adulthood (206). In contrast to amplitude and number of occurrences within an electroencephalogram (EEG), their duration and frequency within the burst does not change as a function of age after early childhood. However, duration varies somewhat among occurrences. After early childhood, spindles have durations that range from 0.5 and 2 seconds and usually are between 0.5 and 1 second.

Extreme spindles are a rare spindle variant that occurs in EEGs of about 0.05% of children and are associated with cerebral palsy and mental retardation (13,306,308). They are most common at 3 years and very rare after 12 years. Extreme spindles differ from typical spindles by having a higher amplitude, longer duration, broader central field, and either a faster or slower frequency. They may occur almost continuously during sleep and have a frequency within the range of 6 to 18 Hz (27).

Distinguishing Features
Versus Frontal-Central Beta Activity

Only beta activity that is localized to the vertex or midline frontal region appears similar to spindles, and this similarity is fostered by midline beta's association with drowsiness. However, midline beta differs from spindles by not demonstrating abrupt beginning and ending. Such beta does not typically occur in bursts and instead usually builds up over seconds and persists for seconds before attenuating over seconds. Therefore, it does not have the characteristic spindle-like morphology. Furthermore, midline beta frequency activity almost always has a predominant frequency greater than 15 Hz.

Versus Paroxysmal Fast Activity

Spindles and paroxysmal fast activity (PFA) overlap in appearance in their abrupt, focal, and brief burst of faster frequencies, but differ in their frequency. PFA characteristically contain a faster frequency, which is usually more than 15 Hz. Morphology and state are other differentiating features. Spindle morphology includes a variable amplitude during an occurrence with maximal amplitude at the midpoint. Spindles also are limited to one state, NREM sleep. Although more common in sleep, PFA may occur in wakefulness. PFA also sometimes includes frequency evolution with a minor slowing in frequency during a burst.

Co-occurring Waves

As an indicator of stage II NREM sleep, spindles are accompanied by other signs of NREM sleep which include vertex sharp transients, positive occipital sharp transients of sleep (POSTS), and a mixture of theta and delta frequency range activity. As the other indicator of Stage II NREM sleep, K complexes also accompany spindles.

Clinical Significance

Spindles are a normal pattern and one that is used in polysomnography for staging sleep. They do not occur in rapid eye movement (REM) or stage I NREM sleep. Unlike vertex sharp transients and K complexes, spindles are not clearly an arousal phenomenon. However, they often occur at times that also demonstrate these other two patterns. Spindles are a resilient pattern that may persist in a normal fashion despite diffuse cerebral dysfunction, even when such dysfunction is severe enough to cause coma (309). When they accompany a coma or a persistent vegetative state, the state is sometimes called spindle coma, and the spindles may be a sign of a better prognosis than similar coma without spindles because their presence indicates the sparing of normal thalamocortical physiologic pathways. Similarly, asymmetric spindles after age 2 years are evidence for unilateral thalamocortical dysfunction. Before 2 years, such dysfunction is manifested by a preponderance of unilateral or asymmetric spindles.

Rarely, spindles may occur during wakefulness. This most often is in the context of a thalamic and internal capsule structural abnormality, hypersomnia, and hyperserotonergic states (310,311). When spindles occur in wakefulness, they usually are accompanied by K complexes in wakefulness, and both also occur in REM sleep.

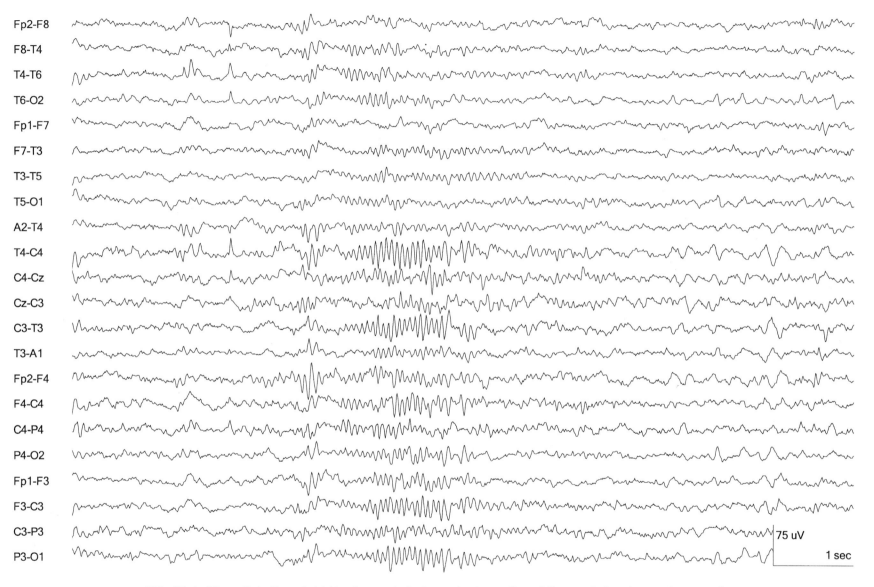

FIG. 27–1. Sleep Spindles. A 14-Hz sleep spindle is maximal over the midline central and posterior central region and has the typical increasing amplitude of the spindle morphology. A 200-msec sleep spindle fragment immediately precedes the 1.5-second sleep spindle. A benign epileptiform transient of sleep with phase reversal at the F8 electrode occurs earlier in the segment (LFF 1 Hz, HFF 70 Hz).

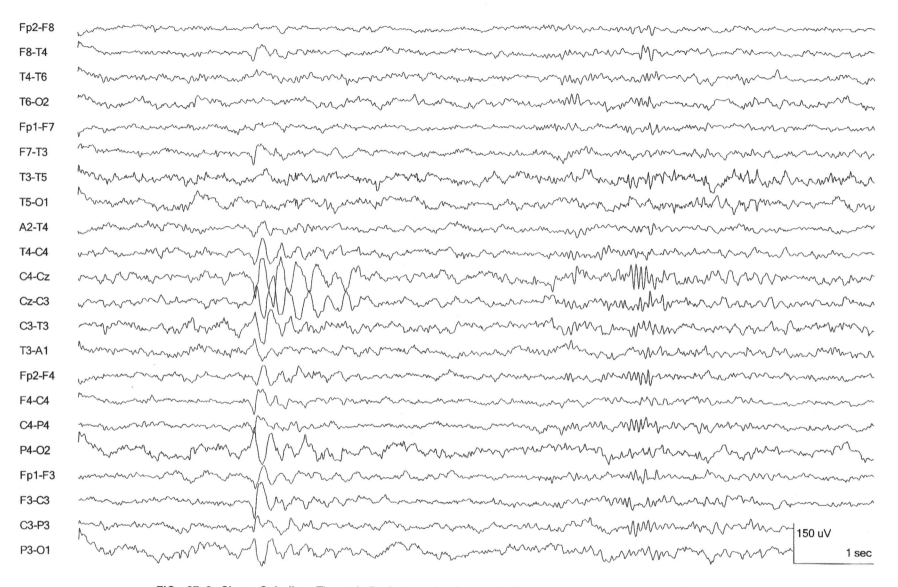

FIG. 27–2. Sleep Spindles. The spindle lasts only about a half second but has a typical frequency, morphology, and field. An unusual train of six vertex sharp transients occur earlier in the segment (LFF 1 Hz, HFF 70 Hz).

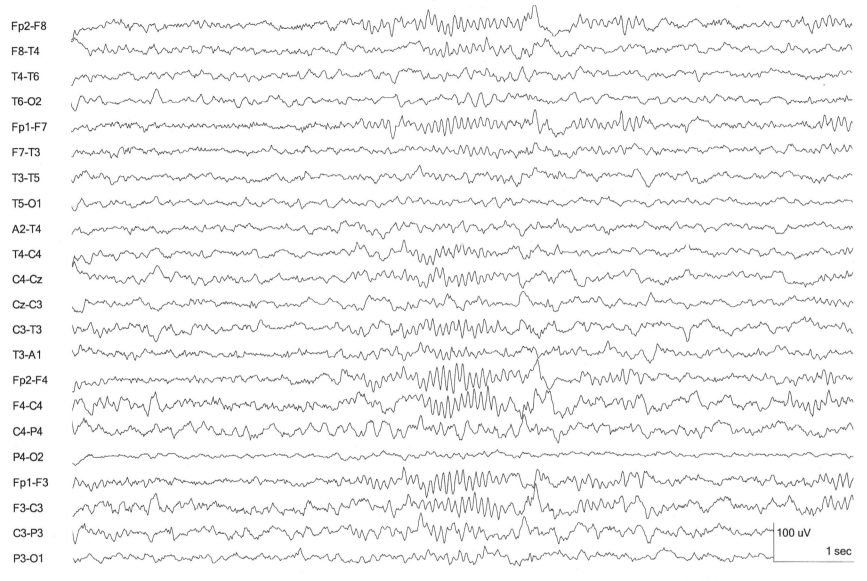

FIG. 27–3. Sleep Spindles. The frontal location and 12-Hz frequency for this otherwise typical sleep spindle is common in deeper stages of non–REM (NREM) sleep (LFF 1 Hz, HFF 70 Hz).

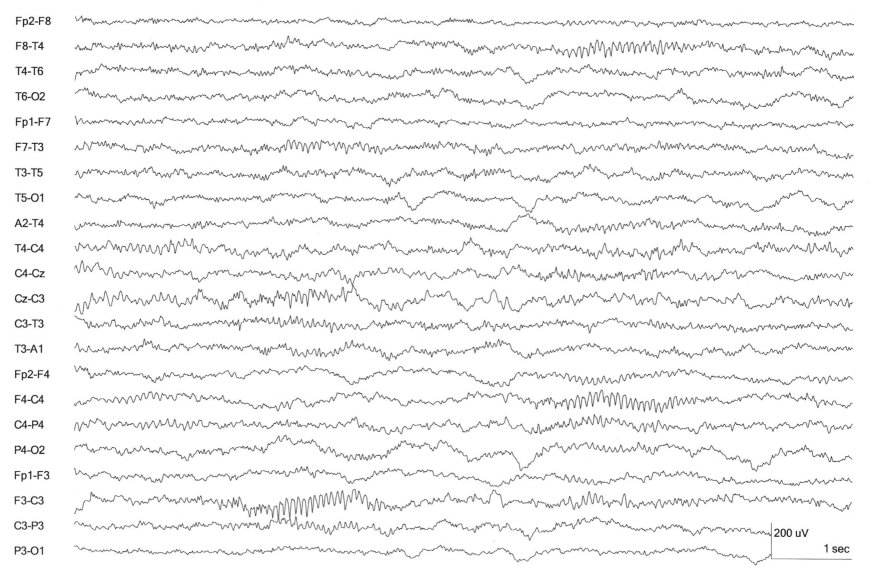

FIG. 27–4. Sleep Spindles. The arciform morphology and unilateral occurrence with shifting asymmetry of these sleep spindles are normal at 1 year old, the age at which this EEG was recorded. Even at this age, these spindles have durations of less than 2 seconds and the central locations of more mature spindles (LFF 1 Hz, HFF 70 Hz).

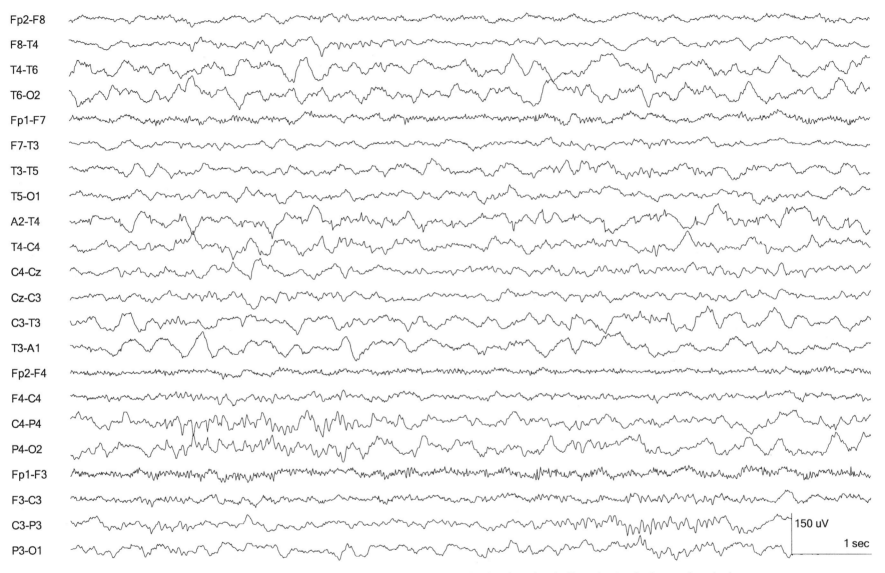

FIG. 27–5. Sleep Spindles. Typical of early infancy's poorly developed spindles, the beginning and end of these two sleep spindles are not as clear as in Figs. 27–1 to 27–4. Also typical are their unilateral fields and durations of 2 to 3 seconds. The first spindle also includes subharmonics. The EEG was recorded from a 3-month-old (LFF 1 Hz, HFF 70 Hz).

CHAPTER 28

Subclinical Rhythmic Electrographic Discharge of Adults

SUBCLINICAL RHYTHMIC ELECTROGRAPHIC DISCHARGE OF ADULTS

Other Names
SREDA

Decharges paroxystiques du carrefour

Description
SREDA is a rare pattern composed of a rhythm that is broadly distributed across the parietal and posterior temporal regions and that demonstrates frequency evolution from the delta range to the theta range (312) (Fig. 28–1). Occasionally, the vertex is included in the field. Throughout its occurrence, it replaces the co-localized background activity, but it does not alter the posterior dominant rhythm when the posterior regions are not included in its distribution. SREDA's onset may be the abrupt development of a delta frequency range rhythm or the gradual coalescing of individual high-amplitude, monophasic or diphasic sharp waves into a delta rhythm. Once the delta frequency rhythm is present, there is frequency evolution into the theta range and the wave persists as sharply contoured 5- to 7-Hz activity for an average of 40 to 80 seconds but may last as short as 10 seconds or as long as 5 minutes (313). The amplitude usually is between 40 and 100 μV but may be as high as 500 μV. Other aspects of the rhythm, including morphology and distribution, do not evolve or have any significant change. The rhythm is almost always bilateral and synchronous and is also symmetric in about 65% of instances. Resolution may be either abrupt or gradual. On resolution, the background activity immediately returns to its prior state. Specifically, the region in which SREDA occurs does not demonstrate focal slowing. SREDA occurs most commonly in the elderly and usually in individuals older than 50 years. However, younger individuals also may demonstrate it, including children (314). Individuals who demonstrate SREDA once are likely to demonstrate it again, either within the same electroencephalogram (EEG) or in future EEGs. Overall, it has an incidence of about 0.05% (315). The only known trigger for SREDA is hyperventilation. It usually occurs during wakefulness or light drowsiness but may occur during stage II non–REM (NREM) sleep. Less common SREDA variants include rhythms that remain in the delta frequency range, have a notched contour, or are frontally localized (312).

Distinguishing Features
Versus Rhythmic Midtemporal Theta Activity

SREDA has a field that is much broader than that of rhythmic midtemporal theta (RMT) activity and with a center that is displaced from the center of RMT's typical field. RMT usually is confined to the temporal lobe and centered in the midtemporal region. RMT also differs by being in the theta frequency range throughout each occurrence and having occurrences that rarely last more than 10 seconds.

Versus Ictal Patterns for Partial Seizures

Unlike typical ictal patterns, SREDA does not demonstrate evolution in its distribution across the scalp or in its wave morphology and does not lead to slowing following its resolution. Furthermore, the alpha rhythm usually is unaffected by SREDA, which rarely occurs with bilateral ictal patterns. Most importantly, SREDA is not associated with any alteration in awareness or any behavioral change.

Versus Fourteen and Six Positive Bursts

Both SREDA and the fourteen and six positive bursts (14&6) may manifest as paroxysmal rhythmic theta frequency activity with a broad field across the posterior scalp during drowsiness. Furthermore, 14&6 sometimes demonstrates frequency evolution. The two patterns may be differentiated by the frequencies within the evolving pattern. SREDA progresses from theta to delta, and 14&6 is from beta to theta. The duration of the pattern also differentiates them. SREDA lasts as short as 10 seconds, and 14&6 lasts as long as 2 seconds. The age of the EEG's subject may be helpful, because SREDA is most common in the elderly and 14&6 is most common in children.

Co-occurring Waves

Because of the state in which it occurs, the background typically includes a posterior dominant rhythm, but this rhythm may be slowed if it accompanies the onset of drowsiness. SREDA is not associated with any specific EEG features.

Clinical Significance

Despite its abrupt onset and subsequently evolving rhythm, SREDA is not an epileptiform pattern. Its propensity to occur in the elderly and during hyperventilation has led to the theory that it is due to regional cerebral hypoxia or vascular insufficiency. A single-photon emission computed tomography (SPECT) study with the injection of 99m Tc-hexamethylpropyleneamine oxime (HMPAO) during SREDA supports this theory and the belief that SREDA is not epileptic. This study did not identify a region of hyperperfusion during SREDA and instead identified hypoperfusion of bilateral temporo-parieto-occipital regions during both the SREDA and baseline scans (316). Regardless of its cause, SREDA is probably benign and of little diagnostic significance.

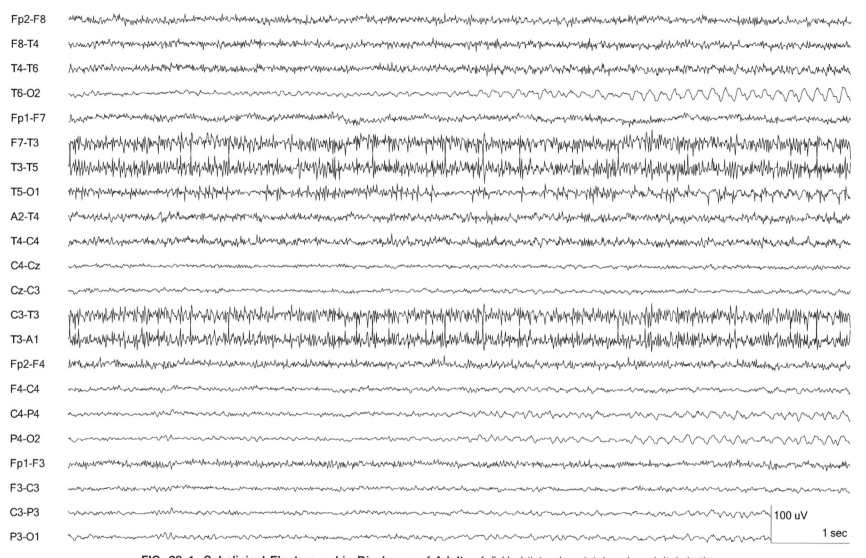

FIG. 28–1. Subclinical Electrographic Discharge of Adults. A 5-Hz bilateral parietal and occipital rhythm emerges from the background and persists for about 32 seconds without topographic evolution. The morphology demonstrates minor evolution into more sharply contoured component waves, but, unlike typical SREDA, evolution from delta frequency range activity does not occur. No behavioral change accompanied the pattern, which was recorded from a 43-year-old without a history of seizures (LFF 1 Hz, HHF 70 Hz).

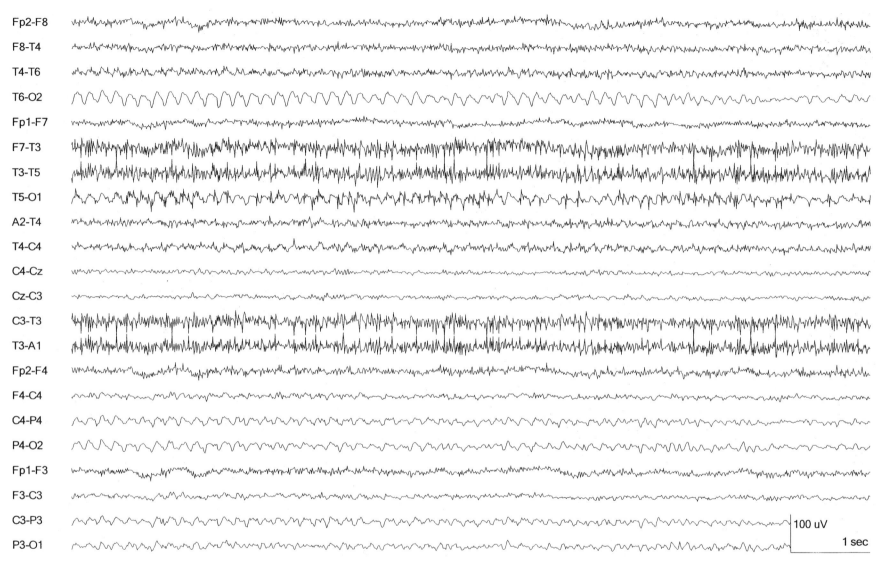

FIG. 28–1. (continued)

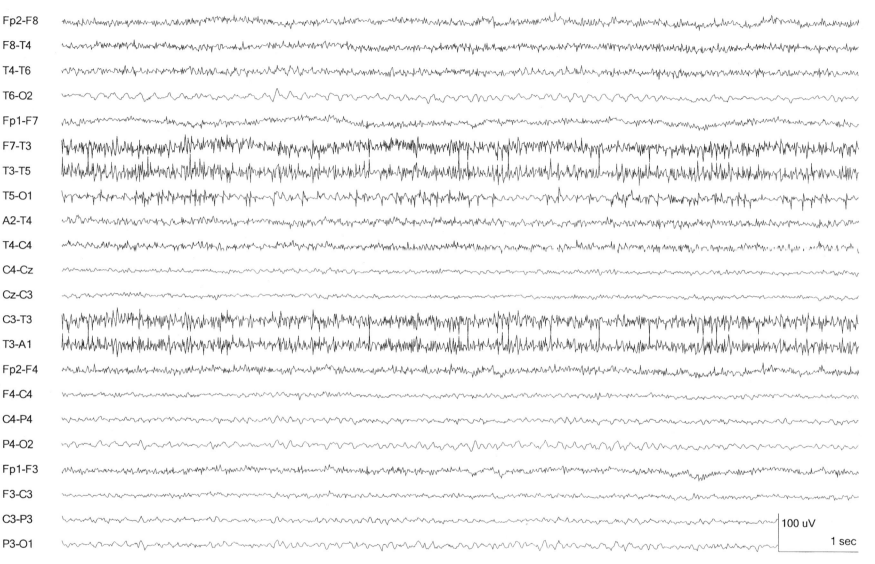

FIG. 28–1. *(continued)*

CHAPTER 29

Theta Activity

CIGÁNEK RHYTHM

Other Names
Episodic anterior drowsy theta
Frontal midline theta rhythm
Midline theta rhythm

Description
Descriptions of the simply termed Cigánek rhythm are highly consistent with regard to frequency range, location, and morphology but less in agreement about duration (Figs. 29–1 and 29–2). A Cigánek rhythm's frequency is almost always between 5 and 7 Hz (43,150). The field is centered at the midline with a maximum that usually is near the vertex (Cz) but may be displaced by one electrode distance anteriorly (Fz) or posteriorly (Pz). An anterior displacement occurs much more commonly than a posterior displacement. The field's distribution may or may not include the immediately parasagittal electrodes. The morphology includes a rising and falling amplitude over the wave's occurrence with a maximum amplitude that usually is greater than 50 µV and wave elements that usually are sinusoidal but may be arciform. Other than the rising and falling amplitude, the rhythm does not evolve. Although some reports include a duration definition of greater than 3 seconds similar rhythms lasting less than 3 seconds have been reported. Cigánek rhythms may last as long as 20 seconds (55,317,318).

Distinguishing Features
Versus Mu Rhythm

The central location and occasional arciform morphology are the overlapping features of the mu and Cigánek rhythms. However, these two rhythms are easily distinguishable by frequency and field. The mu rhythm is within the alpha frequency range and is usually asymmetrically placed with a parasagittally centered field. Attenuation with upper extremity movement is not always reliable as a distinguishing feature because such movement may be accompanied by arousal, which causes the Cigánek rhythm to attenuate (55). The mu rhythm attenuates in this circumstance as result of the specific motor task.

Versus Hypnopompic and Hypnagogic Hypersynchrony

Occurrence during a transition out of or into wakefulness, building amplitude of theta frequency range activity, and duration are similarities between state change related hypersynchrony and the Cigánek rhythm; however, the two are most easily differentiated by distribution. The hypersynchrony is an essentially generalized phenomenon.

Versus Polymorphic Theta Activity

Polymorphic theta frequency range activity may resemble the Cigánek rhythm because of its occurrence in similar conditions, but it is distinguished most readily through its morphology, duration, and broader field. Because it usually is not a discrete rhythm, polymorphic theta typically includes several frequencies, does not have as clear a start and stop, and extends beyond the central region.

Versus Saw-tooth Waves of REM Sleep

The Cigánek rhythm shares a central localization with saw-tooth waves of rapid eye movement (REM) sleep and has a typical frequency that overlaps with the upper end of the saw-tooth wave frequency range, but it may be distinguished based on morphology and the behavioral state in which the waves occur. The sharp component of saw-tooth waves do not produce a typical arciform morphology; thus, they differ from the waves of a Cigánek rhythm even when the Cigánek waves are arciform. Furthermore, the Cigánek rhythm occurs in drowsiness; thus, it may be distinguished by the accompanying waves that indicate this state, including an intermittent alpha rhythm, central beta frequency activity, slow eye movements, and occasional blinks. Moreover, the Cigánek rhythm does not occur in REM sleep; thus, unlike REM sleep, it may be accompanied by muscle artifact.

Co-occurring Waves

Drowsiness and concentration are the states in which a Cigánek rhythm occurs; thus, the accompanying waves reflect these conditions (319). When occurring in drowsiness, the Cigánek rhythm may be accompanied by generalized theta activity, artifact from slow eye movements, central beta activity, vertex sharp transients, and the absence of an alpha rhythm. The Cigánek rhythm does not occur in non–REM (NREM) sleep beyond stage I and, thus, is not accompanied by sleep spindles or K complexes (318). Its occurrence with concentration is accompanied by other signs of wakefulness, including artifact from eye blinks and an intermittent alpha rhythm.

Clinical Significance

Although Cigánek's original description of this rhythm in 1961 included the assertion that it is abnormal and associated with epilepsy, subsequent publications have more conclusively demonstrated that it is a normal finding (51,313). The reported prevalence of this rhythm varies as a function of how strictly it is defined and depending on whether the population is one of patients or healthy controls. Overall, it is usually close to or less than 1% for patient series and about 6% for healthy controls (55,317,321). Based on multiple reports, its prevalence appears to peak in early adulthood, but it has only a minor decrease through adulthood into late life.

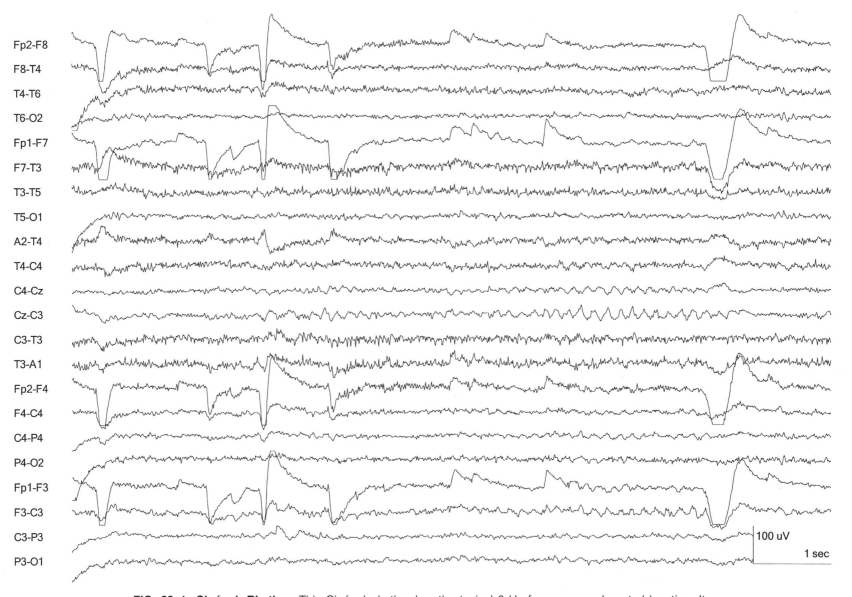

FIG. 29–1. Cigánek Rhythm. This Cigánek rhythm has the typical 6-Hz frequency and central location. Its 2-second duration, slight asymmetry, and somewhat arciform morphology are acceptable variants. The rhythm is accompanied by frequent eye blink artifact, which may co-occur (LFF 1 Hz, HFF 70 Hz).

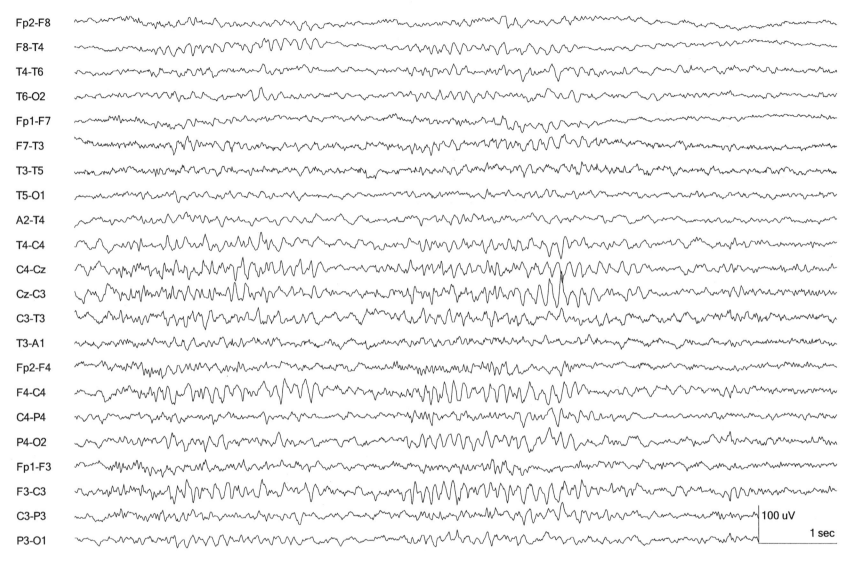

FIG. 29–2. Cigánek Rhythm. Compared to Fig. 29–1, the Cigánek rhythm in this segment is more symmetric and has a greater amount of intermixed faster frequencies, both of which make it less apparent. The central beta activity and slow roving eye movement artifact are signs of drowsiness, a state in which the Cigánek rhythm commonly occurs (LFF 1 Hz, HFF 70 Hz).

POLYMORPHIC THETA ACTIVITY

Other Names
Slowing

Description
The electroencephalogram (EEG) during wakefulness and sleep includes a mixture of activity, often including theta activity. Theta activity comprises rhythms with frequencies within the theta range and individual waves with the durations of elements of theta frequency range rhythms. By definition, a theta rhythm has a frequency of 4.0 Hz to, but not including, 8 Hz (4 Hz $\leq \Theta <$ 8 Hz). Therefore, a theta wave has a duration of 250 msec or less, down to, but not including, 125 msec (125 msec $< \Theta \leq$ 250 msec). Fragments of theta activity occur within the waking EEG of 30% of healthy adults (10). This occurs diffusely or with a shifting asymmetry, increases with drowsiness, and usually has bursting features (9,14). Such theta activity does not typically occur as a rhythm and is irregular with adjacent waves varying in duration and contour. Sustained polymorphic theta activity lasting more than a few seconds is a common sign of drowsiness, and, with greater drowsiness, the duration of the theta activity increases and its frequency decreases (Fig. 29–3). In early drowsiness, it occurs within the alpha rhythm, thereby putting the activity within the alpha rhythm below the alpha frequency range. With greater drowsiness, it occurs more diffusely but with less persistence than within the alpha rhythm. Theta activity that does not disappear with increased wakefulness or that demonstrates a consistent asymmetry is abnormal (14).

Distinguishing Features
Versus Polymorphic Delta Activity

Irregular slowing may occur across a spectrum of frequencies and includes both the theta and delta frequency ranges. The division between these two ranges is arbitrary but useful for quickly communicating an EEG's general appearance. Nevertheless, the duration of the individual waves is the essential distinguishing feature; waves of longer than 250 msec indicate delta activity.

Co-occurring Waves
Diffuse polymorphic theta corresponding to drowsiness may accompany diffuse or central beta frequency activity, artifact from slow eye movements, a Cigánek rhythm, rhythmic mid-temporal theta, and vertex sharp transients. Focal theta activity may demonstrate co-localized slowing into the delta frequency range, amplitude abnormality, or interictal epileptiform discharges. Any of these findings further the evidence that the region demonstrating the focal theta activity is abnormal.

Clinical Significance
Bilateral or generalized polymorphic theta activity is normal in infants. In adults, it is evidence of either normal drowsiness or of encephalopathy. It is a nonspecific finding within encephalopathy; thus, it may be produced by any of encephalopathy's causes, including reversible states associated with sedatives such as barbiturates, neuroleptics, and alcohol (322,323). Persistent and generalized polymorphic theta activity during severe encephalopathy is termed theta coma and has clinical significance similar to that of alpha coma. Both are most likely to occur after a hypoxic-ischemic cerebral injury. Beyond the same clinical context, the theta activity may exist within the same EEG as the pattern indicating alpha coma. This exists with a background alternating between the two frequency ranges. Regardless of whether it is accompanied by alpha activity, theta coma is a temporary pattern and rarely is present more than 5 days after the onset of coma (44).

Focal or persistently asymmetric theta activity is evidence for a focal region of cerebral dysfunction, but it is nonspecific even to the extent of being potentially caused by either a structural lesion or a region of purely physiologic dysfunction (Fig. 29–4). Structural lesions that produce slowing may produce activity in both the delta and theta frequency ranges and implicate subcortical pathology with or without associated cortical pathology (324). Moreover, imaging and EEG comparison studies find that the size of the lesion correlates with the delta activity and the amount of surrounding edema correlates best with the theta activity (325). Independent of size, rapidly growing lesions produce greater slowing.

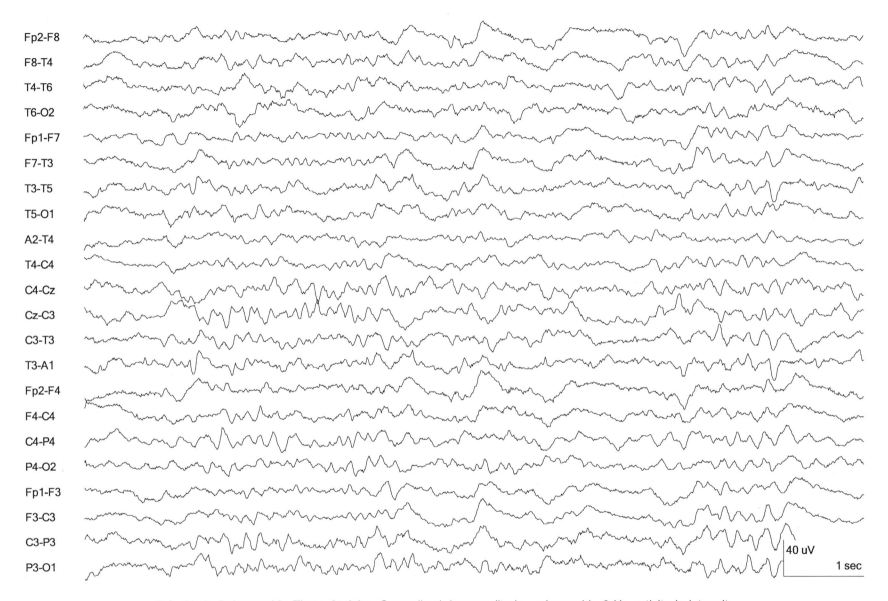

FIG. 29–3. Polymorphic Theta Activity. Generalized, low-amplitude, polymorphic 6-Hz activity is intermittently interrupted by slower activity. This EEG corresponds to severe encephalopathy due to a 10-minute cardiac arrest (LFF 1 Hz, HFF 70 Hz).

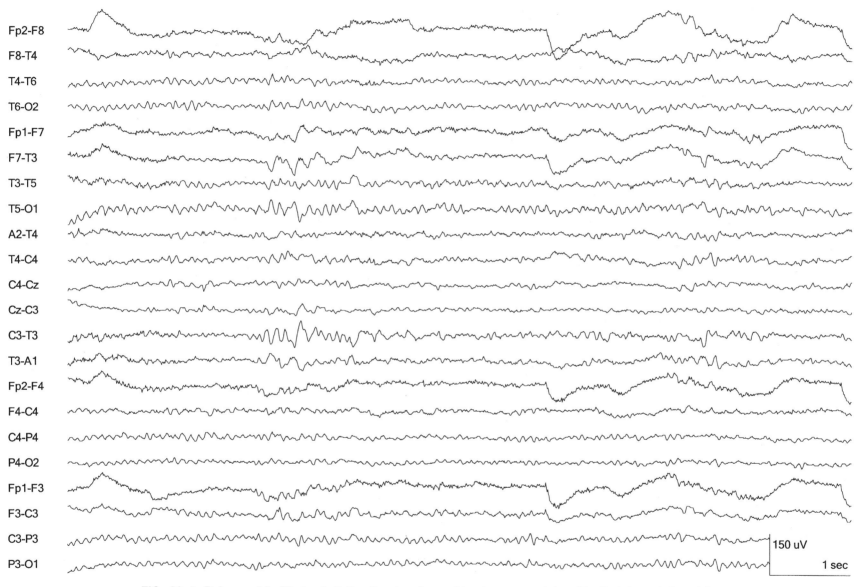

FIG. 29–4. Polymorphic Theta Activity. Focal, polymorphic slow waves intermittently interrupt the alpha rhythm on the left side. This EEG corresponds to 25 year old with normal neurologic examination and brain magnetic resonance imaging (MRI). Bifrontal ocular artifact also is present (LFF 1 Hz, HFF 70 Hz).

RHYTHMIC MIDTEMPORAL THETA

Other Names
Psychomotor variant
Rhythmic midtemporal discharge
Rhythmical theta bursts of drowsiness
Sylvian theta activity
Flat top waves

Description
Rhythmic midtemporal theta (RMT) activity usually contrasts strongly with the surrounding background activity with its burst of rhythmic slowing. Its frequency typically is between 5 and 6 Hz but may be from 4 to 7 Hz (7,61) (Figs. 29–5 and 29–6). Centered in a midtemporal region with spread that may include the anterior temporal, posterior temporal, inferior temporal, and parasagittal regions, the pattern is monomorphic with a contour that may be flat, sharp, or notched, depending on a superimposed, and not easily discernible, 10- to 12-Hz harmonic (7,9,43,326). The monomorphic pattern has medium to high amplitude (50 to 200 µV) and is truly regular, without significant variation in frequency throughout an occurrence. Only the amplitude varies, and this corresponds to the rise and fall with the beginning and ending of a burst. Occurrences are often unilateral but may be bisynchronous. The unilateral occurrences have a shifting asymmetry that may either be even between the sides or have a mild left-sided predominance (7). The bursts commonly last 5 to 10 seconds and occasionally may be longer than 1 minute or as short as 1 second (7,61).

Distinguishing Features
Versus Alpha Activity, Wicket Rhythm

RMT and wicket rhythms are similar in their location and occurrence in drowsiness. Furthermore, the wicket rhythm may occur in the theta frequency range, although it most commonly occurs in the alpha frequency range. The essential difference between the patterns is morphology. RMT does not have the wicket morphology, even when it is sharply contoured. RMT and wicket rhythms also differ in duration; wicket rhythms typically do not last the typical RMT duration of 5 or 10 seconds. However, these two patterns may overlap.

Versus Ictal Epileptiform Patterns for Partial Seizures

Like an ictal pattern, RMT manifests as an abrupt replacement of the preceding background with rhythmic activity. Moreover, it occurs over the temporal lobe, which is a region that commonly produces ictal patterns within the theta frequency range. The key distinguishing feature is RMT's lack of evolution in frequency or distribution. Each occurrence begins and ends without a significant change in frequency or localization.

Versus Polymorphic Theta Activity

Distinguishing whether an occurrence of focal temporal slowing in the theta frequency range is polymorphic theta or RMT is essential because RMT is a normal variant and focal polymorphic theta is an abnormality. This differentiation is especially difficult when the occurrences of slowing are brief, with each one lasting less than a second. Identifying wave regularity and bilateral independence is the key means to identifying the pattern as RMT. An indirect distinguishing feature is the co-localization of abnormality because polymorphic theta is more likely to occur within a region that is abnormal. Interictal epileptiform discharges are one type of abnormality. However, whether the pattern is monomorphic or polymorphic is the pivotal distinguishing feature.

Co-occurring Waves
RMT usually occurs in relaxed wakefulness and drowsiness; thus, it is accompanied by other signs of these states, including an intermittent alpha rhythm; occasional blink artifact; and a mixture of background frequencies, central beta frequency activity, and sometimes a Cigánek rhythm.

Clinical Significance
Although initially believed to be an epileptiform abnormality, RMT now is considered a variant of unknown significance and without clear association with epilepsy (61). Its prevalence is estimated as less than 10% of healthy, awake adults who are older than 60 years and about 1% of children and adolescents

(9,327). Opinions about whether its prevalence in the elderly is greater than in younger adults are divided, with the belief that its prevalence is greater in the elderly accompanied by evidence through imaging or medical histories that it is more significantly associated with cerebral injury or vascular insufficiency (7,61). However, support for this belief that RMT is a sign of pathology is complicated by evidence that sometimes has not distinguished between RMT and polymorphic temporal theta, evidence that it may occur in the healthy young, and other evidence that its prevalence peaks between 50 and 70 years then decreases despite further increases in each associated disease's prevalence (327–329).

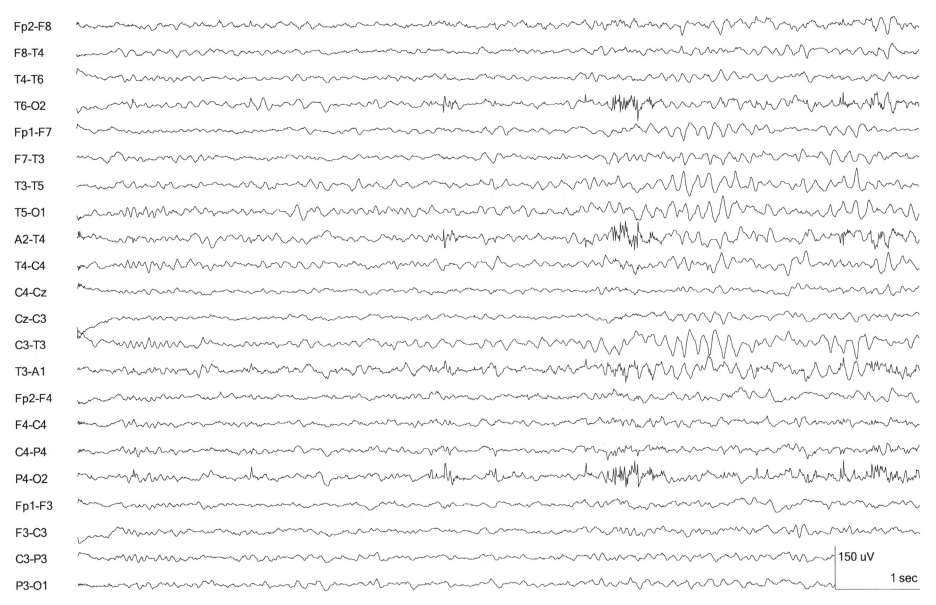

FIG. 29–5. Rhythmic Midtemporal Theta. Monomorphic 6.5-Hz activity is bilateral temporal with a greater amplitude on the left. The individual waves have a sharp contour and notching, which is one typical form for rhythmic midtemporal theta. Bursts of right-sided, lateral electromyographic (EMG) artifact also occur in this segment (LFF 1 Hz, HFF 70 Hz).

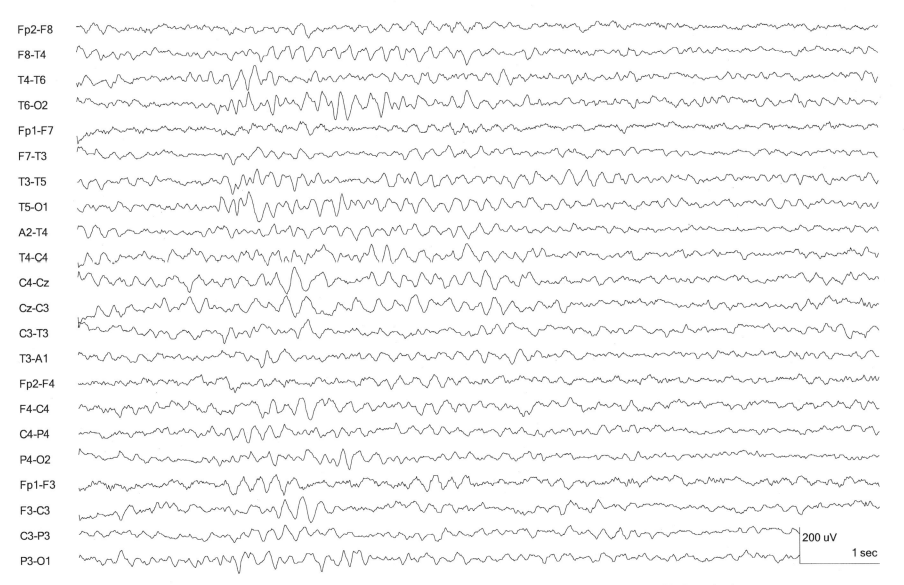

FIG. 29–6. Rhythmic Midtemporal Theta. The 5-Hz rhythm is bisynchronous with a right-sided predominance and consists of flat and notched waves. The rhythm is occurring in drowsiness just before the transition to sleep (LFF 1 Hz, HFF 70 Hz).

CHAPTER 30

Triphasic Waves

TRIPHASIC WAVES

Other Names
Blunt spike-wave

Description
The term triphasic waves (TW) as a title for a specific pattern denotes more than wave morphology. It indicates rhythmic trains of bisynchronous and symmetric waves with a triphasic waveform that occur in adults with one of several pathologic conditions (Figs. 30–1, 30–2, and 30–3). TW rarely occur in those younger than 20 years. Waves with triphasic morphology may occur across all ages and in many particular instances, including as interictal epileptiform discharges and periodic epileptiform discharges. Such waves may be described as having a triphasic morphology but should not be called TW because of the resulting miscommunication in the pattern that is present and its associated clinical significance.

Blunt spike-wave is a less commonly used alternative name for TW that provides an appropriate description for the waveform. TW classically have a lower amplitude, less sharply contoured initiating spike than epileptiform waves of triphasic morphology. The three elements of the overall morphology typically present as the sharpest wave followed by the tallest wave followed by the longest wave. The middle phase, the most prominent of the three, has a positive (downward) deflection in montages with chains that progress anterior to posterior, and its amplitude typically is 200 to 300 µV (52). The other two phases are negative. The three phases also may be characterized as demonstrating progressively increasing durations.

The anterior head region usually manifests the most predominant TW with waves that have higher amplitude and a more clearly defined morphology, but a posterior predominance also may occur. Regardless of whether the predominance is anterior or posterior, a phase lag often is present with the predominant region temporally leading the less predominant one. When channels are organized in the anterior-to-posterior (AP) direction, the lag is evident as a minor, incremental displacement of the TW with each successive channel. The absence of an AP lag is an accepted variation in the manifestation of TW.

The repetition pattern of TW is another characteristic feature. Although they occasionally occur individually, TW usually occur in trains of successive waves without intervening background activity. These trains typically have TW repeating at a frequency of 1.5 to 3 per second with the train as a whole lasting about 0.5 to 3 seconds. The trains start and stop abruptly without changes in waveform or frequency. They typically occur intermittently and without a pattern or periodicity.

Distinguishing Features
Versus Bilateral Periodic Epileptiform Discharges

Although bilateral periodic epileptiform discharges (BiPEDs) are typically generalized, they usually have a frontal predominance that is similar to the frontal field of TW. The wave morphology and the recurrence pattern are the two principal differentiating features. As epileptiform discharges (EDs), BiPEDs are triphasic in morphology; however, their waveform is more similar to epileptic discharges than is the waveform of TW. As such, BiPEDs have a more sharply contoured initiating spike or sharp wave and an overall shorter duration. They also differ from TW by recurring with brief intervals of background activity separating the individual waves. Thus, BiPEDs recur as individual discharges, which differs from the trains of repetitions found with TW. Furthermore, the intervals between the individual waves that constitute BiPEDs tend to be similar in duration. This gives BiPEDs their periodicity. The intervals between trains of TW are inconsistent. TWs' usual occurrence with an AP lag is another differentiating feature. This is manifested by a slightly earlier occurrence of each wave in the more anterior channels.

Versus Frontal Intermittent Rhythmic Delta Activity

Frontal intermittent rhythmic delta activity (FIRDA) and TW have similar distributions and recurrence patterns. Both recur in repetitions that typically last several seconds. Differentiation between the patterns rests essentially on morphology. FIRDA is composed of monophasic slow waves, and each TW clearly include multiple phases. The distinction may be more difficult if FIRDA has superimposed faster frequencies that give the appearance of notched slow waves because subtle initiating spikes or sharps also may cause notching of a slow wave. Distinguishing notched FIRDA due to a mixture of frequencies from TW relies on identifying a consistent location of the notch along the slow wave's slope. A mixture of frequencies will produce notching that is more random. A subtle spike or sharp wave always will be present at the same location with regard to the slow wave's apex.

Versus Ictal or Interictal Epileptiform Discharges

Generalized ictal or interictal EDs have a triphasic morphology and often occur in trains of several complexes. Especially when they are the slow spike and wave form of generalized EDs, their repetition rate may be similar to TW. Morphologic differences provide one means for differentiation. EDs usually are centered at the frontal midline and have a more sharply contoured initiating spike or sharp wave. However, the initiating discharge of slow spike and wave may be similar to that of TW. The occurrence of frequent trains is marginally helpful because an abundance of waves is uncommon for interictal EDs. However, frequent waves may represent either TW or the ictal EDs of nonconvulsive status epilepticus due to symptomatic generalized epilepsy (330). In reality, the patient's history is the best way to determine if the discharges are TW or EDs, but the background activity also may help. TW usually occur in the context of significant generalized slowing, especially when they are due to hepatic disease (331). The background activity for symptomatic generalized epilepsies usually is only moderately slowed. Resolution of the wave with the administration of a benzodiazepine is not an indicator of whether the wave is a TW or an ED because both may respond electrographically to this treatment

(332). Improvement in mentation following antiepileptic treatment is a more specific means to differentiate the two (333). The presence of focal or consistently unilateral TW is unusual for TW and may indicate that the pattern represents interictal EDs.

Versus Ocular Artifact

Eye movements produce several types of artifact, and eye flutter is the one that most closely resembles anterior TW. Eye flutter occurs as paroxysmal slow waves with sharp contours that sometimes appear diphasic. However, they are not triphasic. The extent of their field also distinguishes them from TW because they do not occur beyond the frontal region. Furthermore, the field of ocular artifact ends abruptly. TW have a field that often includes the central region and gradually diminishes with distance from the frontal pole.

Co-occurring Waves

TW occur in the context of diffuse cerebral dysfunction; thus, they are accompanied by generalized slowing. The slowing usually is a mixture of theta and delta frequency range activity with the relative amount of delta activity paralleling the extent of encephalopathy. Generalized attenuation is present in severe encephalopathy. When the cause is metabolic, especially hepatic, fourteen and six positive bursts may be present.

Clinical Significance

Overall, TW most commonly occur in the context of significant impairment in mentation, such as from encephalopathy, dementia, stupor, or coma. Uncommonly, they occur in normal wakefulness. Hepatic encephalopathy is the classic and most common clinical correlate to TW, but numerous causes of encephalopathy may produce TW. Hepatic insufficiency is responsible in about 25% of instances of TW (334). Other reported causes include renal insufficiency, intoxication (lithium among others), hypoxia, serum sodium and calcium concentration abnormalities, malignant hypertension, sepsis, cerebral carcinomatosis, cerebral vasculitis, Alzheimer's disease, brainstem infarction, diencephalic masses, and subdural hematomas (89,96,258,335). Although focal lesions are included in the broad differential diagnosis, the cause is more commonly metabolic or a diffuse degenerative condition (328). Assessing the patient's level of alertness may establish whether the etiology is a metabolic abnormality or a dementing illness. TW are not associated with changes in alertness when dementia is the cause.

Although encephalopathies that are caused by metabolic illness often are reversible with correction of the underlying metabolic abnormality, the likelihood for reversal is poor when TW are present. This is due to the association of TW with more severe forms of metabolic illnesses. In one group of 24 consecutive patients with TW due to metabolic illnesses, only 4 were well 2 years later (328). Thus, the possibility of TW occurrence in the absence of structural injury to the brain may be clinically irrelevant with regard to long-term prognosis. Encephalopathies due to less severe metabolic illness are accompanied by only diffuse slowing on the electroencephalogram (EEG). Regardless of the triphasic morphology, TW are not associated with seizures except as possibly a postictal pattern with a significance that is similar to postictal slowing (7,337).

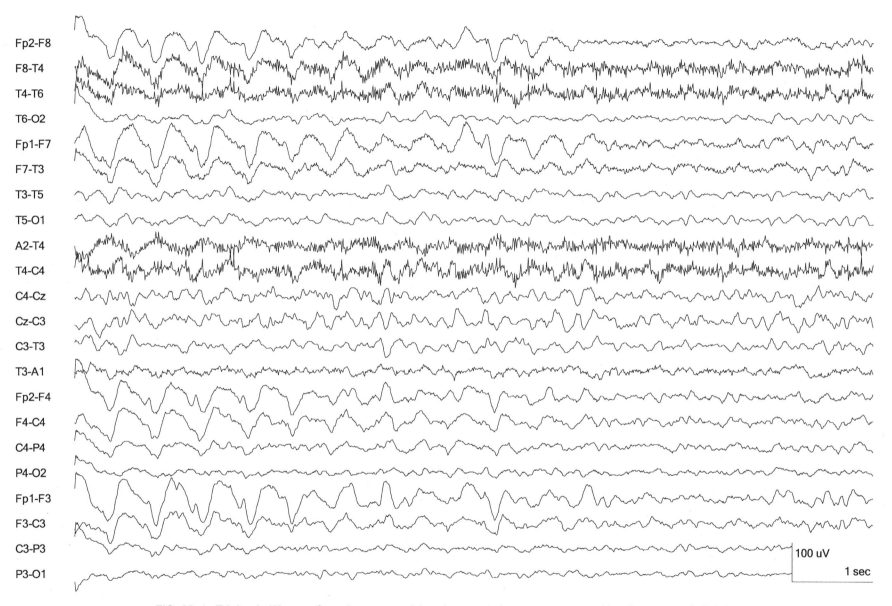

FIG. 30–1. Triphasic Waves. Complexes comprising sharp and slow waves repeat with a frequency of slightly less than 2 Hz and occur with gradual emergence and resolution. The background is generalized slowing. The EEG corresponds to delirium due to neuroleptic toxicity (LFF 1 Hz, HFF 70 Hz).

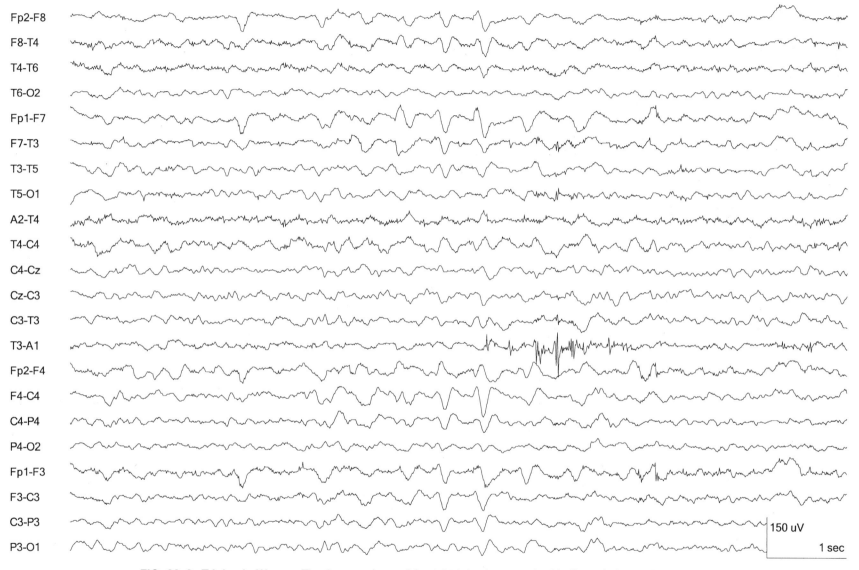

FIG. 30–2. Triphasic Waves. The 2 second run of frontal triphasic waves in this figure is less evident than in Fig. 30–1 because of lower amplitude, but the three phases and fixed morphology across occurrences are clear. The EEG corresponds to a 63-year-old with 3 days of hepatic encephalopathy following a successful liver transplant 3 months earlier. Left-sided muscle artifact is present (LFF 1 Hz, HFF 70 Hz).

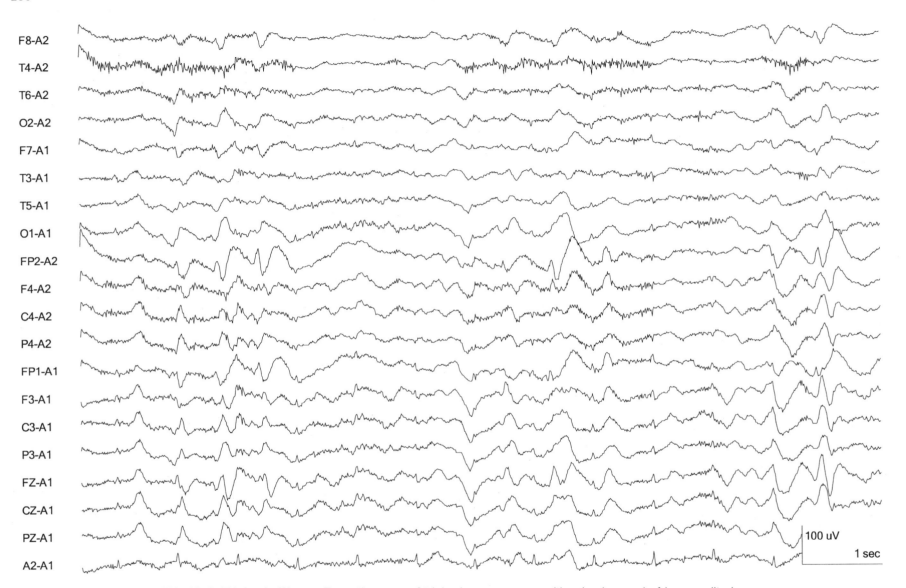

FIG. 30–3. Triphasic Waves. Repeating runs of triphasic waves occur with a background of low-amplitude slowing. An anterior to posterior phase lag is evident in this referential montage. The EEG corresponds to a 54-year-old with acutely worsening autoimmune hepatitis who became comatose 3 days before this recording (LFF 1 Hz, HFF 70 Hz).

CHAPTER 31

Vertex Sharp Transients

VERTEX SHARP TRANSIENT

Other Names
Vertex wave
V wave
Biparietal hump

Description
The vertex sharp transient (VST) is a surface negative sharp wave that phase reverses at or near the vertex and occurs in drowsiness and non–REM (NREM) sleep (Fig. 31–1). It often has a broad distribution with extension into the frontal, parietal, and sometimes temporal regions. Although it usually appears monophasic or diphasic, it often is triphasic on closer inspection. The three phases are defined by two small positive spikes and the larger negative sharp wave that they precede and follow. The sharp wave typically is 100 msec in duration in adulthood and often is slightly longer in duration in childhood. Although the sharp wave may not be high amplitude, it usually is taller than the surrounding background activity. The sharp wave's phase reversal is the center of the VST's field and most often is at Cz. However, it also commonly occurs at C3 and C4 with a shifting asymmetry that does not favor one side in normal recordings. VSTs occur individually or in trains of successive waves that rarely last longer than several seconds and have up to about 3 VSTs per second (Figs. 31–2 and 31–3). When trains occur, the small spikes become less apparent, and the pattern may appear to be a run of repeating monophasic sharp waves.

During development, VSTs first occur with a clear morphology at 5 to 6 months (338). Although they are not as sharp as they become in early childhood, their amplitude during infancy and the toddler years is higher than at any other age and may reach 250 µV. During childhood, the amplitude gradually de-creases, and this decline continues though adulthood at a slower rate. By late adulthood, VSTs may be blunted and low amplitude or completely absent. The localization of the wave's phase reversal during early childhood may be at or near either the central or parietal midline. The electroencephalograms (EEGs) of children with parietal VSTs demonstrate a gradual migration of the VST to the central region over several years. Biparietal hump is an old term for the VST that does not refer to possible parietal localization during childhood. It refers to the appearance of VSTs when they are recorded without midline or central electrodes, as they were in the early years after EEG's invention.

Distinguishing Features
Versus Interictal Epileptiform Discharge

Although they are rare, interictal epileptiform discharges (IEDs) at the vertex occur. Parasagittal IEDs are more common and occur within the region of off-center VSTs. Regardless of their localization, IEDs typically have a sharper contour and lower amplitude than VSTs. They do not stand above the background activity as a characteristic feature but instead stand out because of their sharpness against the slowing of drowsiness or sleep. When the IED is a rolandic spike, it has the additional differentiating feature of its characteristic morphology. Like the VST, classic rolandic spikes are triphasic; however, the first and third phases are less symmetric. Polarity also may distinguish rolandic spikes from VSTs. When a rolandic spike's tangential dipole is present, the positive end is central, which is the opposite polarity of the VST. Lastly, rolandic spikes that occur in repetitions do not appear monophasic. They keep their triphasic morphology, and, furthermore, they often are separated by brief periods of background EEG activity.

Versus K Complex

The morphology of a K complex is more complicated than that of a VST, and this is the most differentiating feature. Although K complexes also have a negative phase reversal at the vertex, their morphology is polyphasic, longer in duration, less sharply contoured, and without as great an amplitude difference between the phases as VSTs have. Indeed, the polyphasic pattern of K complexes is more evident than the triphasic pattern of a VST because more than one of its phases has an amplitude greater than the background. Also like VSTs, K complexes occur individually; but unlike VSTs, they do not occur in trains and often are immediately followed by a sleep spindle.

Co-occurring Waves

VSTs first occur in late stage I NREM sleep and persist through the other stages of NREM sleep. In lighter sleep, they may be accompanied by central theta or beta activity, temporal theta activity, diffuse theta activity, and ocular artifact indicating slow roving eye movements. The posterior dominant rhythm (PDR) is absent in late stage I NREM. With deeper sleep, VSTs are accompanied by K complexes, positive occipital sharp transients of sleep (POSTS), sleep spindles, and generalized delta frequency range activity.

Clinical Significance

VSTs are a normal and common phenomenon that likely represent a long latency evoked potential. Most often they occur spontaneously, but they may be evoked by sudden stimulation through multiple modalities. Auditory stimulation is the modality that most easily elicits VSTs, and similar but smaller electronegative waves may occur in wakefulness after a sudden noise. VSTs are resilient and may be present in a normal fashion even when focal pathology is present at the vertex.

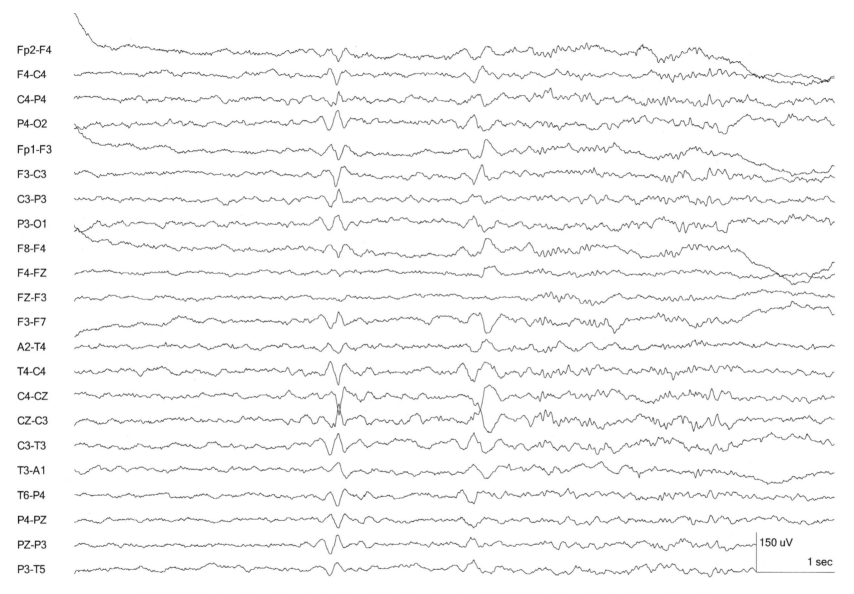

FIG. 31–1. Vertex Sharp Transients. The first vertex sharp transient is triphasic and better formed than the second. It also better demonstrates the extent of the midline field, which phase reverses at the C3 and C4 electrodes in the parasagittal chain and, in this segment, is isoelectric at the Fz electrode. A lower amplitude sleep spindle occurs a half second after the second vertex sharp transient (LFF 1 Hz, HFF 70 Hz).

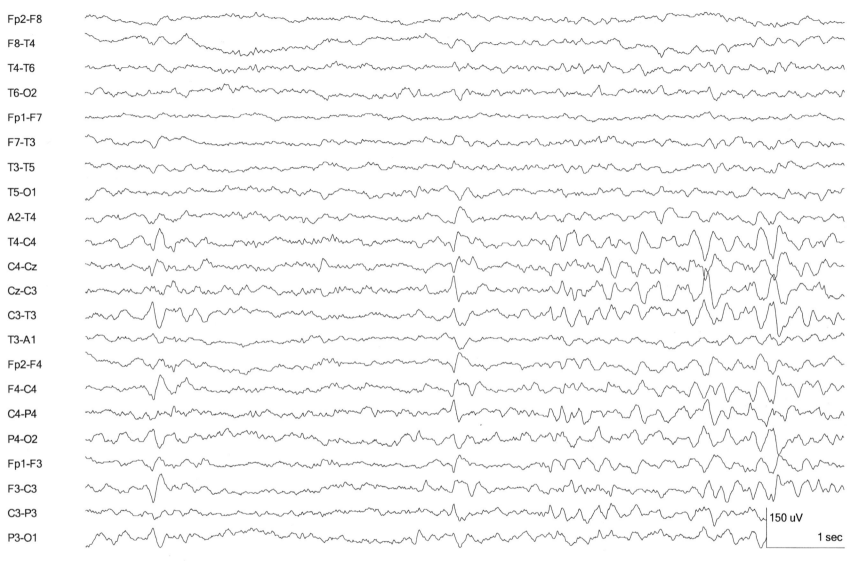

FIG. 31–2. Vertex Sharp Transients. Two individual vertex sharp transients occur in the first half of this segment, and multiple vertex sharp transients occur as a train during the segment's final 4 seconds (LFF 1 Hz, HFF 70 Hz).

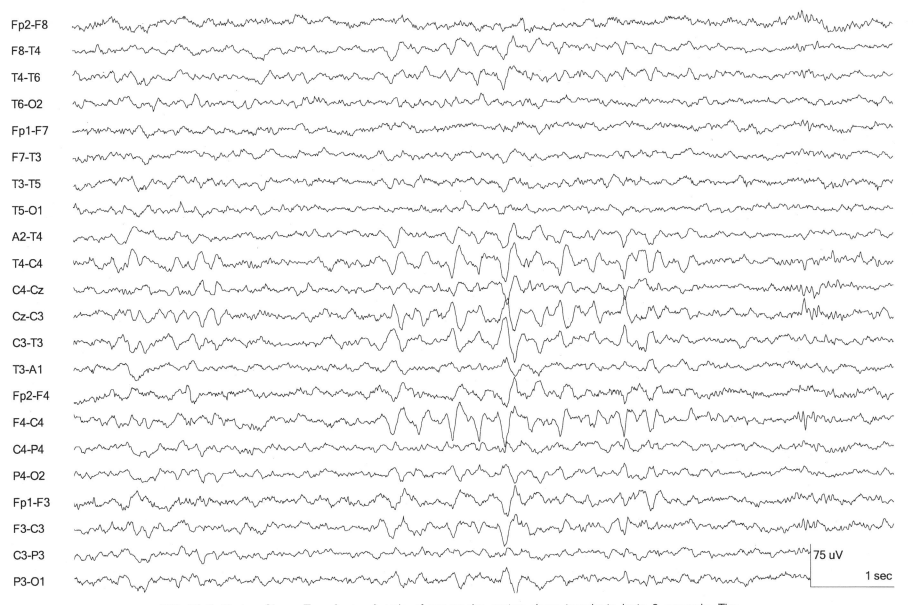

FIG. 31–3. Vertex Sharp Transients. A train of successive vertex sharp transients lasts 3 seconds. The morphology of the individual waves and their phase reversals distinguishes the train from a run of rhythmic slowing. A sleep spindle occurs at the end of the segment (LFF 1 Hz, HFF 70 Hz).

References

1. Chatrian GE, Bergamini L, Dondey M, Klass DW, Lennox-Buchtal M, Petersen I. A glossary of terms most commonly used by clinical electroencephalographers. *Electroencephalogr Clin Neurophysiol* 1974;37:538–553.
2. Jasper HH. The ten-twenty electrode system of the International Federation. *Electroencephalogr Clin Neurophysiol* 1958;10:371–373.
3. Sharbrough FW. Electrical fields and recording techniques. In: Daly DD, Pedley TA, eds. *Current practice of clinical electroencephalography,* 2nd ed. New York: Raven Press, 1990:29–49.
4. Blume WT, Kaibara M, Young GB. *Atlas of adult electroencephalography,* 2nd ed. New York: Lippincott Williams & Wilkins, 2002: pp.1,140.
5. Guideline thirteen: guidelines for standard electrode position nomenclature. American Electroencephalographic Society. *J Clin Neurophysiol* 1994;11:111–113.
6. Niedermeyer E. The normal EEG of the waking adult. In: Niedermeyer E, Lopes da Silva F, eds. *Electroencephalography, basic principles, clinical applications, and related fields.* Baltimore: Williams & Wilkins, 1999:149–173.
7. Fisch BJ. *Fisch and Spehlmann's EEG primer.* 3rd ed. Amsterdam: Elsevier, 1999.
8. Erwin CW, Somerville ER, Radtke RA. A review of electroencephalographic features of normal sleep. *J Clin Neurophysiol* 1984;1:253–274.
9. Blume WT, Kaibara M, Young GB. *Atlas of adult electroencephalography,* 2nd ed. Philadelphia: Lippincott Williams & Wilkins, 2002.
10. Kiloh LG, McComas AJ, Osselton JW, Upton ARM. *Clinical electroencephalography,* 4th ed. London: Butterworths, 1981.
11. Westmoreland BF, Klass DW. Defective alpha reactivity with mental concentration. *J Clin Neurophysiol* 1998;15:424–428.
12. Bancaud J, Hecan H, Lairy GC. Modifications de la reactivite EEG, troubles des fonctions symboliques et troubles confusionnels dans les lesions hemishperiques localisies. *Electroencephalogr Clin Neurophysiol* 1955;7:179–192.
13. Niedermeyer E. Maturation of the EEG: development of waking and sleep patterns. In: Niedermeyer E, Lopes da Silva F, eds. *Electroencephalography, basic principles, clinical applications, and related fields.* Baltimore: Williams & Wilkins, 1999:189–214.
14. Kellaway P. An orderly approach to visual analysis: characteristics of the normal EEG of adults and children. In: Daly DD, Pedley TA, eds. *Current practice of clinical electroencephalography,* 2nd ed. New York: Raven Press, 1990:139–199.
15. Hari R. Magnetoencephalography as a tool of clinical neurophysiology. In: Niedermeyer E, Lopes da Silva F, eds. *Electroencephalography, basic principles, clinical applications, and related fields.* Baltimore: Williams & Wilkins, 1999:1107–1134.
16. Birbaumer N. The EEG of congenitally blind adults. *Electroencephalogr Clin Neurophysiol* 1970;29:318.
17. Anokhin A, Steinlein O, Fischer C, Mao Y, Vogt P, Schalt E, et al. A genetic study of the human low-voltage electroencephalogram. *Hum Genet* 1992;90(1–2):99–112.
18. Kellaway P. An orderly approach to visual analysis: parameters of the normal EEG in adults and children. In: Klass DW, Daly DD, eds. *Current practice of clinical electroencephalography.* New York: Raven Press, 1979:69–147.
19. Markand ON. Alpha rhythms. *J Clin Neurophysiol* 1990;7:163–189.
20. Hubbard O, Sunde D, Goldensohn ES. The EEG in centenarians. *Electroencephalogr Clin Neurophysiol* 1976;40:407–417.
21. Shigeta M, Julin P, Almkvist O, Basun H, Rudberg U, Wahlund LO. EEG in successful aging; a 5 year follow-up study from the eighth to ninth decade of life. *Electroencephalogr Clin Neurophysiol* 1995;95(2):77–83.
22. Torres F, Faoro A, Loewenson R, Johnson E. The electroencephalogram of elderly subjects revisited. *Electroencephalogr Clin Neurophysiol* 1983;56:391–398.
23. Storm van Leeuwen W, Bekkering DH. Some results obtained with the EEG spectrograph. *Electroencephalogr Clin Neurophysiol* 1958;10:563–570.
24. Kellaway P, Maulsby RL. The normative electroencephalographic data reference library. Final report. In. Houston: Baylor University College of Medicine, 1966:50–52.
25. Santamaria J, Chiappa KH. The EEG of drowsiness in normal adults. *J Clin Neurophysiol* 1987;4:327–382.
26. Niedermeyer E. Sleep and EEG. In: Niedermeyer E, Lopes da Silva F, eds. *Electroencephalography, basic principles, clinical applications, and related fields.* Baltimore: Williams & Wilkins, 1999:174–188.
27. Westmoreland BF, Klass DW. Unusual EEG patterns. *J Clin Neurophysiol* 1990;7:209–228.
28. Belsh JM, Chokroverty S, Barabas G. Posterior rhythmic slow activity in EEG after eye closure. *Electroencephalogr Clin Neurophysiol* 1983;56:562–568.
29. Lopes da Silva FH, Hoeks A, Smits H, Zetterberg LH. Model of brain rhythmic activity. The alpha-rhythm of the thalamus. *Kybernetik* 1974;15(1):27–37.
30. Lopes da Silva F. Neural mechanisms underlying brain waves: from neural membranes to networks. *Electroencephalogr Clin Neurophysiol* 1991;79:81–93.
31. Basar E, Schurmann M, Basar-Eroglu C, Karakas S. Alpha oscillations in brain functioning: an integrative theory. *Int J Psychophysiol* 1997;26(1–3):5–29.
32. Ciulla C, Takeda T, Endo H. MEG characterization of spontaneous alpha rhythm in the human brain. *Brain Topogr* 1999;11(3):211–222.
33. Sadato N, Nakamura S, Oohashi T, Nishina E, Fuwamoto Y, Waki A, et al. Neural networks for generation and suppression of alpha rhythm: a PET study. *Neuroreport* 1998;9: 893–897.
34. Goldman RI, Stern JM, Engel Jr J, Cohen MS. Simultaneous EEG and fMRI of the alpha rhythm. *Neuroreport* 2002;13:2487–2492.
35. Foxe JJ, Simpson GV, Ahlfors SP. Parieto-occipital approximately 10 Hz activity reflects anticipatory state of visual attention mechanisms. *Neuroreport* 1998;9:3929–3933.
36. Strauss H, Ostow M, Greenstein L. *Diagnostic electroencephalography.* New York: Grune and Stratton, 1952.
37. Salinsky MC, Binder LM, Oken BS, Storzbach D, Aron CR, Dodrill CB. Effects of gabapentin and carbamazepine on the EEG and cognition in healthy volunteers. *Epilepsia* 2002;43:482–490.
38. Loeb C, Poggio CF. Electroencephalogram in a case of pontomesencephalic haemorrhage. *Electroencephalogr Clin Neurophysiol* 1953;5:295–296.
39. Loeb C, Rosadini G, Poggio CF. Electroencephalograms during coma. *Neurology* 1959; 9:910–918.
40. Aichner F, Bauer G. Cerebral anoxia: clinical aspects. In: Niedermeyer E, Lopes da Silva F, eds. *Electroencephalography, basic principles, clinical applications, and related fields.* Baltimore: Williams & Wilkins, 1999:445–458.
41. Cantero JL, Atienza M. Alpha burst activity during human REM sleep: descriptive study and functional hypotheses. *Clin Neurophysiol* 2000;111:909–915.

42. Sharbrough FW. Nonspecific abnormal EEG patterns. In: Niedermeyer E, Lopes da Silva F, eds. *Electroencephalography, basic principles, clinical applications, and related fields.* Baltimore: Williams & Wilkins, 1999:215–234.

43. Westmoreland BF. Benign EEG variants and patterns of uncertain clinical significance. In: Daly DD, Pedley TA, eds. *Current practice of clinical electroencephalography,* 2nd ed. New York: Raven Press, 1990:243–252.

44. Young GB, Blume WT, Campbell VM, Demelo JD, Leung LS, McKeown MJ, et al. Alpha, theta and alpha-theta coma: a clinical outcome study utilizing serial recordings. *Electroencephalogr Clin Neurophysiol* 1994;91(2):93–99.

45. Niedermeyer E. Alpha rhythms as physiological and abnormal phenomena. *Int J Psychophysiol* 1997;26(1–3):31–49.

46. Guterman B, Sebastian P, Sodha N. Recovery from alpha coma after lorazepam overdose. *Clin Electroencephalogr* 1981;12(4):205–208.

47. Westmoreland BF, Klass DW, Sharbrough FW, Reagan TJ. Alpha-coma. Electroencephalographic, clinical, pathologic, and etiologic correlations. *Arch Neurol* 1975;32:713–718.

48. Grindal AB, Suter C. "Alpha-pattern coma" in high voltage electrical injury. *Electroencephalogr Clin Neurophysiol* 1975;38:521–526.

49. Berkhoff M, Donati F, Bassetti C. Postanoxic alpha (theta) coma: a reappraisal of its prognostic significance. *Clin Neurophysiol* 2000;111:297–304.

50. Gastaut H, Pinsard N, Raybaud C, Aicardi J, Zifkin B. Lissencephaly (agyria-pachygyria): clinical findings and serial EEG studies. *Dev Med Child Neurol* 1987;29(2):167–180.

51. Chatrian GE. Coma, other states of altered responsivness, and brain death. In: Daly DD, Pedley TA, eds. *Current practice of clinical electroencephalography,* 2nd ed. New York: Raven Press, 1990:425–487.

52. Markand ON. Electroencephalography in diffuse encephalopathies. *J Clin Neurophysiol* 1984;1:357–407.

53. Yamada T, Stevland N, Kimura J. Alpha-pattern coma in a 2-year-old child. *Arch Neurol* 1979;36:225–227.

54. Kozelka JW, Pedley TA. Beta and mu rhythms. *J Clin Neurophysiol* 1990;7:191–207.

55. Westmoreland BF, Klass DW. Midline theta rhythm. *Arch Neurol* 1986;43:139–141.

56. Koshino Y, Isaki K. Familial occurrence of the mu rhythm. *Clin Electroencephalogr* 1986;17(1):44–50.

57. Hari R, Salmelin R, Makela JP, Salenius S, Helle M. Magnetoencephalographic cortical rhythms. *Int J Psychophysiol* 1997;26(1–3):51–62.

58. van Sweden B, Wauquier A, Niedermeyer E. Normal aging and transient cognitive disorders in the elderly. In: Niedermeyer E, Lopes da Silva F, eds. *Electroencephalography, basic principles, clinical applications, and related fields.* Baltimore: Williams & Wilkins, 1999: 340–348.

59. Niedermeyer E. Alpha-like rhythmical activity of the temporal lobe. *Clin Electroencephalogr* 1990;21:210–224.

60. Asokan G, Pareja J, Niedermeyer E. Temporal minor slow and sharp EEG activity and cerebrovascular disorder. *Clin Electroencephalogr* 1987;18:201–210.

61. Niedermeyer E. Abnormal EEG patterns: epileptic and paroxysmal. In: Niedermeyer E, Lopes da Silva F, eds. *Electroencephalography, basic principles, clinical applications, and related fields.* Baltimore: Williams & Wilkins, 1999:235–260.

62. Niedermeyer E. The "third rhythm": further observations. *Clin Electroencephalogr* 1991; 22(2):83–96.

63. Reiher J, Lebel M. Wicket spikes: clinical correlates of a previously undescribed EEG pattern. *Can J Neurol Sci* 1977;4(1):39–47.

64. Shinomiya S, Fukunaga T, Nagata K. Clinical aspects of the "third rhythm" of the temporal lobe. *Clin Electroencephalogr* 1999;30(4):136–142.

65. Batista MS, Coelho CF, de Lima MM, Silva DF. A case-control study of a benign electroencephalographic variant pattern. *Arq Neuropsiquiatr* 1999;57(3A):561–565.

66. Tiihonen J, Hari R, Kajola M, Karhu J, Ahlfors S, Tissari S. Magnetoencephalographic 10-Hz rhythm from the human auditory cortex. *Neurosci Lett* 1991;129:303–305.

67. Reilly EL. EEG recording and operation of the apparatus. In: Niedermeyer E, Lopes da Silva F, eds. *Electroencephalography, basic principles, clinical applications, and related fields.* Baltimore: Williams & Wilkins, 1999:122–142.

68. Cooper R, Osselton JW, Shaw JC. *EEG technology,* 2nd ed. London: Butterworths, 1974.

69. Brittenham DM. Artifacts, activities not arising from the brain. In: Daly DD, Pedley TA, eds. *Current practice of clinical electroencephalography,* 2nd ed. New York: Raven Press, 1990: 85–105.

70. Bennett. *Atlas of electroencephalography in coma and cerebral death.* New York: Raven Press, 1976:111.

71. Egol AB, Guntupalli KK. Intravenous infusion device artifact in the EEG-confusion in the diagnosis of electrocerebral silence. *Intensive Care Med* 1983;9(1):29–32.

72. Mowery G. Artifacts. *Am J EEG Technology* 1962;2(2):41–58.

73. Reiher J, Klass DW. "Small sharp spikes" (SSS): electroencephalographic characteristics and clinical significance. *Electroencephalogr Clin Neurophysiol* 1970;28(1):94.

74. Hughes JR, Gruener G. Small sharp spikes revisited: further data on this controversial pattern. *Clin Electroencephalogr* 1984;15(4):208–213.

75. Saito F, Fukushima Y, Kubota S. Small sharp spikes: possible relationship to epilepsy. *Clin Electroencephalogr* 1987;18(3):114–119.

76. Molaie M, Santana HB, Otero C, Cavanaugh WA. Effect of epilepsy and sleep deprivation on the rate of benign epileptiform transients of sleep. *Epilepsia* 1991;32(1):44–50.

77. White JC, Langston JW, Pedley TA. Benign epileptiform transients of sleep. Clarification of the small sharp spike controversy. *Neurology* 1977;27:1061–1068.

78. Westmoreland BF, Reiher J, Klass DW. Recording small sharp spikes with depth electroencephalography. *Epilepsia* 1979;20:599–606.

79. Berger H. On the electroencephalogram of man, second report. In: Gloor P, ed. *Hans Berger on the electroencephalogram of man.* Amsterdam: Elsevier, 1969:75–93.

80. Kellaway P, Fox B. Electroencephalographic diagnosis of cerebral pathology in infants during sleep. I. Rationale, technique, and the characteristics of normal sleep in infants. *J Pediatr* 1952;41:262–287.

81. Kinoshita T, Michel CM, Yagyu T, Lehmann D, Saito M. Diazepam and sulpiride effects on frequency domain EEG source locations. *Neuropsychobiology* 1994;30(2–3):126–131.

82. Brenner RP, Atkinson R. Generalized paroxysmal fast activity: electroencephalographic and clinical features. *Ann Neurol* 1982;11:386–390.

83. Speckmann E-J, Elger CE. Introduction to the neurophysiological basis of the EEG and DC potentials. In: Niedermeyer E, Lopes da Silva F, eds. *Electroencephalography, basic principles, clinical applications, and related fields.* Baltimore: Williams & Wilkins, 1999:15–27.

84. Glaze DG. Drug effects. In: Daly DD, Pedley TA, eds. *Current practice of clinical electroencephalography,* 2nd ed. New York: Raven Press, 1990:489–512.

85. Schmidt D. The influence of antiepileptic drugs on the electroencephalogram: a review of controlled clinical studies. *Electroencephalogr Clin Neurophysiol Suppl* 1982;36:453–466.

86. Pohunkova D, Sulc J, Vana S. Influence of thyroid hormone supply on EEG frequency spectrum. *Endocrinol Exp* 1989;23(4):251–258.

87. Cobb WA, Guiloff RJ, Cast J. Breach rhythm: the EEG related to skull defects. *Electroencephalogr Clin Neurophysiol* 1979;47:251–271.

88. Jaffe R, Jacobs LD. Focal high voltage beta activity: clinical correlations. *Electroencephalogr Clin Neurophysiol* 1970;29:323.

89. Bauer G. Coma and brain death. In: Niedermeyer E, Lopes da Silva F, eds. *Electroencephalography, basic principles, clinical applications, and related fields.* Baltimore: Williams & Wilkins, 1999:459–475.

90. Hughes JR. Extreme stereotypy in the burst suppression pattern. *Clin Electroencephalogr* 1986;17(4):162–168.

91. Reeves AL, Westmoreland BF, Klass DW. Clinical accompaniments of the burst-suppression EEG pattern. *J Clin Neurophysiol* 1997;14:150–153.

92. Pourmand R. Burst-suppression pattern with unusual clinical correlates. *Clin Electroencephalogr* 1994;25(4):160–163.

93. Young GB. The EEG in coma. *J Clin Neurophysiol* 2000;17:473–485.

94. Stecker MM, Cheung AT, Pochettino A, Kent GP, Patterson T, Weiss SJ, et al. Deep hypothermic circulatory arrest: I. Effects of cooling on electroencephalogram and evoked potentials. *Ann Thorac Surg* 2001;71:14–21.

95. Bauer G, Bauer R. EEG, drug effects, and central nervous system poisoning. In: Niedermeyer E, Lopes da Silva F, eds. *Electroencephalography, basic principles, clinical applications, and related fields*. Baltimore: Williams & Wilkins, 1999:671–691.

96. Rumpl E. Craniocerebral trauma. In: Niedermeyer E, Lopes da Silva F, eds. *Electroencephalography, basic principles, clinical applications, and related fields*. Baltimore: Williams & Wilkins, 1999:393–415.

97. Synek VM. Prognostically important EEG coma patterns in diffuse anoxic and traumatic encephalopathies in adults. *J Clin Neurophysiol* 1988;5(2):161–174.

98. Magnus O, Van der Holst M. Zeta waves: a special type of slow delta waves. *Electroencephalogr Clin Neurophysiol* 1987;67:140–146.

99. Ganji S, Hellman S, Stagg S, Furlow J. Episodic coma due to acute basilar artery migraine: correlation of EEG and brainstem auditory evoked potential patterns. *Clin Electroencephalogr* 1993;24(1):44–48.

100. Ramelli GP, Sturzenegger M, Donati F, Karbowski K. EEG findings during basilar migraine attacks in children. *Electroencephalogr Clin Neurophysiol* 1998;107:374–378.

101. Ammirati F, Colivicchi F, Di Battista G, Garelli FF, Santini M. Electroencephalographic correlates of vasovagal syncope induced by head-up tilt testing. *Stroke* 1998;29:2347–2351.

102. Visser GH, Wieneke GH, van Huffelen AC. Carotid endarterectomy monitoring: patterns of spectral EEG changes due to carotid artery clamping. *Clin Neurophysiol* 1999;110:286–294.

103. Sebel PS, Bovill JG, Wauquier A, Rog P. Effects of high-dose fentanyl anesthesia on the electroencephalogram. *Anesthesiology* 1981;55:203–211.

104. Gibbs F, Gibbs E. *Atlas of electroencephalography.* Cambridge, MA: Lew A. Cummings, 1941.

105. Niedermeyer E. Cerebrovascular disorders and EEG. In: Niedermeyer E, Lopes da Silva F, eds. *Electroencephalography, basic principles, clinical applications, and related fields.* Baltimore: Williams & Wilkins, 1999:317–339.

106. Naidu S, Niedermeyer E. Degenerative disorders of the central nervous system. In: Niedermeyer E, Lopes da Silva F, eds. *Electroencephalography, basic principles, clinical applications, and related fields.* Baltimore: Williams & Wilkins, 1999:360–382.

107. Inui K, Motomura E, Kaige H, Nomura S. Temporal slow waves and cerebrovascular diseases. *Psychiatry Clin Neurosci* 2001;55:525–531.

108. Matsuura M, Yoshino M, Ohta K, Onda H, Nakajima K, Kojima T. Clinical significance of diffuse delta EEG activity in chronic schizophrenia. *Clin Electroencephalogr* 1994;25(3):115–121.

109. Thumasupapong S, Tin T, Sukontason K, Sawaddichi C, Karbwang J. Electroencephalography in cerebral malaria. *Southeast Asian J Trop Med Public Health* 1995;26(1):34–37.

110. Schauble B, Castillo PR, Boeve BF, Westmoreland BF. EEG findings in steroid-responsive encephalopathy associated with autoimmune thyroiditis. *Clin Neurophysiol* 2003;114(1):32–37.

111. Westmoreland BF. The EEG in cerebral inflammatory processes. In: Niedermeyer E, Lopes da Silva F, eds. *Electroencephalography, basic principles, clinical applications, and related fields.* Baltimore: Williams & Wilkins, 1999:302–316.

112. Zifkin BG, Cracco RQ. An orderly approach ot the abnormal EEG. In: Daly DD, Pedley TA, eds. *Current practice of clinical electroencephalography,* 2nd ed. New York: Raven Press, 1990:253–267.

113. Whittle IR, Clarke M, Gregori A, Piper IR, Miller JD. Interstitial white matter brain oedema does not alter the electroencephalogram. *Br J Neurosurg* 1992;6:433–437.

114. Schaul N. Pathogenesis and significance of abnormal nonepileptiform rhythms in the EEG. *J Clin Neurophysiol* 1990;7:229–248.

115. Huppertz HJ, Hof E, Klisch J, Wagner M, Lucking CH, Kristeva-Feige R. Localization of interictal delta and epileptiform EEG activity associated with focal epileptogenic brain lesions. *Neuroimage* 2001;13(1):15–28.

116. Maytal J, Novak GP, Knobler SB, Schaul N. Neuroradiological manifestations of focal polymorphic delta activity in children. *Arch Neurol* 1993;50:181–184.

117. Martinius J, Matthes A, Lombroso CT. Electroencephalographic features in posterior fossa tumors in children. *Electroencephalogr Clin Neurophysiol* 1968;25:128–139.

118. Fischer-Williams M, Dike G. Brain tumors and other space-occupying lesions. In: Niedermeyer E, Lopes da Silva F, eds. *Electroencephalography, basic principles, clinical applications, and related fields.* Baltimore: Williams & Wilkins, 1999:285–301.

119. Dunne JW, Silbert PL. Zeta waves: a distinctive type of intermittent delta wave studied prospectively. *Clin Exp Neurol* 1991;28:238–243.

120. Fariello RG, Orrison W, Blanco G, Reyes PF. Neuroradiological correlates of frontally predominant intermittent rhythmic delta activity (FIRDA). *Electroencephalogr Clin Neurophysiol* 1982;54:194–202.

121. Koshino Y, Murata I, Murata T, Omori M, Hamada T, Miyagoshi M, et al. Frontal intermittent delta activity in schizophrenic patients receiving antipsychotic drugs. *Clin Electroencephalogr* 1993;24(1):13–18.

122. Calzetti S, Bortone E, Negrotti A, Zinno L, Mancia D. Frontal intermittent rhythmic delta activity (FIRDA) in patients with dementia with Lewy bodies: a diagnostic tool? *Neurol Sci* 2002;23[Suppl 2]:S65–66.

123. Nakano M, Abe K, Ono J, Yanagihara T. Intermittent rhythmic delta activity (IRDA) in a patient with band heterotopia. *Clin Electroencephalogr* 1998;29(3):138–141.

124. Pietrini V, Terzano MG, D'Andrea G, Parrino L, Cananzi AR, Ferro-Milone F. Acute confusional migraine: clinical and electroencephalographic aspects. *Cephalalgia* 1987;7(1):29–37.

125. Frequin ST, Linssen WH, Pasman JW, Hommes OR, Merx HL. Recurrent prolonged coma due to basilar artery migraine. A case report. *Headache* 1991;31(2):75–81.

126. Neufeld MY, Chistik V, Chapman J, Korczyn AD. Intermittent rhythmic delta activity (IRDA) morphology cannot distinguish between focal and diffuse brain disturbances. *J Neurol Sci* 1999;164(1):56–59.

127. Hansen HC, Zschocke S, Sturenburg HJ, Kunze K. Clinical changes and EEG patterns preceding the onset of periodic sharp wave complexes in Creutzfeldt-Jakob disease. *Acta Neurol Scand* 1998;97(2):99–106.

128. Markand ON, Panszi JG. The electroencephalogram in subacute sclerosing panencephalitis. *Arch Neurol* 1975;32:719–726.

129. Watemberg N, Alehan F, Dabby R, Lerman-Sagie T, Pavot P, Towne A. Clinical and radiologic correlates of frontal intermittent rhythmic delta activity. *J Clin Neurophysiol* 2002;19:535–539.

130. Gullapalli D, Fountain NB. Clinical correlation of occipital intermittent rhythmic delta activity. *J Clin Neurophysiol* 2003;20:35–41.

131. Normand MM, Wszolek ZK, Klass DW. Temporal intermittent rhythmic delta activity in electroencephalograms. *J Clin Neurophysiol* 1995;12:280–284.

132. Geyer JD, Bilir E, Faught RE, Kuzniecky R, Gilliam F. Significance of interictal temporal lobe delta activity for localization of the primary epileptogenic region. *Neurology* 1999;52:202–205.

133. Di Gennaro G, Quarato PP, Onorati P, Colazza GB, Mari F, Grammaldo LG, et al. Localizing significance of temporal intermittent rhythmic delta activity (TIRDA) in drug-resistant focal epilepsy. *Clin Neurophysiol* 2003;114(1):70–78.

134. Eeg-Olofsson O. The development of the electroencephalogram in normal children from the age of 1 through 15 years. 14 and 6 Hz positive spike phenomenon. *Neuropadiatrie* 1971;2(4):405–427.

135. Reiher J, Carmant L. Clinical correlates and electroencephalographic characteristics of two additional patterns related to 14 and 6 per second positive spikes. *Can J Neurol Sci* 1991;18: 488–491.

136. Beydoun A, Drury I. Unilateral 14 and 6 Hz positive bursts. *Electroencephalogr Clin Neurophysiol* 1992;82:310–312.

137. Silverman D. Phantom spike-waves and the fourteen and six per second positive spike pattern: a consideration of their relationship. *Electroencephalogr Clin Neurophysiol* 1967; 23:207–213.

138. Lombroso CT, Schwartz IH, Clark DM, Muench H, Barry PH, Barry J. Ctenoids in healthy youths. Controlled study of 14- and 6-per-second positive spiking. *Neurology* 1966;16:1152–1158.

139. Schwartz IH, Lombroso CT. 14 and 6/second positive spiking (ctenoids) in the electroencephalograms of primary school pupils. *J Pediatr* 1968;72:678–682.

140. Yamada T, Tucker RP, Kooi KA. Fourteen and six c/sec positive bursts in comatose patients. *Electroencephalogr Clin Neurophysiol* 1976;40:645–653.

141. Drury I. 14-and-6 Hz positive bursts in childhood encephalopathies. *Electroencephalogr Clin Neurophysiol* 1989;72:479–485.

142. Okuma T, Kuba K, Matsushita T, Nakao T, Fujii S, Shimoda Y. Study on 14 and 6 per second positive spikes during nocturnal sleep. *Electroencephalogr Clin Neurophysiol* 1968;25: 140–149.

143. Takahashi H. Activation methods. In: Niedermeyer E, Lopes da Silva F, eds. *Electroencephalography, basic principles, clinical applications, and related fields.* Baltimore: Williams & Wilkins, 1999:261–284.

144. Zysno AE, Buttner G. The EEG in experimental changes in the acid-base metabolism. *Electroencephalogr Clin Neurophysiol* 1971;30:273–274.

145. Yamatani M, Konishi T, Murakami M, Okuda T. Hyperventilation activation on EEG recording in childhood. *Epilepsia* 1994;35:1199–1203.

146. Epstein MA, Duchowny M, Jayakar P, Resnick TJ, Alvarez LA. Altered responsiveness during hyperventilation-induced EEG slowing: a non-epileptic phenomenon in normal children. *Epilepsia* 1994;35:1204–1207.

147. Yamashiro Y, Takahashi H, Takahashi K. Cerebrovascular Moyamoya disease. *Eur J Pediatr* 1984;142(1):44–50.

148. Kurlemann G, Fahrendorf G, Krings W, Sciuk J, Palm D. Characteristic EEG findings in childhood moyamoya syndrome. *Neurosurg Rev* 1992;15(1):57–60.

149. Kuroda S, Kamiyama H, Isobe M, Houkin K, Abe H, Mitsumori K. Cerebral hemodynamics and "re-build-up" phenomenon on electroencephalogram in children with moyamoya disease. *Childs Nerv Syst* 1995;11(4):214–219.

150. Niedermeyer E. Epileptic seizure disorders. In: Niedermeyer E, Lopes da Silva F, eds. *Electroencephalography, basic principles, clinical applications, and related fields.* Baltimore: Williams & Wilkins, 1999:476–585.

151. Amit R, Crumrine PK. Ictal midline epileptiform discharges. *Clin Electroencephalogr* 1993; 24(2):67–69.

152. Sharbrough FW. Scalp-recorded ictal patterns in focal epilepsy. *J Clin Neurophysiol* 1993;10: 262–267.

153. Worrell GA, So EL, Kazemi J, O'Brien TJ, Mosewich RK, Cascino GD, et al. Focal ictal beta discharge on scalp EEG predicts excellent outcome of frontal lobe epilepsy surgery. *Epilepsia* 2002;43:277–282.

154. Risinger MW, Engel Jr J, Van Ness PC, Henry TR, Crandall PH. Ictal localization of temporal lobe seizures with scalp/sphenoidal recordings. *Neurology* 1989;39:1288–1293.

155. Foldvary N, Klem G, Hammel J, Bingaman W, Najm I, Luders H. The localizing value of ictal EEG in focal epilepsy. *Neurology* 2001;57:2022–2028.

156. Lee SK, Kim JY, Hong KS, Nam HW, Park SH, Chung CK. The clinical usefulness of ictal surface EEG in neocortical epilepsy. *Epilepsia* 2000;41:1450–1455.

157. Devinsky O, Kelley K, Porter RJ, Theodore WH. Clinical and electroencephalographic features of simple partial seizures. *Neurology* 1988;38:1347–1352.

158. Bare MA, Burnstine TH, Fisher RS, Lesser RP. Electroencephalographic changes during simple partial seizures. *Epilepsia* 1994;35:715–720.

159. Drury I, Henry TR. Ictal patterns in generalized epilepsy. *J Clin Neurophysiol* 1993;10: 268–280.

160. Lee SI, Kirby D. Absence seizure with generalized rhythmic delta activity. *Epilepsia* 1988;29:262–267.

161. Gibbs F, Gibbs E, Lennox W. Epilepsy: a paroxysmal cerebral dysrhythmia. *Brain* 1937;60: 377–388.

162. Lombroso CT. Sylvian seizures and midtemporal spike foci in children. *Arch Neurol* 1967;17:52–59.

163. Graf M, Lischka A. Topographical EEG analysis of rolandic spikes. *Clin Electroencephalogr* 1998;29(3):132–137.

164. Legarda S, Jayakar P, Duchowny M, Alvarez L, Resnick T. Benign rolandic epilepsy: high central and low central subgroups. *Epilepsia* 1994;35:1125–1129.

165. van der Meij W, Wieneke GH, van Huffelen AC. Dipole source analysis of rolandic spikes in benign rolandic epilepsy and other clinical syndromes. *Brain Topogr* 1993;5(3):203–213.

166. van der Meij W, Huiskamp GJ, Rutlen GJ, Wieneke GH, van Huffelen AC, van Nieuwenhuizen O. The existence of two sources in rolandic epilepsy: confirmation with high resolution EEG, MEG and fMRI. *Brain Topogr* 2001;13(4):275–282.

167. Archer JS, Briellman RS, Abbott DF, Syngeniotis A, Wellard, RM, Jackson, GD. Benign epilepsy with centro-temporal spikes: spike triggered fMRI shows somato-sensory cortex activity. *Epilepsia* 2003;44:200–204.

168. Degen R, Degen HE. Contribution to the genetics of rolandic epilepsy: waking and sleep EEGs in siblings. *Epilepsy Res Suppl* 1992;6:49–52.

169. Nicholl JS, Willis JK, Rice J. The effect of hyperventilation on the frequency of Rolandic spikes. *Clin Electroencephalogr* 1998;29(4):181–182.

170. Kellaway P. The electroencephalographic features of benign centrotemporal (rolandic) epilepsy of childhood. *Epilepsia* 2000;41:1053–1056.

171. van der Meij W, Wieneke GH, van Huffelen AC, Schenk-Rootlieb AJ, Willemse J. Identical morphology of the rolandic spike-and-wave complex in different clinical entities. *Epilepsia* 1993;34:540–550.

172. Kurth C, Bittermann HJ, Wegerer V, Bleich S, Steinhoff BJ. Fixation-off sensitivity in an adult with symptomatic occipital epilepsy. *Epilepsia* 2001;42:947–949.

173. Talwar D, Rask CA, Torres F. Clinical manifestations in children with occipital spike-wave paroxysms. *Epilepsia* 1992;33:667–674.

174. Engel Jr J, Rapin I, Giblin DR. Electrophysiological studies in two patients with cherry red spot—myoclonus syndrome. *Epilepsia* 1977;18:73–87.

175. Malow BA, Selwa LM, Ross D, Aldrich MS. Lateralizing value of interictal spikes on overnight sleep-EEG studies in temporal lobe epilepsy. *Epilepsia* 1999;40:1587–1592.

176. Gilbert DL, Sethuraman G, Kotagal U, Buncher CR. Meta-analysis of EEG test performance shows wide variation among studies. *Neurology* 2003;60:564–570.

177. Jabbari B, Russo MB, Russo ML. Electroencephalogram of asymptomatic adult subjects. *Clin Neurophysiol* 2000;111(1):102–105.

178. Trojaborg W. EEG abnormalities in 5,893 jet pilot applicants registered in a 20-year period. *Clin Electroencephalogr* 1992;23(2):72–78.

179. Gregory RP, Oates T, Merry RT. Electroencephalogram epileptiform abnormalities in candidates for aircrew training. *Electroencephalogr Clin Neurophysiol* 1993;86:75–77.

180. Sam MC, So EL. Significance of epileptiform discharges in patients without epilepsy in the community. *Epilepsia* 2001;42:1273–1278.

181. Zivin L, Marsan CA. Incidence and prognostic significance of "epileptiform" activity in the EEG of non-epileptic subjects. *Brain* 1968;91:751–778.

182. Goodin DS, Aminoff MJ. Does the interictal EEG have a role in the diagnosis of epilepsy? *Lancet* 1984;1:837–839.
183. Drury I, Beydoun A. Interictal epileptiform activity in elderly patients with epilepsy. *Electroencephalogr Clin Neurophysiol* 1998;106:369–373.
184. Hedstrom A, Olsson I. Epidemiology of absence epilepsy: EEG findings and their predictive value. *Pediatr Neurol* 1991;7(2):100–104.
185. Westmoreland BF. Epileptiform electroencephalographic patterns. *Mayo Clin Proc* 1996;71: 501–511.
186. de Weerd AW, Arts WF. Significance of centro-temporal spikes on the EEG. *Acta Neurol Scand* 1993;87:429–433.
187. Noriega-Sanchez A, Markand ON. Clinical and electroencephalographic correlation of independent multifocal spike discharges. *Neurology* 1976;26:667–672.
188. Kotagal P. Multifocal independent Spike syndrome: relationship to hypsarrhythmia and the slow spike-wave (Lennox-Gastaut) syndrome. *Clin Electroencephalogr* 1995;26(1):23–29.
189. Brunquell P, Tezcan K, DiMario Jr FJ. Electroencephalographic findings in ornithine transcarbamylase deficiency. *J Child Neurol* 1999;14:533–536.
190. Stern JM. The epilepsy of trisomy 9p. *Neurology* 1996;47:821–824.
191. Lombroso CT. Consistent EEG focalities detected in subjects with primary generalized epilepsies monitored for two decades. *Epilepsia* 1997;38:797–812.
192. Markand ON. Slow spike-wave activity in EEG and associated clinical features: often called 'Lennox' or 'Lennox-Gastaut' syndrome. *Neurology* 1977;27:746–757.
193. Silva DF, Lima MM, Anghinah R, Zanoteli E, Lima JG. Atypical EEG pattern in children with absence seizures. *Arq Neuropsiquiatr* 1995;53(2):258–261.
194. Burr W, Stefan H, Kuhnen C, Hoffmann F, Penin H. Effect of valproic acid treatment on spike-wave discharge patterns during sleep and wakefulness. *Neuropsychobiology* 1983;10(1): 56–59.
195. Yenjun S, Harvey AS, Marini C, Newton MR, King MA, Berkovic SF. EEG in adult-onset idiopathic generalized epilepsy. *Epilepsia* 2003;44:252–256.
196. Tukel K, Jasper H. The electroencephalogram in parasagittal lesions. *Electroencephalogr Clin Neurophysiol* 1952;4:481–494.
197. Blume WT, Pillay N. Electrographic and clinical correlates of secondary bilateral synchrony. *Epilepsia* 1985;26:636–641.
198. Scher MS. Electroencephalography of the newborn: normal and abnormal features. In: Niedermeyer E, Lopes da Silva F, eds. *Electroencephalography, basic principles, clinical applications, and related fields.* Baltimore: Williams & Wilkins, 1999:896–946.
199. Watanabe K, Negoro T, Aso K, Matsumoto A. Reappraisal of interictal electroencephalograms in infantile spasms. *Epilepsia* 1993;34:679–685.
200. Browne TR, Penry JK, Proter RJ, Dreifuss FE. Responsiveness before, during, and after spike-wave paroxysms. *Neurology* 1974;24:659–665.
201. Binnie CD, Marston D. Cognitive correlates of interictal discharges. *Epilepsia* 1992;33[Suppl 6]:S11–17.
202. Licht EA, Fujikawa DG. Nonconvulsive status epilepticus with frontal features: quantitating severity of subclinical epileptiform discharges provides a marker for treatment efficacy, recurrence and outcome. *Epilepsy Res* 2002;51(1–2):13–21.
203. Drury I, Beydoun A, Garofalo EA, Henry TR. Asymmetric hypsarrhythmia: clinical electroencephalographic and radiological findings. *Epilepsia* 1995;36:41–47.
204. Kramer U, Sue WC, Mikati MA. Hypsarrhythmia: frequency of variant patterns and correlation with etiology and outcome. *Neurology* 1997;48:197–203.
205. Rechtschaffen A, Kales A, eds. *A manual of standardized terminology, techniques and scoring system for sleep stages of human subjects.* Bethesda, MD: U.S. Dept. of Health, Education, and Welfare, PHS-NIH, 1968.
206. Crowley K, Trinder J, Kim Y, Carrington M, Colrain I. The effects of normal aging on sleep spindle and K-complex production. *Clin Neurophysiol* 2002;113:1615–1622.
207. Niiyama Y, Satoh N, Kutsuzawa O, Hishikawa Y. Electrophysiological evidence suggesting that sensory stimuli of unknown origin induce spontaneous K-complexes. *Electroencephalogr Clin Neurophysiol* 1996;98:394–400.
208. Fushimi M, Niiyama Y, Fujiwara R, Satoh N, Hishikawa Y. Some sensory stimuli generate spontaneous K-complexes. *Psychiatry Clin Neurosci* 1998;52(2):150–152.
209. Ehrhart J, Ehrhart M, Muzet A, Schieber JP, Naitoh P. K-complexes and sleep spindles before transient activation during sleep. *Sleep* 1981;4:400–407.
210. Wauquier A, Aloe L, Declerck A. K-complexes: are they signs of arousal or sleep protective? *J Sleep Res* 1995;4(3):138–143.
211. Bastien CH, Ladouceur C, Campbell KB. EEG characteristics prior to and following the evoked K-Complex. *Can J Exp Psychol* 2000;54(4):255–265.
212. Numminen J, Makela JP, Hari R. Distributions and sources of magnetoencephalographic K-complexes. *Electroencephalogr Clin Neurophysiol* 1996;99:544–555.
213. Amzica F, Steriade M. The K-complex: its slow (<1-Hz) rhythmicity and relation to delta waves. *Neurology* 1997;49:952–959.
214. Billings RJ. The origin of the occipital lambda wave in man. *Electroencephalogr Clin Neurophysiol* 1989;72:95–113.
215. Shih JJ, Thompson SW. Lambda waves: incidence and relationship to photic driving. *Brain Topogr* 1998;10(4):265–272.
216. Silverman D, Masland RL, Saunders MG, Schwab RS. Irreversible coma associated with electrocerebral silence. *Neurology* 1970;20:525–533.
217. American EEG Society- Guideline three: Minimum technical standards for EEG recording in suspected cerebral death. *J Clin Neurophysiol* 1994;11:10–13.
218. Brenner RP, Schwartzman RJ, Richey ET. Prognostic significance of episodic low amplitude or relatively isoelectric EEG patterns. *Dis Nerv Syst* 1975;36:582–587.
219. Rae-Grant AD, Strapple C, Barbour PJ. Episodic low-amplitude events: an under-recognized phenomenon in clinical electroencephalography. *J Clin Neurophysiol* 1991;8:203–211.
220. Pourmand R. The significance of amplitude asymmetry in clinical electroencephalography. *Clin Electroencephalogr* 1994;25(2):76–80.
221. Markand ON. Organic brain syndromes and dementias. In: Daly DD, Pedley TA, eds. *Current practice of clinical electroencephalography,* 2nd ed. New York: Raven Press, 1990:401–423.
222. van Sweden B. The EEG in chronic alcoholism. *Clin Neurol Neurosurg* 1983;85(1):3–20.
223. Connelly CS, O'Donovan CA, McCall WV, Bell WL, Quinlivan L. Electrocerebral inactivity associated with obstructive sleep apnea. *Neurology* 1997;48:1464–1466.
224. Ko DY. Electrocerebral inactivity associated with obstructive sleep apnea. *Neurology* 1998;50: 1934.
225. Reilly EL. Electrocerebral inactivity as a temperature effect: unlikely as an isolated etiology. *Clin Electroencephalogr* 1981;12(2):69–71.
226. Green JB, Lauber A. Return of EEG activity after electrocerebral silence: two case reports. *J Neurol Neurosurg Psychiatry* 1972;35(1):103–107.
227. Juguilon AC, Reilly EL. Development of EEG activity after ten days of electrocerebral inactivity: ten days of electrocerebral inactivity: a case report in a premature neonate-hydranencephaly or massive ventricular enlargement. *Clin Electroencephalogr* 1982;13(4): 233–240.
228. Castellotti V, Cernibori A, Oliva A. Study of "mitten patterns". *Electroencephalogr Clin Neurophysiol* 1968;25:515.
229. Gibbs EL, Fois A, Gibbs FA. The electroencephalogram in retrolental fibroplasia. *N Engl J Med* 1955;253:1102–1106.
230. Cohen J. EEG and blindness. *Electroencephalogr Clin Neurophysiol* 1969;26:115.
231. Kellaway P, Bloxso A, MacGregor M. Occipital spike foci associated with retrolental fibroplasia and other forms of retinal loss in children. *Electroencephalogr Clin Neurophysiol* 1955;7:469–470.

232. Daly DD. Epilepsy and syncope. In: Daly DD, Pedley TA, eds. *Current practice of clinical electroencephalography,* 2nd ed. New York: Raven Press, 1990:269–334.

233. Catani P, Salzarulo P, Findji F. Occipital spikes and eye movement activity during paradoxical sleep in visually defective children. *Electroencephalogr Clin Neurophysiol* 1978;44: 782–784.

234. Robertson R, Jan JE, Wong PK. Electroencephalograms of children with permanent cortical visual impairment. *Can J Neurol Sci* 1986;13:256–261.

235. Jan JE, Wong PK. Behaviour of the alpha rhythm in electroencephalograms of visually impaired children. *Dev Med Child Neurol* 1988;30:444–450.

236. Altman K, Shewmon D. Local paroxysmal fast activity: significance interictally and in infantile spasms. *Epilepsia* 1990;31:623.

237. Chayasirisobhon S, Cullis P, Sack R, Papavasiliou A. Grand mal discharge. *Clin Electroencephalogr* 1984;15(3):155–158.

238. Hooshmand H, Morganroth R, Corredor C. Significance of focal and lateralized beta activity in the EEG. *Clin Electroencephalogr* 1980;11(3):140–144.

239. Rodin E, Smid N, Mason K. The grand mal pattern of Gibbs, Gibbs and Lennox. *Electroencephalogr Clin Neurophysiol* 1976;40:401–406.

240. Nealis JG, Duffy FH. Paroxysmal beta activity in the pediatric electroencephalogram. *Ann Neurol* 1978;4:112–116.

241. Pohlmann-Eden B, Hoch DB, Cochius JI, Chiappa KH. Periodic lateralized epileptiform discharges—a critical review. *J Clin Neurophysiol* 1996;13:519–530.

242. Westmoreland BF, Frere RC, Klass DW. Periodic epileptiform discharges in the midline. *J Clin Neurophysiol* 1997;14:495–498.

243. Schear HE. Periodic EEG activity. *Clin Electroencephalogr* 1984;15(1):32–39.

244. Striano S, De Falco FA, Zaccaria F, Fels A, Natale S, Vacca G. Paroxysmal lateralized epileptiform discharges (PLEDS). Clinical-EEG correlations in twenty cases. *Acta Neurol (Napoli)* 1986;8(1):1–12.

245. Cobb W, Hill D. Electroencephalogram in subacute progressive encephalitis. *Brain* 1950(73): 392–404.

246. Raroque Jr HG, Gonzales PC, Jhaveri HS, Leroy RF, Allen EC. Defining the role of structural lesions and metabolic abnormalities in periodic lateralized epileptiform discharges. *Epilepsia* 1993;34:279–283.

247. Raroque Jr HG, Purdy P. Lesion localization in periodic lateralized epileptiform discharges: gray or white matter. *Epilepsia* 1995;36:58–62.

248. Neufeld MY, Vishnevskaya S, Treves TA, Reider I, Karepov V, Bornstein NM, et al. Periodic lateralized epileptiform discharges (PLEDs) following stroke are associated with metabolic abnormalities. *Electroencephalogr Clin Neurophysiol* 1997;102:295–298.

249. Gross DW, Quesney LF, Sadikot AF. Chronic periodic lateralized epileptiform discharges during sleep in a patient with caudate nucleus atrophy: insights into the anatomical circuitry of PLEDs. *Electroencephalogr Clin Neurophysiol* 1998;107:434–438.

250. Wheless JW, Holmes GL, King DW, Gallagher BB, Murro AM, Flanigin HF, et al. Possible relationship of periodic lateralized epileptiform discharges to thalamic stroke. *Clin Electroencephalogr* 1991;22(4):211–216.

251. Janati A, Chesser MZ, Husain MM. Periodic lateralized epileptiform discharges (PLEDs): a possible role for metabolic factors in pathogenesis. *Clin Electroencephalogr* 1986;17(1): 36–43.

252. Raroque Jr HG, Wagner W, Gonzales PC, Leroy RF, Karnaze D, Riela AR, et al. Reassessment of the clinical significance of periodic lateralized epileptiform discharges in pediatric patients. *Epilepsia* 1993;34:275–278.

253. Chen KS, Kuo MF, Wang HS, Huang SC. Periodic lateralized epileptiform discharges of pediatric patients in Taiwan. *Pediatr Neurol* 2003;28(2):100–103.

254. Westmoreland BF, Klass DW, Sharbrough FW. Chronic periodic lateralized epileptiform discharges. *Arch Neurol* 1986;43:494–496.

255. Garcia-Morales I, Garcia MT, Galan-Davila L, Gomez-Escalonilla C, Saiz-Diaz R, Martinez-Salio A, et al. Periodic lateralized epileptiform discharges: etiology, clinical aspects, seizures, and evolution in 130 patients. *J Clin Neurophysiol* 2002;19:172–177.

256. Westmoreland BF. Periodic lateralized epileptiform discharges after evacuation of subdural hematomas. *J Clin Neurophysiol* 2001;18:20–24.

257. Mehryar GR, McIntyre HB. Periodic lateralized epileptiform discharges associated with subdural hematoma. *Bull Los Angeles Neurol Soc* 1975;40(1):8–12.

258. Brenner RP. EEG and dementia. In: Niedermeyer E, Lopes da Silva F, eds. *Electroencephalography, basic principles, clinical applications, and related fields.* Baltimore: Williams & Wilkins, 1999:349–359.

259. Brick JF, Gutierrez AR, Cheek JC, Breen L. Transient appearance of periodic EEG discharges in senile dementia. *Clin Electroencephalogr* 1991;22(2):108–111.

260. Chabolla DR, Moore JL, Westmoreland BF. Periodic lateralized epileptiform discharges in multiple sclerosis. *Electroencephalogr Clin Neurophysiol* 1996;98:5–8.

261. Funakawa I, Yasuda T, Terao A. Periodic lateralized epileptiform discharges in mitochondrial encephalomyopathy. *Electroencephalogr Clin Neurophysiol* 1997;103:370–375.

262. Baykan B, Kinay D, Gokyigit A, Gurses C. Periodic lateralized epileptiform discharges: association with seizures. *Seizure* 2000;9:402–406.

263. Brenner RP, Schaul N. Periodic EEG patterns: classification, clinical correlation, and pathophysiology. *J Clin Neurophysiol* 1990;7:249–267.

264. Lai CW, Gragasin ME. Electroencephalography in herpes simplex encephalitis. *J Clin Neurophysiol* 1988;5:87–103.

265. Gross DW, Wiebe S, Blume WT. The periodicity of lateralized epileptiform discharges. *Clin Neurophysiol* 1999;110:1516–1520.

266. Kurita A, Furushima H, Yamada H, Inoue K. Periodic lateralized epileptiform discharges in influenza B-associated encephalopathy. *Intern Med* 2001;40:813–816.

267. Sokol DK, Kleiman MB, Garg BP. LaCrosse viral encephalitis mimics herpes simplex viral encephalitis. *Pediatr Neurol* 2001;25:413–415.

268. Au WJ, Gabor AJ, Vijayan N, Markand ON. Periodic lateralized epileptiform complexes (PLEDs) in Creutzfeldt- Jakob disease. *Neurology* 1980;30:611–617.

269. Aguglia U, Gambardella A, Le Piane E, Messina D, Farnarier G, Oliveri RL, et al. Disappearance of periodic sharp wave complexes in Creutzfeldt-Jakob disease. *Neurophysiol Clin* 1997;27(4):277–282.

270. Chatrian GE, Shaw C-M, Leffman H. The significance of periodic lateralized epileptiform discharges in EEG: an electrographic, clinical and pathological study. *Electroencephalogr Clin Neurophysiol* 1964;17:177–193.

271. Handforth A, Cheng JT, Mandelkern MA, Treiman DM. Markedly increased mesiotemporal lobe metabolism in a case with PLEDs: further evidence that PLEDs are a manifestation of partial status epilepticus. *Epilepsia* 1994;35:876–881.

272. Ali, II, Pirzada NA, Vaughn BV. Periodic lateralized epileptiform discharges after complex partial status epilepticus associated with increased focal cerebral blood flow. *J Clin Neurophysiol* 2001;18:565–569.

273. Assal F, Papazyan JP, Slosman DO, Jallon P, Goerres GW. SPECT in periodic lateralized epileptiform discharges (PLEDs): a form of partial status epilepticus? *Seizure* 2001;10(4): 260–265.

274. Ono S, Chida K, Fukaya N, Yoshihashi H, Takasu T. Dysphasia accompanied by periodic lateralized epileptiform discharges. *Intern Med* 1997;36(1):59–61.

275. Garzon E, Fernandes RM, Sakamoto AC. Serial EEG during human status epilepticus: evidence for PLED as an ictal pattern. *Neurology* 2001;57:1175–1183.

276. Nei M, Lee JM, Shanker VL, Sperling MR. The EEG and prognosis in status epilepticus. *Epilepsia* 1999;40:157–163.

277. Reeves RR, Thompson SW. Trifocal independent periodic lateralized epileptiform discharges. *Clin Electroencephalogr* 1993;24(3):114–117.

278. Hughes JR, Taber J, Uppal H. TRI-PLEDs: a case report. *Clin Electroencephalogr* 1998;29(2): 106–108.

279. Nicolai J, van Putten MJ, Tavy DL. BIPLEDs in akinetic mutism caused by bilateral anterior cerebral artery infarction. *Clin Neurophysiol* 2001;112:1726–1728.

280. Lawn ND, Westmoreland BF, Sharbrough FW. Multifocal periodic lateralized epileptiform discharges (PLEDs): EEG features and clinical correlations. *Clin Neurophysiol* 2000;111: 2125–2129.

281. de la Paz D, Brenner RP. Bilateral independent periodic lateralized epileptiform discharges. Clinical significance. *Arch Neurol* 1981;38:713–715.

282. Vas GA, Cracco JB. Diffuse encephalopathies. In: Daly DD, Pedley TA, eds. *Current practice of clinical electroencephalography*, 2nd ed. New York: Raven Press, 1990:371–399.

283. Lombroso CT. Remarks on the EEG and movement disorder in SSPE. *Neurology* 1968; 18(1 Pt 2):69–75.

284. Gurses C, Ozturk A, Baykan B, Gokyigit A, Eraksoy M, Barlas M, et al. Correlation between clinical stages and EEG findings of subacute sclerosing panencephalitis. *Clin Electroencephalogr* 2000;31(4):201–206.

285. Yemisci M, Gurer G, Saygi S, Ciger A. Generalised periodic epileptiform discharges: clinical features, neuroradiological evaluation and prognosis in 37 adult patients. *Seizure* 2003;12: 465–472.

286. Synek VM, Shaw NA. Epileptiform discharges in presence of continuous background activity in anoxic coma. *Clin Electroencephalogr* 1989;20(2):141–146.

287. Hughes JR. Two forms of the 6/sec spike and wave complex. *Electroencephalogr Clin Neurophysiol* 1980;48:535–550.

288. Tharp BR. The 6-per-second spike and wave complex. The wave and spike phantom. *Arch Neurol* 1966;15:533–537.

289. Kerxhalli JS, Vogel W, Broverman DM, Klaiber EL. Effect of ascorbic acid on the human electroencephalogram. *J Nutr* 1975;105:1356–1358.

290. Vogel W, Broverman DM, Klaiber EL, Kobayashi Y. EEG driving responses as a function of monoamine oxidase. *Electroencephalogr Clin Neurophysiol* 1974;36:205–207.

291. Niedermeyer E. The EEG in patients with migraine and other forms of headache. In: Niedermeyer E, Lopes da Silva F, eds. *Electroencephalography, basic principles, clinical applications, and related fields*. Baltimore: Williams & Wilkins, 1999:595–602.

292. Takahashi Y, Fujiwara T, Yagi K, Seino M. Wavelength specificity of photoparoxysmal responses in idiopathic generalized epilepsy. *Epilepsia* 1995;36:1084–1088.

293. Jayakar P, Chiappa KH. Clinical correlations of photoparoxysmal responses. *Electroencephalogr Clin Neurophysiol* 1990;75:251–254.

294. So EL, Ruggles KH, Ahmann PA, Olson KA. Prognosis of photoparoxysmal response in nonepileptic patients. *Neurology* 1993;43:1719–1722.

295. de Falco FA, Roberti R, Florio C, Franzese G. Photoparoxysmal response on eye closure in photosensitive patients. *Acta Neurol* (Napoli) 1992;14(4–6):290–296.

296. Radhakrishnan K, Nayak SD, Nandini VS, Venugopal A. Prevalence of photoparoxysmal response among South Indian epilepsy patients. *Seizure* 1998;7:397–401.

297. Quirk JA, Fish DR, Smith SJ, Sander JW, Shorvon SD, Allen PJ. Incidence of photosensitive epilepsy: a prospective national study. *Electroencephalogr Clin Neurophysiol* 1995;95: 260–267.

298. Wolf P, Goosses R. Relation of photosensitivity to epileptic syndromes. *J Neurol Neurosurg Psychiatry* 1986;49:1386–1391.

299. Shiraishi H, Fujiwara T, Inoue Y, Yagi K. Photosensitivity in relation to epileptic syndromes: a survey from an epilepsy center in Japan. *Epilepsia* 2001;42:393–397.

300. Wright EA, Gilmore RL. Features of the geriatric EEG: age-dependent incidence of POSTS. *Clin Electroencephalogr* 1985;16(1):11–15.

301. Egawa I, Yoshino K, Hishikawa Y. Positive occipital sharp transients in the human sleep EEG. *Folia Psychiatr Neurol Jpn* 1983;37(1):57–65.

302. Brenner RP, Zauel DW, Carlow TJ. Positive occipital sharp transients of sleep in the blind. *Neurology* 1978;28:609–612.

303. Mizrahi EM. Avoiding the pitfalls of EEG interpretation in childhood epilepsy. *Epilepsia* 1996;37[Suppl 1]:S41–51.

304. Yasoshima A, Hayashi H, Iijima S, Sugita Y, Teshima Y, Shimizu T, et al. Potential distribution of vertex sharp wave and saw-toothed wave on the scalp. *Electroencephalogr Clin Neurophysiol* 1984;58:73–76.

305. Berger RJ, Olley P, Oswald I. The EEG, eye-movements and dreams of the blind. *Q J Exp Psychol* 1962;14:183–186.

306. Gibbs F, Gibbs E. *Atlas of electroencephalography*. Redding, MA: Addison-Wesley Publishing Company, 1964.

307. Principe JC, Smith JR. Sleep spindle characteristics as a function of age. *Sleep* 1982;5(1): 73–84.

308. Gibbs E, Gibbs F. Extreme spindles: correlation of electroencephalographic sleep pattern with mental retardation. *Science* 1962;138:1106–1107.

309. Dadmehr N, Pakalnis A, Drake Jr ME. Spindle coma in viral encephalitis. *Clin Electroencephalogr* 1987;18(1):34–37.

310. Janati A, Hester RL. Spindle activity in the waking electroencephalogram: report of a case with hemispheric glioblastoma. *Clin Electroencephalogr* 1986;17(1):1–5.

311. Niedermeyer E, Singer HS, Folstein SE, Allen RP, Miranda F, Fineyre F, et al. Hypersomnia with simultaneous waking and sleep patterns in the electroencephalogram. A case report with neurotransmitter studies. *J Neurol* 1979;221:1–13.

312. Westmoreland BF, Klass DW. Unusual variants of subclinical rhythmic electrographic discharge of adults (SREDA). *Electroencephalogr Clin Neurophysiol* 1997;102:1–4.

313. Westmoreland BF, Klass DW. A distinctive rhythmic EEG discharge of adults. *Electroencephalogr Clin Neurophysiol* 1981;51:186–191.

314. Nagarajan L, Gregory PB, Hewitt IK, Gubbay SS, Parry TS. Subclinical rhythmic EEG discharge of adults: SREDA in two children. *Pediatr Neurol* 2001;24:313–316.

315. de Falco FA, Vacca G, Fels A, Natale S, Striano S. An unusual EEG pattern in elderly subjects: subclinical rhythmic EEG discharge of adults ("SREDA"). Electroclinical study of six cases. *Acta Neurol* (Napoli) 1983;5:373–379.

316. Thomas P, Migneco O, Darcourt J, Chatel M. Single photon emission computed tomography study of subclinical rhythmic electrographic discharge in adults. *Electroencephalogr Clin Neurophysiol* 1992;83:223–227.

317. Okada S, Urakami Y. Midline theta rhythm revisited. *Clin Electroencephalogr* 1993;24(1): 6–12.

318. Janati A, Kidwai S, Nowack WJ. Episodic anterior drowsy theta in adults. *Clin Electroencephalogr* 1986;17(3):135–138.

319. Inanaga K. Frontal midline theta rhythm and mental activity. *Psychiatry Clin Neurosci* 1998;52:555–566.

320. Ciganek L. Theta-discharges in the middle-line — EEG symptom of temporal lobe epilepsy. *Electroencephalogr Clin Neurophysiol* 1961;13:669–673.

321. Shinomiya S, Urakami Y, Nagata K, Takahashi N, Inoue R. Frontal midline theta rhythm: differentiating the physiological theta rhythm from the abnormal discharge. *Clin Electroencephalogr* 1994;25(1):30–35.

322. Rangaswamy M, Porjesz B, Chorlian DB, Choi K, Jones KA, Wang K, et al. Theta power in the EEG of alcoholics. *Alcohol Clin Exp Res* 2003;27:607–615.

323. Schuld A, Kuhn M, Haack M, Kraus T, Hinze-Selch D, Lechner C, et al. A comparison of the effects of clozapine and olanzapine on the EEG in patients with schizophrenia. *Pharmacopsychiatry* 2000;33(3):109–111.

324. Kappelle LJ, van Huffelen AC, van Gijn J. Is the EEG really normal in lacunar stroke? *J Neurol Neurosurg Psychiatry* 1990;53(1):63–66.

325. Fernandez-Bouzas A, Harmony T, Bosch J, Aubert E, Fernandez T, Valdes P, et al. Sources of abnormal EEG activity in the presence of brain lesions. *Clin Electroencephalogr* 1999;30(2): 46–52.

326. Lin YY, Wu ZA, Hsieh JC, Yu HY, Kwan SY, Yen DJ, et al. Magnetoencephalographic study of rhythmic mid-temporal discharges in non-epileptic and epileptic patients. *Seizure* 2003;12: 220–225.

327. Eeg-Olofsson O, Petersen I. Rhythmic mid-temporal discharges in the EEG of normal children and adolescents. *Clin Electroencephalogr* 1982;13(1):40–45.

328. Oken BS, Kaye JA. Electrophysiologic function in the healthy, extremely old. *Neurology* 1992;42(3 Pt 1):519–526.

329. Maynard SD, Hughes JR. A distinctive electrographic entity: bursts of rhythmical temporal theta. *Clin Electroencephalogr* 1984;15(3):145–150.

330. Sheridan PH, Sato S. Triphasic waves of metabolic encephalopathy versus spike-wave stupor. *J Neurol Neurosurg Psychiatry* 1986;49(1):108–109.

331. Fisch BJ, Klass DW. The diagnostic specificity of triphasic wave patterns. *Electroencephalogr Clin Neurophysiol* 1988;70:1–8.

332. Fountain NB, Waldman WA. Effects of benzodiazepines on triphasic waves: implications for nonconvulsive status epilepticus. *J Clin Neurophysiol* 2001;18(4):345–352.

333. Nowack WJ, King JA. Triphasic waves and spike wave stupor. *Clin Electroencephalogr* 1992;23(2):100–104.

334. Niedermeyer E. Metabolic central nervous system disorders. In: Niedermeyer E, Lopes da Silva F, eds. *Electroencephalography, basic principles, clinical applications, and related fields.* Baltimore: Williams & Wilkins, 1999:416–431.

335. Tomer Y, Neufeld MY, Shoenfeld Y. Coma with triphasic wave pattern in EEG as a complication of temporal arteritis. *Neurology* 1992;42:439–440.

336. Sundaram MB, Blume WT. Triphasic waves: clinical correlates and morphology. *Can J Neurol Sci* 1987;14:136–140.

337. Ogunyemi A. Triphasic waves during post-ictal stupor. *Can J Neurol Sci* 1996;23:208–212.

338. Hughes JR. The development of the vertex sharp transient. *Clin Electroencephalogr* 1998; 29(4):183–187.

339. Schaul N, Lueders H, Sachdev K. Generalized, bilaterally synchronous bursts of slow waves in the EEG. *Arch Neurol* 1981;38(11):690–692.

340. Schaul N, Gloor P, Gotman J. The EEG in deep midline lesions. *Neurology* 1981;31(2): 157–167.

Subject Index